DRUG
DISCOVERY AND
DEVELOPMENT

TECHNOLOGY IN TRANSITION

Commissioning Editor: Timothy Horne
Development Editor: Barbara Simmons
Project Manager: Nancy Arnott
Designer: Erik Bigland
Illustration Manager: Bruce Hogarth
Illustrator: Graeme Chambers

DRUG DISCOVERY AND DEVELOPMENT

TECHNOLOGY IN TRANSITION

Edited by

H P Rang MB BS MA DPhil FMedSci FRS

Emeritus Professor of Pharmacology, University College, London;
Formerly Director, Novartis Institute for Medical Sciences, London

Foreword by

Daniel Vasella MD

President and CEO, Novartis International

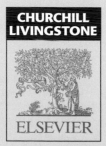

EDINBURGH LONDON NEW YORK PHILADELPHIA ST LOUIS SYDNEY TORONTO 2006

CHURCHILL
LIVINGSTONE
ELSEVIER

First published 2006

ISBN 0443 064202

British Library Cataloguing in Publication Data
A catalogue record for this book is available from the British Library

Library of Congress Cataloging in Publication Data
A catalog record for this book is available from the Library of Congress

Notice
Knowledge and best practice in this field are constantly changing. As new research and experience broaden our knowledge, changes in practice, treatment and drug therapy may become necessary or appropriate. Readers are advised to check the most current information provided (i) on procedures featured or (ii) by the manufacturer of each product to be administered, to verify the recommended dose or formula, the method and duration of administration, and contraindications. It is the responsibility of the practitioner, relying on their own experience and knowledge of the patient, to make diagnoses, to determine dosages and the best treatment for each individual patient, and to take all appropriate safety precautions. To the fullest extent of the law, neither the Publisher nor the Editor assumes any liability for any injury and/or damage to persons or property arising out or related to any use of the material contained in this book.
The Publisher

The publisher's policy is to use **paper manufactured from sustainable forests**

Printed in China

Foreword

There has been a revolution in biomedical science over the past 20 years, and there is every reason to believe that a therapeutic revolution may follow in its wake. Breakthroughs such as the mapping of the human genome greatly advanced science, but considerable work must now be completed to unravel the function and pathways of these genes. Conventional synthetic small molecule drugs, which are the main theme in this book, are likely to remain the dominant form of therapeutic intervention in the near- and mid-term. The book details how the scientific revolution is changing the ways in which we look for new therapies.

Close to 1000 individual substances are approved for medical use, the majority being custom-designed synthetic compounds produced by the drug discovery efforts of pharmaceutical companies. In recent years, about 30 new compounds have been approved yearly. Drug therapy has decreased morbidity improving quality of life, reduced hospitalizations, helped patients avoid surgery, and reduced mortality.

This book, written by a team of scientists and managers with long experience in the pharmaceutical business, takes the process of drug discovery from start to finish. It emphasizes the importance of multi-disciplinary teamwork, which has become increasingly important today. In an age of specialists, a molecular biologist may find it hard to understand the importance of pharmacokinetics, and a computational chemist may feel daunted by discussions of toxicology, pharmaceutical formulation or clinical trials design. Yet all these specialists must work together and understand each other's concerns in order to solve the problems that are invariably encountered in the research and development process. Tenacity is key, and it can be best achieved when the members of the team genuinely understand each other. Close cooperation from discovery to launch also reduces time to market, which is crucial for patients in need of innovative medicines.

Gaining an overview of each stage of research and development, from the earliest planning of a new project to the endpoint of successfully registering a new medicine, can be a slow and difficult business for young scientists or managers with an ambition to make their mark on therapeutics. This book will be a useful tool. There are many sources of detailed technical information about particular aspects of pharmaceutical research and development, which are used by specialists, but this book aims to provide a solid overview of all steps, in a style that is simple to understand and serves as an easy reference for non-specialists.

Daniel Vasella, MD

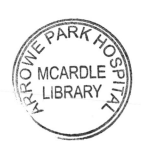

Preface

A large pharmaceutical company is an exceptionally complex organization. Several features stand out. First, like any company, it must make a profit, and handle its finances efficiently in order to survive. Modern pharmaceutical companies are so large that they are financially comparable to a small nation, and the average cost of bringing a new drug to market – about $800m – is a sum that any government would think twice about committing.

Second, there is an underlying altruism in the mission of a pharmaceutical company, in the sense that its aim is to provide therapies that meet a significant medical need, and thereby relieve human suffering. Though cynics will point to examples where the profit motive seems to have prevailed over ethical and altruistic concerns, the fact remains that the modern pharmacopeia has enormous power to alleviate disease, and owes its existence almost entirely to the work of the pharmaceutical industry.

Third, the industry is research-based to an unusual extent. Biomedical science has arguably advanced more rapidly than any other domain of science in the last few decades, and new discoveries naturally create expectations that they will lead on improved therapies. Though discoveries in other fields may have profound implications for our understanding of the natural world, their relevance for improving the human condition is generally much less direct. For this reason, the pharmaceutical industry has to stay abreast of leading-edge scientific progress to a greater extent than most industries.

Finally, the products of the pharmaceutical industry have considerable social impact, producing benefits in terms of life expectancy and relief of disability, risks of adverse effects, changes in lifestyle – for example, the contraceptive pill – and financial pressures which affect healthcare policy on a national and international scale. In consequence, an elaborate, and constantly changing, regulatory system exists to control the approval of new drugs, and companies need to devote considerable resources to negotiating this tricky interface.

This book provides an introduction to the way a pharmaceutical company goes about its business of discovering and developing new drugs. The first part gives a brief historical account of the evolution of the industry from its origins in the mediaeval apothecaries' trade, and discusses the changing understanding of what we mean by disease, and what therapy aims to achieve, as well as summarizing case histories of the discovery and development of some important drugs.

The second part focuses on the science and technology involved in the discovery process, that is the stages by which a promising new chemical entity is identified, from the starting point of a medical need and an idea for addressing it. A chapter on biopharmaceuticals, whose discovery and development tend to follow routes somewhat different from synthetic compounds, is included here, as well as accounts of patent issues that arise in the discovery phase, and a chapter on research management in this environment. Managing drug discovery scientists can be likened in some ways to managing a team of huskies on a polar journey. Huskies provide the essential driving force, but are somewhat wayward and unpredictable creatures, prone to fighting each other, occasionally running off on their own, and inclined to bite the expedition leader. Success in husky terms means gaining the respect of other huskies, not of humans. (We must not, of course, push the analogy too far. Scientists, unlike huskies, do care about reaching the goal, and the project management plan – in my experience at least – does not involve killing them to feed their colleagues.)

The third section of the book deals with drug development, that is the work that has to be undertaken to turn the drug candidate that emerges from the discovery process into a product on the market, and a final chapter presents some facts and figures about the way the whole process operates in practice.

No small group on its own can produce a drug, and throughout the book there is strong emphasis on the need for interdisciplinary team-work. The main reason for writing it was to help individual specialists to understand better the work of colleagues who address different aspects of the problem. The incentive came from my own experience when, after a career in academic pharmacology, I joined Sandoz as a research director in 1985, motivated by a wish to see whether my knowledge of pharmacology could be put to use in developing useful new medicines. It was a world startlingly different from what I was used to, full of people – mostly very friendly and forthcoming – whose work I really did not understand. Even the research laboratories worked in a different way. Enjoyable though it was to explore this new territory, and to come to understand the language and preoccupations of colleagues in other disciplines, it would have been a lot quicker and more painless had I been able to read a book about it first! No such book existed, nor has any appeared since. Hence this book, which is aimed not only at scientists who want to understand better the broad range of activities involved in producing a new drug, but also non-scientists who want to understand the realities of drug discovery research. Inevitably, in covering such a broad range, the treatment has to be superficial, concentrating on general principles rather than technical details, but further reading is suggested for those seeking more detail. I am much indebted to my many friends and colleagues, especially to those who have taken the time to write chapters, but also to those with whom I have worked over the years and who taught me many valuable lessons.

It is hoped that those seeking a general guide to pharmaceutical R & D will find the book helpful.

H P Rang   London, 2006

Contributors

Julie Ducharme BPharm MSc PhD
Adjunct Professor, Faculté de Pharmacie, Université de Montréal; Director, Department of Drug Metabolism and Pharmacokinetics, AstraZeneca R & D Montreal, Montreal, Quebec, Canada

Adam J Dudley PhD
Department of Drug Metabolism and Pharmacokinetics, AstraZeneca Pharmaceuticals, Wilmington, Delaware, USA

Christine Easdale BSc (Hons)
Senior Director, Integrated Services, Quintiles Ltd, Bracknell, UK

Philip Grubb European Patent Attorney
Formerly Intellectual Property Counsel, Novartis International, Basel, Switzerland

Hubert Haag PhD
Lead Identification Technologies, Sanofi-Aventis, Frankfurt, Germany

Inger Hägglöf MSc (Pharm)
Project Leader, AstraZeneca AB Operations, Supply & Capability, Dossier Management Group, Södertälje, Sweden

Paul Herrling PhD
Head of Corporate Research, Novartis International, Basel, Switzerland

Åsa Holmgren MSc (Pharm)
Regulatory Affairs Director, AstraZeneca R & D, Södertälje, Sweden

Richard K Howell BSc (Hons)
Project Director, Driver Safety and Well-being, AstraZeneca Global SHE, Macclesfield, Cheshire, UK

Harry LeVine, III PhD
Associate Professor, University of Kentucky, Center on Aging, Department of Molecular & Cellular Biochemistry, Lexington, Kentucky, USA

H P Rang MB BS MA DPhil FMedSci FRS
Emeritus Professor of Pharmacology, University College, London;
Formerly Director, Novartis Institute for Medical Sciences, London.

Kurt A Stoeckli PhD
Lead Identification Technologies, Sanofi-Aventis, Frankfurt, Germany

R A Thompson PhD
Department of DMPK & Bioanalytical Chemistry, AstraZeneca R & D, Mölndal, Sweden

Colin W Vose PhD CChem, FRSC
Director, Strategic Business Development, Quintiles Ltd, Edinburgh, UK

Christopher S J Walpole DPhil
Director, Chemistry, AstraZeneca R & D Montreal, Montreal, Quebec, Canada

Contents

Contents

SECTION 1
INTRODUCTION AND BACKGROUND

1 The development of the pharmaceutical industry

H P Rang

Antecedents and origins

Our task in this book is to give an account of the principles underlying drug discovery as it happens today, and to provide pointers to the future. The present situation, of course, represents merely the current frame of a long-running movie. To understand the significance of the different elements that appear in the frame, and to predict what is likely to change in the next few frames, we need to know something about what has gone before. In this chapter we give a brief and selective account of some of the events and trends that have shaped the pharmaceutical industry. Most of the action in our metaphorical movie happened in the last century, despite the film having started at the birth of civilization, some 10 000 years ago. The next decade or two will certainly see at least as much change as the past century.

Many excellent and extensive histories of medicine and the pharmaceutical industry have been published, to which readers seeking more detailed information are referred (Mann, 1984; Sneader, 1985; Weatherall, 1990; Porter, 1997; see also Drews, 2000, 2003).

Disease has been recognized as an enemy of humankind since civilization began, and plagues of infectious diseases arrived as soon as humans began to congregate in settlements about 5000 years ago. Early writings on papyrus and clay tablets describe many kinds of disease, and list a wide variety of herbal and other remedies used to treat them. The earliest such document, the famous Ebers papyrus, dating from around 1550BC, describes more than 800 such remedies. Disease was in those times regarded as an affliction sent by the gods; consequently, the remedies were aimed partly at neutralizing or purging the affliction, and partly at appeasing the deities. Despite its essentially theistic basis, early medicine nevertheless discovered, through empiricism and common sense, many plant extracts whose pharmacological properties we recognize and still use today; their active principles include opium alkaloids, ephedrine, emetine, cannabis, senna and many others[1].

In contrast to the ancient Egyptians, who would, one feels, have been completely unsympathetic to medical

---

[1]There were, it should be added, far more – such as extracts of asses' testicles, bats' eyes and crocodile dung – that never found their way into modern pharmacology.

science had they been time-warped into the 21st century, the ancient Greeks might have felt much more at home in the present era. They sought to understand nature, work out its rules and apply them to alleviate disease, just as we aim to do today. The Hippocratic tradition had little time for theistic explanations. However, the Greeks were not experimenters, and so the basis of Greek medicine remained essentially theoretical. Their theories were philosophical constructs, whose perceived validity rested on their elegance and logical consistency; the idea of testing theory by experiment came much later, and this aspect of present-day science would have found no resonance in ancient Greece. The basic concept of four humours – black bile, yellow bile, blood and phlegm – proved, with the help of Greek reasoning, to be an extremely versatile framework for explaining health and disease. Given the right starting point – cells, molecules and tissues instead of humours – they would quickly have come to terms with modern medicine. From a therapeutic perspective, Greek medicine placed rather little emphasis on herbal remedies; they incorporated earlier teachings on the subject, but made few advances of their own. The Greek traditions formed the basis of the prolific writings of Galen in the 2nd century AD, whose influence dominated the practice of medicine in Europe well into the Renaissance. Other civilizations, notably Indian, Arabic and Chinese, similarly developed their own medical traditions, which – unlike those of the Greeks – still flourish independently of the western ones.

Despite the emphasis on herbal remedies in these early medical concepts, and growing scientific interest in their use as medicines from the 18th century onwards, it was only in the mid-19th century that chemistry and biology advanced sufficiently to give a scientific basis to drug therapy, and it was not until the beginning of the 20th century that this knowledge actually began to be applied to the discovery of new drugs. In the long interim, the apothecaries' trade flourished; closely controlled by guilds and apprenticeship schemes, it formed the supply route for the exotic preparations that were used in treatment. The early development of therapeutics – based, as we have seen, mainly on superstition and on theories that have been swept away by scientific advances – represents prehistory as far as the development of the pharmaceutical industry is concerned, and there are few, if any, traces of it remaining[2].

---

[2]Plenty of traces remain outside the pharmaceutical industry, in the form of a wide variety of 'alternative' and 'complementary' therapeutic procedures, such as herbalism, moxibustion, reflexology and acupuncture, whose underlying principles originated in the prescientific era and remain largely beyond the boundaries of science. It may not be long, given the growing appeal of such approaches in the public's eye, before the mainstream pharmaceutical industry decides that it must follow this trend. That will indeed be a challenge for drug discovery research.

Therapeutics in the 19th century

Although preventive medicine had made some spectacular advances, for example in controlling scurvy (Lind, 1763) and in the area of infectious diseases, vaccination (Jenner, 1798), curtailment of the London cholera epidemic of 1854 by turning off the Broad Street Pump (Snow), and control of childbirth fever and surgical infections using antiseptic techniques (Semmelweis, 1861; Lister, 1867), therapeutic medicine was virtually non-existent until the end of the 19th century.

Oliver Wendell Holmes – a pillar of the medical establishment – wrote in 1860: '....I firmly believe that if the whole materia medica, as now used, could be sunk to the bottom of the sea, it would be all the better for mankind – and the worse for the fishes' (see Porter, 1997). This may have been a somewhat ungenerous appraisal, for some contemporary medicines – notably digitalis, famously described by Withering in 1785, extract of willow bark (salicylic acid), and *Cinchona* extract (quinine) – had beneficial effects that were well documented. But on balance, Holmes was right – medicines did more harm than good.

We can obtain an idea of the state of therapeutics at the time from the first edition of the *British Pharmacopoeia*, published in 1864, which lists 311 preparations. Of these, 187 were plant-derived materials, only nine of which were purified substances. Most of the plant products – lemon juice, rose hips, yeast etc. – lacked any components we would now regard as therapeutically relevant, but some – digitalis, castor oil, ergot, colchicum – were pharmacologically active. Of the 311 preparations, 103 were 'chemicals' mainly inorganic – iodine, ferrous sulfate, sodium bicarbonate, and many toxic salts of bismuth, arsenic, lead and mercury – but also a few synthetic chemicals, such as diethyl ether and chloroform. The remainder were miscellaneous materials and a few animal products, such as lard, cantharidin and cochineal.

An industry begins to emerge

For the pharmaceutical industry, the transition from prehistory to actual history occurred late in the 19th century (3Q19C, as managers of today might like to call it), when three essential strands came together. These were: the evolving science of biomedicine (and especially pharmacology); the emergence of synthetic organic chemistry; and the development of a chemical industry in Europe, coupled with a medical supplies trade – the result of buoyant entrepreneurship, mainly in America.

Developments in biomedicine

Science began to be applied whole-heartedly to medicine – as to almost every other aspect of life – in the 19th century. Among the most important milestones from the point of view of drug discovery was the elaboration in 1858 of cell theory, by the German pathologist Rudolf Virchow. Virchow was a remarkable man: pre-eminent as a pathologist, he also designed the Berlin sewage system and instituted hygiene inspections in schools, and later became an active member of the Reichstag. The tremendous reductionist leap of the cell theory gave biology – and the pharmaceutical industry – the scientific foundation it needed. It is only by thinking of living systems in terms of the function of their cells that one can begin to understand how molecules affect them.

A second milestone was the birth of pharmacology as a scientific discipline when the world's first Pharmacological Institute was set up in 1847 at Dorpat by Rudolf Buchheim – literally by Buchheim himself, as the Institute was in his own house and funded by him personally. It gained such recognition that the university built him a new one 13 years later. Buchheim foresaw that pharmacology as a science was needed to exploit the knowledge of physiology, which was being advanced by pioneers such as Magendie and Claude Bernard, and link it to therapeutics. When one remembers that this was at a time when organic chemistry and physiology were both in their cradles, and therapeutics was ineffectual, Buchheim's vision seems bold, if not slightly crazy. Nevertheless, his Institute was a spectacular success. Although he made no truly seminal discoveries, Buchheim imposed on himself and his staff extremely high standards of experimentation and argument, which eclipsed the empiricism of the old therapeutic principles and attracted some exceptionally gifted students. Among these was the legendary Oswald Schmiedeberg, who later moved to Strasbourg, where he set up an Institute of Pharmacology of unrivalled size and grandeur, which soon became the Mecca for would-be pharmacologists all over the world.

A third milestone came with Louis Pasteur's germ theory of disease, proposed in Paris in 1878. A chemist by training, Pasteur's initial interest was in the process of fermentation of wine and beer, and the souring of milk. He showed, famously, that airborne infection was the underlying cause, and concluded that the air was actually alive with microorganisms. Particular types, he argued, were pathogenic to humans, and accounted for many forms of disease, including anthrax, cholera and rabies. Pasteur successfully introduced several specific immunization procedures to give protection against infectious diseases. Robert Koch, Pasteur's rival and near-contemporary, clinched the infection theory by observing anthrax and other bacilli in the blood of infected animals.

The founder of chemotherapy – some would say the founder of molecular pharmacology – was Paul Ehrlich (see Drews, 2004 for a mini-biography). Born in 1854 and trained in pathology, Ehrlich became interested in histological stains and tested a wide range of synthetic chemical dyes that were being produced at that time. He invented 'vital staining' – staining by dyes injected into living animals – and described how the chemical properties of the dyes, particularly their acidity and lipid solubility, influenced the distribution of dye to particular tissues and cellular structures. Thence came the idea of specific binding of molecules to particular cellular components, which directed not only Ehrlich's study of chemotherapeutic agents, but much of pharmacological thinking ever since. 'Receptor' and 'magic bullets' are Ehrlich's terms, though he envisaged receptors as targets for toxins, rather than physiological mediators. Working in Koch's Institute, Ehrlich developed diphtheria antitoxin for clinical use, and put forward a theory of antibody action based on specific chemical recognition of microbial macromolecules, work for which he won the 1908 Nobel Prize. Ehrlich became director of his own Institute in Frankfurt, close to a large dye works, and returned to his idea of using the specific binding properties of synthetic dyes to develop selective antimicrobial drugs.

At this point, we interrupt the biological theme at the end of the 19th century, with Ehrlich in full flood, on the verge of introducing the first designer drugs, and turn to the chemical and commercial developments that were going on simultaneously.

Developments in chemistry

The first synthetic chemicals to be used for medical purposes were, ironically, not therapeutic agents at all, but anaesthetics. Diethyl ether ('sweet oil of vitriol') was first made and described in 1540. Early in the 19th century, it and nitrous oxide (prepared by Humphrey Davy in 1799 and found – by experiments on himself – to have stupefacient properties) were used to liven up parties and sideshows; their usefulness as surgical anaesthetics was demonstrated, amid much controversy, only in the 1840s[3], by which time chloroform had also made its appearance. Synthetic chemistry at the time could deal only with very simple molecules, made

---

[3] An event welcomed, in his inimitable prose style, by Oliver Wendell Holmes in 1847: 'The knife is searching for disease, the pulleys are dragging back dislocated limbs – Nature herself is working out the primal curse which doomed the tenderest of her creatures to the sharpest of her trials, but the fierce extremity of suffering has been steeped in the waters of forgetfulness, and the deepest furrow in the knotted brow of agony has been smoothed forever'.

by recipe rather than reason, as our understanding of molecular structure was still in its infancy. The first therapeutic drug to come from synthetic chemistry was amyl nitrite, prepared in 1859 by Guthrie and introduced, on the basis of its vasodilator activity, for treating angina by Brunton in 1864 – the first example of a drug born in a recognizably 'modern' way, through the application of synthetic chemistry, physiology and clinical medicine. This was a landmark indeed, for it was nearly 40 years before synthetic chemistry made any further significant contribution to therapeutics, and not until well into the 20th century that physiological and pharmacological knowledge began to be applied to the invention of new drugs.

It was during the latter half of the 19th century that the foundations of synthetic organic chemistry were laid, the impetus coming from work on aniline, a copious byproduct of the coal-tar industry. An English chemist, Perkin, who in 1856 succeeded in preparing from aniline a vivid purple compound, *mauvein*, laid the foundations. This was actually a chemical accident, as Perkin's aim had been to synthesize quinine. Nevertheless, the discovery gave birth to the synthetic dyestuffs industry, which played a major part in establishing the commercial potential of synthetic organic chemistry – a technology which later became a linchpin of the evolving pharmaceutical industry. A systematic approach to organic synthesis went hand in hand with improved understanding of chemical structure. Crucial steps were the establishment of the rules of chemical equivalence (valency), and the elucidation of the structure of benzene by Von Kekulé in 1865. The first representation of a structural formula depicting the bonds between atoms in two dimensions, based on valency rules, also appeared in 1865[4].

The reason why Perkin had sought to synthesize quinine was that the drug, prepared from *Cinchona* bark, was much in demand for the treatment of malaria, one of whose effects is to cause high fever. So quinine was (wrongly, as it turned out) designated as an antipyretic drug, and used to treat fevers of all kinds. Because quinine itself could not be synthesized, fragments of the molecule were made instead. These included antipyrine, phenacetin and various others, which were introduced with great success in the 1880s and 1890s, the first drugs to be 'designed' on chemical principles[5].

The apothecaries' trade

Despite the lack of efficacy of the pharmaceutical preparations that were available in the 19th century, the apothecaries' trade flourished; then, as now, physicians felt themselves obliged to issue prescriptions to satisfy the expectations of their patients for some token of remedial intent. Early in the 19th century, when many small apothecary businesses existed to satisfy the demand on a local basis, a few enterprising chemists undertook the task of isolating the active substances from these plant extracts. This was a bold and inspired leap, and one that attracted a good deal of ridicule. Although the old idea of 'signatures', which held that plants owed their medicinal properties to their biological characteristics[6], was falling into disrepute, few were willing to accept that individual chemical substances could be responsible for the effects these plants produced, such as emesis, narcosis, purgation or fever. The trend began with Friedrich Sertürner, a junior apothecary in Westphalia, who in 1805 isolated and purified morphine, barely surviving a test of its potency on himself. This was the first 'alkaloid', so named because of its ability to neutralize acids and form salts. This discovery led to the isolation of several more plant alkaloids, including emetine, strychnine, caffeine and quinine, mainly by two remarkably prolific chemists, Caventou and Pelletier, working in Paris in the period 1810–1825. The recognition that medicinal plants owed their properties to their individual chemical constituents, rather than to some intangible property associated with their living nature, marks a critical point in the history of the pharmaceutical industry. It can be seen as the point of origin of two of the three strands from which the industry grew – namely the beginnings of the 'industrialization' of the apothecaries' trade, and the emergence of the science of pharmacology. And by revealing the chemical nature of medicinal preparations, it hinted at the future possibility of making medicines artificially. Even though, at that time, synthetic organic chemistry was barely out of its cradle, these discoveries provided the impetus that later caused the chemical industry to turn, at a very early stage in its history, to making drugs.

The first local apothecary business to move into large-scale production and marketing of pharmaceuticals was the old-established Darmstadt firm Merck,

---

[4]Its author, the Edinburgh chemist Alexander Crum Brown, was also a pioneer of pharmacology, and was the first person to use a chemical reaction – quaternization of amines – to modify naturally occurring substances such as strychnine and morphine. With Thomas Fraser, in 1868, he found that this drastically altered their pharmacological properties, changing strychnine, for example, from a convulsant to a paralysing agent. Although they knew neither the structures of these molecules nor the mechanisms by which they acted, theirs was the first systematic study of structure–activity relationships.
[5]These drugs belong pharmacologically to the class of non-steroidal anti-inflammatories (NSAIDs), the most important of which is aspirin (acetylsalicylic acid). Ironically, aspirin itself had been synthesized many years earlier, in 1855, with no pharmacological purpose in mind. Aspirin was not developed commercially until 1899, subsequently generating huge revenues for Bayer, the company responsible.

[6]According to this principle, pulmonaria (lungwort) was used to treat respiratory disorders because its leaves resembled lungs, saffron to treat jaundice, and so on.

founded in 1668. This development, in 1827, was stimulated by the advances in purification of natural products. Merck was closely followed in this astute business move by other German- and Swiss-based apothecary businesses, giving rise to some which later also became giant pharmaceutical companies, such as Schering and Boehringer. The American pharmaceutical industry emerged in the middle of the 19th century. Squibb began in 1858, with ether as its main product. Soon after came Parke Davis (1866) and Eli Lilly (1876); both had a broader franchise as manufacturing chemists. In the 1890s Parke Davis became the world's largest pharmaceutical company, one of whose early successes was to purify crystalline adrenaline from adrenal glands and sell it in ampoules for injection. The US scientific community contested the adoption of the word 'adrenaline' as a trade name, but industry won the day and the scientists were forced to call the hormone 'epinephrine'.

The move into pharmaceuticals was also followed by several chemical companies such as Bayer, Hoechst, Agfa, Sandoz, Geigy and others, which began, not as apothecaries, but as dyestuffs manufacturers. The dyestuffs industry at that time was also based largely on plant products, which had to be refined, and were sold in relatively small quantities, so the commercial parallels with the pharmaceutical industry were plain. Dye factories, for obvious reasons, were usually located close to large rivers, a fact that accounts for the present-day location of many large pharmaceutical companies in Europe. As we shall see, the link with the dyestuffs industry later came to have much more profound implications for drug discovery.

From about 1870 onwards – following the crucial discovery by Kekulé of the structure of benzene – the dyestuffs industry turned increasingly to synthetic chemistry as a source of new compounds, starting with aniline-based dyes. A glance through any modern pharmacopoeia will show the overwhelming preponderance of synthetic aromatic compounds, based on the benzene ring structure, among the list of useful drugs. Understanding the nature of aromaticity was critical. Though we might be able to dispense with the benzene ring in some fields of applied chemistry, such as fuels, lubricants, plastics or detergents, its exclusion would leave the pharmacopoeia bankrupt. Many of these dyestuffs companies saw the potential of the medicines business from 1880 onwards, and moved into the area hitherto occupied by the apothecaries. The result was the first wave of companies ready to apply chemical technology to the production of medicines. Many of these founder companies remained in business for years. It was only recently, when their cannibalistic urges took over in the race to become large, that mergers and take-overs caused many names to disappear.

Thus the beginnings of a recognizable pharmaceutical industry date from about 1860–1880, its origins being

in the apothecaries and medical supplies trades on the one hand, and the dyestuffs industry on the other. In those early days, however, they had rather few products to sell; these were mainly inorganic compounds of varying degrees of toxicity, and others best described as concoctions. Holmes (see above) dismissed the pharmacopoeia in 1860 as worse than useless.

To turn this ambitious new industry into a source of human benefit, rather than just corporate profit, required two things. First, it had to embrace the principles of biomedicine, and in particular pharmacology, which provided a basis for understanding how disease and drugs, respectively, affect the function of living organisms. Second, it had to embrace the principles of chemistry, going beyond the descriptors of colour, crystallinity, taste, volatility etc. towards an understanding of the structure and properties of molecules, and how to make them in the laboratory. As we have seen, both of these fields had made tremendous progress towards the end of the 19th century, so at the start of the 20th century the time was right for the industry to seize its chance. Nevertheless, several decades passed before the inventions coming from the industry began to make a major impact on the treatment of disease.

The industry enters the 20th century

By the end of the 19th century various synthetic drugs had been made and tested, including the 'antipyretics' (see above) and also various central nervous system depressants. Chemical developments based on chloroform had produced chloral hydrate, the first non-volatile CNS depressant, which was in clinical use for many years as a hypnotic drug. Independently, various compounds based on urea were found to act similarly, and von Mering followed this lead to produce the first barbiturate, *barbitone* (since renamed barbital), which was introduced in 1903 by Bayer and gained widespread clinical use as a hypnotic, tranquillizer and antiepileptic drug – the first blockbuster. Almost simultaneously, Einthorn in Munich synthesized *procaine*, the first synthetic local anaesthetic drug, which followed the naturally occurring alkaloid cocaine. The local anaesthetic action of cocaine on the eye was discovered by Sigmund Freud and his ophthalmologist colleague Koeller in the late 19th century, and was heralded as a major advance for ophthalmic surgery. After several chemists had tried, with limited success, to make synthetic compounds with the same actions, procaine was finally produced and introduced commercially in 1905 by Hoechst. Barbitone and procaine were triumphs for chemical ingenuity, but owed little or nothing to physiology, or indeed pharmacology. The physiological site or sites of action of barbiturates remain unclear to this day, and their mechanism of action at the molecular level was unknown until the 1980s.

From this stage, where chemistry began to make an impact on drug discovery, up to the last quarter of the 20th century, when molecular biology began to emerge as a dominant technology, we can discern three main routes by which new drugs were discovered, namely chemistry-driven approaches, target-directed approaches, and accidental clinical discoveries. In many of the most successful case histories, graphically described by Weatherall (1990), the three were closely interwoven. The remarkable family of diverse and important drugs that came from the original sulfonamide, lead, described below, exemplifies this pattern very well.

Chemistry-driven drug discovery

Synthetic chemistry

The pattern of drug discovery driven by synthetic chemistry – with biology often struggling to keep up – became the established model in the early part of the 20th century, and prevailed for at least 50 years. The balance of research in the pharmaceutical industry up to the 1970s placed chemistry clearly as the key discipline in drug discovery, the task of biologists being mainly to devise and perform assays capable of revealing possible useful therapeutic activity among the many anonymous white powders that arrived for testing. Research management in the industry was largely in the hands of chemists. This strategy produced many successes, including benzodiazepine tranquillizers, several antiepileptic drugs, antihypertensive drugs, antidepressants and antipsychotic drugs. The surviving practice of classifying many drugs on the basis of their chemical structure (e.g. phenothiazines, benzodiazepines, thiazides etc.) rather than on the more logical basis of their site or mode of action stems from this era. The development of antiepileptic drugs exemplifies this approach well. Following the success of barbital (see above) several related compounds were made, including the phenyl derivative *phenobarbital*, first made in 1911. This proved to be an effective hypnotic (i.e. sleep-inducing) drug, helpful in allowing peaceful nights in a ward full of restive patients. By chance, it was found by a German doctor also to reduce the frequency of seizures when tested in epileptic patients – an example of clinical serendipity (see below), and it became widely used for this purpose, being much more effective in this regard than barbital itself. About 20 years later, Putnam, working in Boston, developed an animal model whereby epilepsy-like seizures could be induced in mice by electrical stimulation of the brain via extracranial electrodes. This simple model allowed hundreds of compounds to be tested for potential antiepileptic activity. *Phenytoin* was an early success of this programme, and several more compounds followed, as chemists from several companies embarked on synthetic programmes. None of this relied at all on an understanding of the mechanism of action of these compounds – which is still controversial; all that was needed were teams of green-fingered chemists, and a robust assay that fairly predicted efficacy in the clinic.

Natural product chemistry

We have mentioned the early days of pharmacology, with its focus on plant-derived materials, such as *atropine, tubocurarine, strychnine, digitalis* and *ergot alkaloids*, which were almost the only drugs that existed until well into the 20th century. Despite the rise of synthetic chemistry, natural products remain a significant source of new drugs, particularly in the field of chemotherapy, but also in other applications. Following the discovery of *penicillin* by Fleming in 1929 – described by Mann (1984) as 'the most important medical discovery of all time' – and its development as an antibiotic for clinical use by Chain and Florey in 1938, an intense search was undertaken for antibacterial compounds produced by fungi and other microorganisms, which yielded many useful antibiotics, including *chloramphenicol* (1947), *tetracyclines* (1948), *streptomycin* (1949) and others. The same fungal source that yielded streptomycin also produced *actinomycin D*, used in cancer chemotherapy. Higher plants have continued to yield useful drugs, including *vincristine* and *vinblastine* (1958), and *paclitaxel* (taxol, 1971).

Outside the field of chemotherapy, successful drugs derived from natural products include *ciclosporin* (1972) and *tacrolimus* (1993), both of which come from fungi and are used to prevent transplant rejection. Soon after came *mevastatin* (1976), another fungal metabolite, which was the first of the 'statin' series of cholesterol-lowering drugs which act by inhibiting the enzyme HMG CoA reductase.

Overall, the pharmaceutical industry continues to have something of a love–hate relationship with natural products. They often have weird and wonderful structures that cause hardened chemists to turn pale; they are often near-impossible to synthesize, troublesome to produce from natural sources, and 'optimizing' such molecules to make them suitable for therapeutic use is akin to remodelling Westminster Abbey to improve its acoustics. But the fact remains that Nature unexpectedly provides some of our most useful drugs, and most of its potential remains untapped.

Target-directed drug discovery

Although chemistry was the pre-eminent discipline in drug discovery until the 1970s, the seeds of the biological revolution had long since been sown, and within the chemistry-led culture of the pharmaceutical industry these developments began to bear fruit in certain areas

This happened most notably in the field of chemotherapy, where Ehrlich played such an important role as the first 'modernist' who defined the principles of drug specificity in terms of a specific interaction between the drug molecule and a target molecule – the 'receptive substance' – in the organism, an idea summarized in his famous Latin catchphrase *Corpora non agunt nisi fixata*. Although we now take it for granted that the chemical nature of the target molecule, as well as that of the drug molecule, determines what effects a drug will produce, nobody before Ehrlich had envisaged drug action in this way[7]. By linking chemistry and biology, Ehrlich effectively set the stage for drug discovery in the modern style. But despite Ehrlich's seminal role in the evolution of the pharmaceutical industry, discoveries in his favourite field of endeavour, chemotherapy, remained for many years empirical rather than target directed[8].

The fact is that Ehrlich's preoccupation with the binding of chemical dyes, as exemplified by biological stains, for specific constituents of cells and tissues, turned out to be misplaced, and not applicable to the problem of achieving selective toxicity. Although he soon came to realize that the dye-binding moieties of cells were not equivalent to the supposed drug-binding moieties, neither he nor anyone else succeeded in identifying the latter and using them as defined targets for new compounds. The history of successes in the field of chemotherapy prior to the antibiotic era, some of which are listed in Table 1.1, actually represents a series of striking achievements in synthetic chemistry, coupled to the development of assay systems in animals, according to the chemistry-led model that we have already discussed. The popular image of 'magic bullets' – a phrase famously coined by Ehrlich – designed to home in, like cruise missiles, on defined targets is actually a misleading one in the context of the early days of chemotherapy, but there is no doubt that Ehrlich's thinking prepared the ground for the steady advance of target-directed approaches to drug discovery, a trend that, from the

Table 1.1
Examples of drugs from different sources: natural products, synthetic chemistry and biopharmaceuticals

Natural products	Synthetic chemistry	Biopharmaceuticals produced by recombinant DNA technology
Antibiotics (penicillin, streptomycin, tetracyclines, cephalosporins etc.)	Early successes include: Antiepileptic drugs	Human insulin (the first biotech product, registered 1982)
Anticancer drugs (doxorubicin, bleomycin, actinomycin, vincristine, vinblastine, taxol etc.)	Antihypertensive drugs Antimetabolites	Human growth hormone α-interferon, γ-interferon
Atropine, hyoscine	Barbiturates	Hepatitis B vaccine
Ciclosporin	Bronchodilators	Tissue plasminogen activator (t-PA)
Cocaine	Diuretics	Hirudin
Colchicine	Local anaesthetics	Blood clotting factors
Digitalis (digoxin)	Sulfonamides	Erythropoietin
Ephedrine	*[Since c.1950, synthetic chemistry has*	G-CSF, GM-CSF
Heparin	*accounted for the great majority of new*	
Human growth hormone*	*drugs]*	
Insulin (porcine, bovine)*		
Opium alkaloids (morphine, papaverine)		
Physostigmine		
Rauwolfia alkaloids (reserpine)		
Statins		
Streptokinase		
Tubocurarine		
Vaccines		

*Now largely or entirely replaced by material prepared by recombinant DNA technology.

[7]Others came close at around the same time, particularly the British physiologist J. N. Langley (1905), who interpreted the neuromuscular blocking effect of 'curari' in terms of its interaction with a specific 'receptive substance' at the junction between the nerve terminal and the muscle fibre. This was many years before chemical transmission at this junction was discovered. Langley's student, A. V. Hill (1909), first derived the equations based on the Law of Mass Action, which describe how binding varies with drug concentration. Hill's quantitative theory later formed the basis of 'receptor theory', elaborated by pharmacologists from A. J. Clark (1926) onwards. Although this quantitative approach underlies much of our current thinking about drug–receptor interactions, it was Ehrlich's more intuitive approach that played the major part in shaping drug discovery in the early days.

[8]Even now, important new chemotherapeutic drugs, such as the taxanes, continue to emerge through a combination of a chance biological discovery and high-level chemistry.

1950s onwards, steadily shifted the industry's focus from chemistry to biology (Maxwell and Eckhardt, 1990; Lednicer, 1993). A few selected case histories exemplify this general trend.

The sulfonamide story

Ehrlich's major triumph was the discovery in 1910 of *Salvarsan* (Compound 606), the first compound to treat syphilis effectively, which remained in use for 40 years. Still, bacterial infections, such as pneumonia and wound infections, proved resistant to chemical treatments for many years, despite strenuous effort on the part of the pharmaceutical industry. In 1927, IG Farbenindustrie, which had a long-standing interest in discovering antimicrobial drugs, appointed Gerhard Domagk to direct their research. Among the various leads that he followed was a series of azo dyes, included among which were some sulfonamide derivatives (a modification introduced earlier into dyestuffs to improve their affinity for certain fibres). These were much more effective in animals, and less toxic, than anything that had gone before, and *Prontosil* – a dark-red azo dye – was introduced in 1935. In the same year, it saved the life of Domagk's daughter, who developed septicaemia after a needle prick. It was soon discovered that the azo linkage in the Prontosil molecule was rapidly cleaved in the body, yielding the colourless compound *sulfanilamide*, which accounted for the antibacterial effect of Prontosil[9].

With chemistry still firmly in the driving seat, and little concern about mechanisms or targets, many sulfonamides were made in the next few years and they dramatically improved the prognosis of patients suffering from infectious diseases.

The mechanistic light began to dawn in 1940, when D. D. Woods, a microbiologist in Oxford, discovered that the antibacterial effect of sulfonamides was antagonized by *p*-aminobenzoic acid (PABA), a closely related compound and a precursor in the biosynthesis of folic acid (Figure 1.1). Bacteria, but not eukaryotic cells, have to synthesize their own folic acid to support DNA synthesis. Woods deduced that sulfonamides compete with PABA for a target enzyme, now known to be dihydropteroate synthase, and thus prevent folic acid synthesis.

---

[9]Sulfanilamide, a known compound, could not be patented, and so many companies soon began to make and sell it in various formulations. In 1937 about 80 people who took the drug died as a result of solvent-induced liver and kidney damage. It was this accident that led to the US Food and Drug Act, with the Food & Drug Administration (FDA) to oversee it (see Chapter 20).

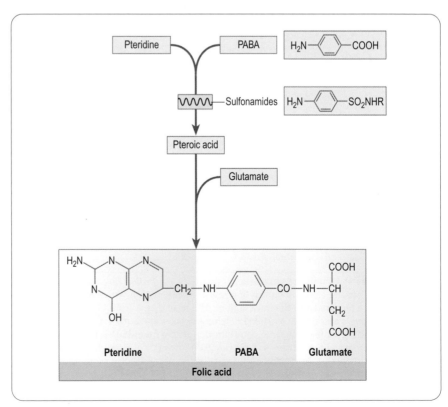

Fig. 1.1
Folic acid synthesis and PABA.

The discovery of sulfonamides and the elucidation of their mechanism of action had great repercussions, scientifically as well as clinically. In the drug discovery field, it set off two major lines of inquiry. First, the sulfonamide structure proved to be a rich source of molecules with many different, and useful, pharmacological properties – an exuberant vindication of the chemistry-led approach to drug discovery. Second, attacking the folic acid pathway proved to be a highly successful strategy for producing therapeutically useful drugs – a powerful boost for the 'targeteers', who were still few in number at this time.

The chemical dynasty originating with sulfanilamide is shown in Figure 1.2. An early spin-off came from the clinical observation that some sulfonamides produced an alkaline diuresis, associated with an increased excretion of sodium bicarbonate in the urine. Carbonic anhydrase, an enzyme which catalyses the interconversion of carbon dioxide and carbonic acid, was described in 1940, and its role in renal bicarbonate excretion was discovered a few years later, which prompted the finding that some, but not all, sulfonamides inhibit this enzyme. Modification of the sulfonamide structure led eventually to *acetazolamide* the first commercially available carbonic anhydrase inhibitor, as a diuretic in 1952. Following the diuretic trail led in turn to *chlorothiazide*

(1957), the first of the thiazide diuretics, which, though devoid of carbonic anhydrase inhibitory activity, was much more effective than acetazolamide in increasing sodium excretion, and much safer than the earlier mercurial diuretics, which had until then been the best drugs available for treating oedema associated with heart failure and other conditions. Still further modifications led first to *frusemide* (1962) and later to *bumetanide* (1984), which were even more effective than the thiazides in producing a rapid diuresis – 'torrential' being the adjective applied by clinicians with vivid imaginations. Other modifications of the thiazide structures led to the accidental but important discovery of a series of hypotensive vasodilator drugs, such as *hydralazine* and *diazoxide*. In yet another development, *carbutamide*, one of the sulfonamides synthesized by Boehringer in 1954 as part of an antibacterial drug programme, was found accidentally to cause hypoglycaemia. This drug was the first of the sulfonylurea series, from which many further derivatives, such as *tolbutamide* and *glibenclamide*, were produced and used successfully to treat diabetes. All of these products of the sulfonamide dynasty are widely used today. Their chemical relationship to sulfonamides is clear, though none of them has antibacterial activity. Their biochemical targets in smooth muscle, the kidney, the pancreas and

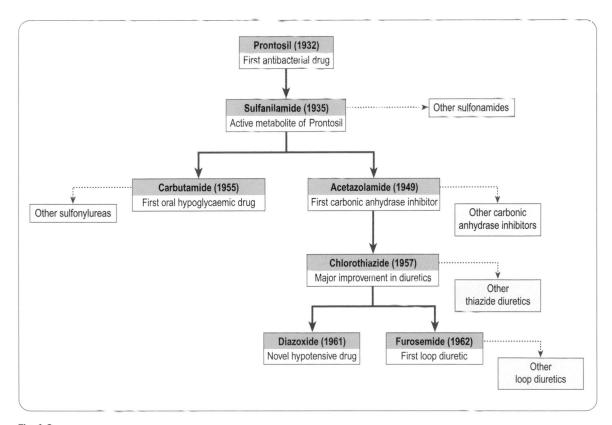

Fig. 1.2
Sulfonamide dynasty.

elsewhere, are all different. Chemistry, not biology, was the guiding principle in their discovery and synthesis.

Target-directed approaches to drug design have played a much more significant role in areas other than antibacterial chemotherapy, the approaches being made possible by advances on two important fronts, separated, as it happens, by the Atlantic Ocean. In the United States, the antimetabolite principle, based on interfering with defined metabolic pathways, proved to be highly successful, due largely to the efforts of George Hitchings and Gertrude Elion at Burroughs Wellcome. In Europe, drug discovery took its lead more from physiology than biochemistry, and sprung from advances in knowledge of chemical transmitters and their receptors. The names of Henry Dale and James Black deserve special mention here.

Hitchings and Elion and the antimetabolite principle

George Hitchings and Gertrude Elion came together in 1944 in the biochemistry department of Burroughs Wellcome in Tuckahoe, New York. Their biochemical interest lay in the synthesis of folic acid, based on the importance of this pathway for the action of sulfonamides, and they set about synthesizing potential 'antimetabolites' of purines and pyrimidines as chemotherapeutic agents. At the time, it was known that this pathway was important for DNA synthesis, but the role of DNA in cell function was uncertain. It turned out to be an inspired choice, and theirs was one of the first drug discovery programmes to focus on a biochemical pathway, rather than on a series of chemical compounds[10].

Starting from a series of purine and pyrimidine analogues, which had antibacterial activity, Hitchings and Rlion identified a key enzyme in the folic acid pathway, namely dihydrofolate reductase, which was necessary for DNA synthesis and was inhibited by many of their antibacterial pyrmidine analogues. Because all cells, not just bacteria, use this reaction to make DNA, they wondered why the drugs showed selectivity in their ability to block cell division, and found that the enzyme showed considerable species variation in its susceptibility to inhibitors. This led them to seek inhibitors that would selectively attack bacteria, protozoa and human neoplasms, which they achieved with great success. Drugs to emerge from this programme included the antituberculosis drug *pyrimethamine*, the antibacterial

trimethoprim, and the anticancer drug *6-mercaptopurine*, as well as *azathioprine*, an immunosuppressant drug that was later widely used to prevent transplant rejection. Another spin-off from the work of Hitchings and Elion was *allopurinol*, an inhibitor of purine synthesis that is used in the treatment of gout. Later on, Elion – her enthusiasm for purines and pyrimidines undiminished – led the research group which in 1977 discovered one of the first effective antiviral drugs, *aciclovir*, an inhibitor of DNA polymerase, and later the first antiretroviral drug, *zidovudine* (AZT), which inhibits reverse transcriptase. Hitchings and Elion, by focusing on the metabolic pathways involved in DNA synthesis, invented an extraordinary range of valuable therapeutic drugs, an achievement unsurpassed in the history of drug discovery.

James Black and receptor-targeted drugs

As already mentioned, the concept of 'receptors' as recognition sites for hormones and other physiological mediators came from J. N. Langley's analysis of the mechanism of action of 'curari'. Henry Dale's work on the distinct 'muscarinic' and 'nicotinic' actions of acetylcholine also pointed to the existence of two distinct types of cholinergic receptor, though Dale himself dismissed the receptor concept as an abstract and unhelpful cloak for ignorance. During the 1920s and 1930s, major discoveries highlighting the role of chemical mediators were made by physiologists, including the discovery of insulin, adrenal steroids and several neurotransmitters, and the realization that chemical signalling was crucial for normal function focused attention on the receptor mechanisms needed to decode these signals. Pharmacologists, particularly A. J. Clark, J. H. Gaddum and H. O. Schild, applied the Law of Mass Action to put ligand–receptor interactions on a quantitative basis. Schild's studies on drug antagonism in particular, which allowed the binding affinity of competitive antagonists to receptors to be estimated from pharmacological experiments, were an important step forward, which provided the first – and still widely used – quantitative basis for classifying drug receptors. On the basis of such quantitative principles, R. P. Ahlquist in 1948 proposed the existence of two distinct classes of adrenergic receptor, α and β, which accounted for the varied effects of epinephrine and norepinephrine on the cardiovascular system. This discovery inspired James Black, working in the research laboratories of Imperial Chemical Industries in the UK, to seek antagonists that would act selectively on β-adrenoceptors and thus block the effects of epinephrine on the heart, which were thought to be

---

[10]They were not alone. In the 1940s, a group at Lederle laboratories made *aminopterin* and *methotrexate*, folic acid antagonists which proved effective in treating leukaemia.

harmful in patients with coronary disease. His chemical starting point was *dichloroisoprenaline*, which had been found by Slater in 1957 to block the relaxant effects of epinephrine on bronchial smooth muscle – of no interest to Slater at the time, as he was looking for compounds with the opposite effect. The result of Black's efforts was the first β-adrenoceptor blocking drug, *pronethalol* (1960), which had the desired effects in humans but was toxic. It was quickly followed by *propranolol* (registered in 1964[11]) – one of the earliest blockbusters, which found many important applications in cardiovascular medicine. This was the first time that a receptor, identified pharmacologically, had been deliberately targeted in a drug discovery project.

Black, after moving to Smith Kline and French, went on from this success to look for novel histamine antagonists that would block the stimulatory effect of histamine on gastric acid secretion, this effect being resistant to the then-known antihistamine drugs. The result of this project, in which the chemistry effort proved much tougher than the β-adrenoceptor antagonist project, was the first H_2-receptor antagonist, *burimamide* (1972). This compound was a major clinical advance, being the first effective drug for treating peptic ulcers, but (like pronethalol) was quickly withdrawn because of toxicity, to be replaced by *cimetidine* (1976). In 1988 Black, along with Hitchings and Elion, was awarded the Nobel Prize.

Black's work effectively opened up the field of receptor pharmacology as an approach to drug discovery, and the pharmaceutical industry quickly moved in to follow his example. Lookalike β-adrenoceptor antagonists and H_2-receptor antagonists followed rapidly during the 1970s and 1980s, and many other receptors were set up as targets for potential therapeutic agents, based on essentially the same approach – though with updated technology – that Black and his colleagues had introduced.

Drews (2000) estimated that of 483 identified targets on which the current set of approved drugs act, G-protein-coupled receptors – of which β-adrenoceptors and H_2-receptors are typical examples – account for 45%. Many other successful drugs have resulted from target-directed projects along the lines pioneered by Black and his colleagues. In recent years, of course, receptors have changed from being essentially figments in an operational scheme devised by pharmacologists to explain their findings, to being concrete molecular entities that can be labelled, isolated as proteins, cloned and expressed, just like many other proteins. As we shall see in later chapters, these advances have completely transformed the techniques employed in drug discovery research.

Accidental clinical discoveries

Another successful route to the discovery of new drugs has been through observations made in the clinic. Until drug discovery became an intentional activity, such serendipitous observations were the only source of knowledge. Withering's discovery in 1785 of the efficacy of digitalis in treating dropsy, and Wenkebach's discovery in 1914 of the antidysrhythmic effect of quinine, when he treated a patient with malaria who also happened to suffer from atrial tachycardia, are two of many examples where the clinical efficacy of plant-derived agents has been discovered by highly observant clinicians. More recently, clinical benefit of unexpected kinds has been discovered with synthetic compounds developed for other purposes. In 1937, for example, Bradley tried *amphetamine* as a means of alleviating the severe headache suffered by children after lumbar puncture (spinal tap), on the grounds that the drug's cardiovascular effects might prove beneficial. The headache was not alleviated, but Bradley noticed that the children became much less agitated. From this chance observation he went on to set up one of the first controlled clinical trials, which demonstrated unequivocally that amphetamine had a calming effect – quite unexpected for a drug known to have stimulant effects in other circumstances. From this developed the widespread use, validated by numerous controlled clinical trials, of amphetamine-like drugs, particularly *methylphenidate* (Ritalin) to treat attention deficit hyperactivity disorder (ADHD) in children. Other well-known examples include the discovery of the antipsychotic effects of phenothiazines by Laborit in 1949. Laborit was a naval surgeon, concerned that patients were dying from 'surgical shock' – circulatory collapse resulting in irreversible organ failure – after major operations. Thinking that histamine might be involved, he tested the antihistamine *promethazine* combined with autonomic blocking drugs to prevent this cardiovascular reaction. Although it was ineffective in treating shock, promethazine caused some sedation and Laborit tried some chemically related sedatives, notably *promazine*, which had little antihistamine activity. Patients treated with it fared better during surgery, but Laborit particularly noticed that they appeared much calmer postoperatively. He therefore persuaded his psychiatrist colleagues to test the drug on psychotic patients, tests that quickly revealed the drug's antipsychotic effects and led to the development of the antipsychotic *chlorpromazine*. In a sequel, other phenothiazine-like tricyclic compounds were tested for antipsychotic activity but were found accidentally to relieve the symptoms of depression. After

---

[11]Ironically, propranolol had been made in 1959 in the laboratories of Boehringer Ingelheim, as part of a different, chemistry-led project. Only when linked to its target could the clinical potential of propranolol be revealed – chemistry alone was not enough!

Bradley and Laborit, psychiatrists had become alert to looking for the unexpected.

Astute clinical observation has revealed many other unexpected therapeutic effects, for example the efficacy of various antidepressant and antiepileptic drugs in treating certain intractable pain states.

The regulatory process

In the mid-19th century restrictions on the sale of poisonous substances were imposed in the USA and UK, but it was not until the early 1900s that any system of 'prescription-only' medicines was introduced, requiring approval by a medical practitioner. Soon afterwards, restrictions began to be imposed on what 'cures' could be claimed in advertisements for pharmaceutical products and what information had to be given on the label; legislation evolved at a leisurely pace. Most of the concern was with controlling frankly poisonous or addictive substances or contaminants, not with the efficacy and possible harmful effects of new drugs.

In 1937, the use of diethylene glycol as a solvent for a sulfonamide preparation caused 107 deaths in the USA, and a year later the 1906 Food and Drugs Act was revised, requiring safety to be demonstrated before new products could be marketed, and also allowing federal inspection of manufacturing facilities. The requirement for proven efficacy, as well as safety, was added in the Kefauver–Harris amendment in 1962.

In Europe, preoccupied with the political events in the first half of the century, matters of drug safety and efficacy were a minor concern, and it was not until the mid-1960s, in the wake of the thalidomide disaster – a disaster averted in the USA by an assiduous officer, who used the provisions of the 1938 Food and Drugs Act to delay licensing approval – that the UK began to follow the US lead in regulatory laws. Until then, the ability of drugs to do harm – short of being frankly poisonous or addictive – was not really appreciated, most of the concern having been about contaminants. In 1959, when thalidomide was first put on the market by the German company Chemie Grünenthal, regulatory controls did not exist in Europe: it was up to the company to decide how much research was needed to satisfy itself that the drug was safe and effective. Grünenthal made a disastrously wrong judgement (see Sjöstrom and Nilsson, 1972, for a full account), which resulted in an estimated 10 000 cases of severe congenital malformation following the company's specific recommendation that the drug was suitable for use by pregnant women. This single event caused an urgent reappraisal, leading to the introduction of much tighter government controls.

In the UK, the Committee on the Safety of Drugs was established in 1963. For the first time, as in the USA, all new drugs (including new mixtures and formulations) had to be submitted for approval before clinical trials could begin, and before they could be marketed. Legally, companies could proceed even if the Committee did not approve, but very few chose to do so. This loophole was closed by the Medicines Act (1968), which made it illegal to proceed without approval. Initially, safety alone was the criterion for approval; in 1970, under the Medicines Act, evidence of efficacy was added to the criteria for approval. It was the realization that all drugs, not just poisons or contaminants, have the potential to cause harm that made it essential to seek proof of therapeutic efficacy to ensure that the net effect of a new drug was beneficial.

In the decade leading up to 1970, the main planks in the regulatory platform – evidence of safety, efficacy and chemical purity – were in place in most developed countries. Subsequently, the regulations have been adjusted in various minor ways, and adopted with local variations in most countries.

A progressive tightening of the restrictions on the licensing of new drugs continued for about two decades after the initial shock of thalidomide, as public awareness of the harmful effects of drugs became heightened, and the regulatory bodies did their best to respond to public demand for assurance that new drugs were 'completely safe'. The current state of licensing regulations is described in Chapter 20.

Concluding remarks

In this chapter we have followed the evolution of ideas and technologies that have led to the state of drug discovery research that existed circa 1970. The main threads, which came together, were:

● Clinical medicine, by far the oldest of the antecedents, which relied largely on herbal remedies right up to the 20th century;
● Pharmacy, which began with the apothecary trade in the 17th century, set up to serve the demand for herbal preparations;
● Organic chemistry, beginning in the mid-19th century and evolving into medicinal chemistry via dyestuffs;
● Pharmacology, also beginning in the mid-19th century and setting out to explain the effects of plant-derived pharmaceutical preparations in physiological terms.

Some of the major milestones are summarized in Table 1.2.

The pharmaceutical industry as big business began around the beginning of the 20th century, and for 60 or more years was dominated by chemistry. Gradually, from the middle of the century onwards, the balance

Table 1.2
Milestones in the development of the pharmaceutical industry

Year	Event	Notes
c. 1550 BC	Ebers papyrus	The earliest known compendium of medical remedies
1540	Diethyl ether synthesized	'Sweet oil of vitriol', arguably the first synthetic drug
1668	Merck (Darmstadt) founded	The apothecary business which later (1827) evolved into the first large-scale pharmaceutical company
1775	Nitrous oxide synthesized	
1785	Withering describes use of digitalis extract to treat 'dropsy'	The first demonstration of therapeutic efficacy
1803	Napoleon established examination and licensing scheme for doctors	
1763	Lind shows that lack of fruit causes scurvy	
1798	Jenner shows that vaccination prevents smallpox	
1799	Humphrey Davy demonstrates anaesthetic effect of nitrous oxide	
1806	Sertürner purifies morphine and shows it to be the active principle of opium	A seminal advance – the first evidence that herbal remedies contain active chemicals. Many other plant alkaloids isolated 1820–1840
1846	Morton administers ether as anaesthetic at Massachusets General Hospital	The first trial of surgical anaesthesia
1847	Chloroform administered to Queen Victoria to control labour pain	
1847	The first Pharmacological Institute set up by Bucheim	
mid-19C	The first pharmaceutical companies formed: Merck (1827) Squibb (1858) Hoechst (1862) Parke Davis (1866) Lilley (1876) Burroughs Wellcome (1880)	In many cases, pharmaceutical companies evolved from dyestuffs companies or apothecaries
1858	Virchow proposes cell theory	
1859	Amyl nitrite synthesized	
1865	Benzene structure elucidated (Kekule), and first use of structural fromulae to describe organic molecules	Essential foundations for the development of organic synthesis
1867	Brunton demonstrates use of amyl nitrite to relieve anginal pain	
1878	Pasteur proposes germ theory of disease	
1898	Heroin (diacetylmorphine) developed by Bayer	The first synthetic derivative of a natural product. Heroin was marketed as a safe and non-addictive alternative to morphine
1899	Aspirin developed by Bayer	
1903	Barbital developed by Bayer	
1904	Elliott demonstrates biological activity of extracts of adrenal glands, and proposes adrenaline release as a physiological mechanism	The first evidence for a chemical mediator – the basis of much modern pharmacology

Table 1.2
Milestones in the development of the pharmaceutical industry—cont'd

Year	Event	Notes
1910	Ehrlich discovers Salvarsan	The first antimicrobial drug, which revolutionized the treatment of syphilis
1912	Starling coins the term 'hormone'	
1921	MacLeod, Banting and Best discover insulin	Produced commercially by Lilly (1925)
1926	Loewi demonstrates release of 'Vagusstoff' from heart	The first clear evidence for chemical neurotransmission
1929	Fleming discovers penicillin	Penicillin was not used clinically until Chain and Florey solved production problems in 1938
1935	Domagk discovers sulfonamides	The first effective antibacterial drugs, and harbingers of the antimetabolite era
1936	Steroid hormones isolated by Upjohn company	
1937	Bovet discovers antihistamines	Subsequently led to discovery of antipsychotic drugs
1946	Gilman and Philips demonstrate anticancer effect of nitrogen mustards	The first anticancer drug
1951	Hitchings and Elion discover mercaptopurine	The first anticancer drug from the antimetabolite approach
1961	Hitchings and Schwartz discover azathioprine	Also from the antimetabolite programme, the first effective immunosuppressant able to prevent transplant rejection
1962	Black and his colleagues discover pronethalol	The first β-adrenoceptor antagonist to be used clinically
1972	Black and his colleagues discover burimamide	The first selective H_2 antagonist
1976	Genentech founded	The first biotech company, based on recombinant DNA technology
c. 1990	Introduction of combinatorial chemistry	

shifted towards pharmacology until, by the mid-1970s, chemistry and pharmacology were evenly balanced. This was a highly productive period for the industry, which saw many new drugs introduced, some of them truly novel but also many copycat drugs, which found an adequate market despite their lack of novelty. The maturation of the scientific and technological basis of the discovery process to its 1970s level coincided with the development of much more stringent regulatory controls, which also reached a degree of maturity at this time, and an acceptable balance seemed to be struck between creativity and restraint.

We ended our historical account in the mid-1970s, when drug discovery seemed to have found a fairly serene and successful equilibrium, and products and profits flowed at a healthy rate. Just around the corner, however, lay the arrival on the drug discovery scene of molecular biology and its commercial wing, the biotechnology industry, which over the next 20 years were to transform the process and diversify its products in a dramatic fashion (see Chapters 3 and 12). Starting in 1976, when the first biotechnology companies (Cetus and Genentech) were founded in the USA, there are now about 1300 such companies in the USA and another 900 in Europe, and the products of such enterprises account for a steadily rising proportion – currently about 25% – of new therapeutic agents registered. As well as contributing directly in terms of products, biotechnology is steadily and radically transforming the ways in which conventional drugs are discovered.

The last quarter of the century has been a turbulent period which has affected quite radically the scientific basis of the development of new medicines, as well as the commercial environment in which the industry operates. The changes that are occurring show no sign of slowing down, and it is too soon to judge which developments will prove genuinely successful in terms of drug discovery, and which will not. In later chapters we discuss in detail the present state of the art with respect to the science and technology of drug discovery. The major discernible trends are as follows:

- Genomics as an approach to identifying new drug targets (Chapters 6 and 7);
- Increasing use of informatics technologies to store and interpret data (Chapter 7);

- High-throughput screening of large compound libraries as a source of chemical leads (Chapter 8);
- Combinatorial chemistry as a means of efficiently and systematically synthesizing collections of related compounds (Chapter 9);
- Increased emphasis on 'drugability' – mainly centred on pharmacokinetics and toxicology – in the selection of lead compounds (Chapter 10);
- Increased use of transgenic animals as disease models for drug testing (Chapter 11);
- The growth of biopharmaceuticals (Chapter 12).

What effect are these changes having on the success of the industry in finding new drugs? Despite the difficulty of defining and measuring such success, the answer seems to be 'not much so far'. Productivity, measured by the flow of new drugs (Figure 1.3) seems, if anything, to have drifted downwards over the last 15 years, and very markedly so since the 1960s, when regulatory controls began to be tightened. This measure, of course, takes no account of whether new drugs have inherent novelty and represent a significant therapeutic advance, or are merely the result of one company copying another. There are reasons for thinking that new drugs are now more innovative than they used to be, but clear evidence for this is hard to find. One sign is the growth of biopharmaceuticals relative to conventional drugs (Figure 1.4; see Chapters 12 and 21); most biopharmaceuticals represent novel therapeutic strategies, and there is less scope for copycat projects, which still account for a substantial proportion of new synthetic drugs. Adding to the disquiet caused by the downward trend in Figure 1.3 is the fact that research and development expenditure has steadily increased over the same period, and that development times – from discovery of a new molecule to market – have remained at 10–12 years since 1982. Costs, times and success rates are discussed in more detail in Chapter 21.

Nobody really understands why the apparent drop in research productivity has occurred, but speculations abound. One factor may be the increasing regulatory hurdles, which mean that development takes longer and costs more than it used to, so that companies have become more selective in choosing which compounds to develop. Another factor may be the trend away from 'me-too' drugs (drugs that differ little, if at all, from those already in use, but which nevertheless provide the company with a profitable share of the market while providing little or no benefit to patients).

The hope is that the downward trend will be reversed as the benefit of new technologies to the drug discovery process works through the system, as long development times mean that technologies introduced since 1990 have not yet had time to make an impact on registrations.

In the remainder of this book, we describe drug discovery at the time of writing (2003) – a time when the molecular biology revolution is in full swing. In a few years' time our account will undoubtedly look as dated as the 1970s scenario seems to us today.

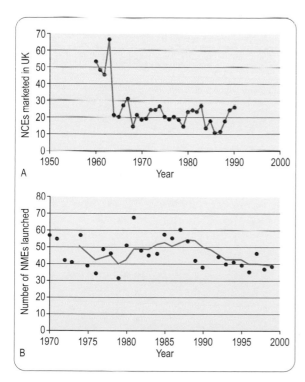

Fig. 1.3
Productivity – new drugs introduced 1970–2000. (a) Number of new chemical entities (NCEs) marketed in the UK 1960–1990, showing the dramatic effect of the thalidomide crisis in 1961. (Data from Griffin (1991) International Journal of Pharmacy 5: 206–209.) (b) Annual number of new molecular entities marketed in 20 countries worldwide 1970–1999. The line represents a 5-year moving average. (Data from Centre for Medicines Research Pharma R&D Compendium, 2000.)

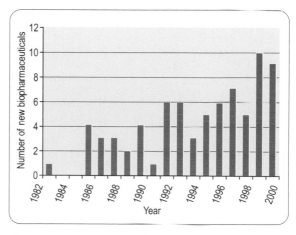

Fig. 1.4
Growth of biopharmaceuticals.

References

Drews J (2000) Drug discovery: a historical perspective. Science 287; 1960–1964.

Drews J (2003) In quest of tomorrow's medicines, 2nd edn. New York: Springer.

Drews J (2004) Paul Ehrlich: magister mundi. Nature Reviews Drug Discovery 3: 797–801.

Lednicer D (ed) (1993) Chronicles of drug discovery. Vol 3. Washington, DC: American Chemical Society.

Mann R D (1984) Modern drug use: an enquiry on historical principles. Lancaster: MTP Press.

Maxwell R A, Eckhardt S B (1990) Drug discovery: a casebook and analysis. Clifton, NJ: Humana Press.

Office of Health Economics (1983) Pharmaceutical innovation: recent trends, future prospects. Report No. 74. London, Office of Health Economics.

Porter R (1997) The greatest benefit to mankind: a medical history of humanity from antiquity to the present. London: Harper Collins.

Sjöstrom H, Nilsson R (1972) Thalidomide and the power of the drug companies. Harmondsworth: Penguin.

Sneader W (1985) Drug discovery: the evolution of modern medicines. Chichester: John Wiley.

Weatherall M (1990) In search of a cure: a history of pharmaceutical discovery. Oxford: Oxford University Press.

The nature of disease and the purpose of therapy

H P Rang

Introduction

In this book, we are concerned mainly with the drug discovery process itself, which those involved in research proudly regard as the mainspring of the pharmaceutical industry. In this chapter we consider the broader context of the human environment into which new drugs and medicinal products are launched, and where they must find their proper place. Most pharmaceutical companies place at the top of their basic mission statement a commitment to improve the public's health, to relieve the human burden of disease. Few would argue with the spirit of this commitment. Nevertheless, we need to look more closely at what it means, how disease is defined, what medical therapy aims to alter, and how – and by whom – the effects of therapy are judged and evaluated. Here we outline some of the basic principles underlying these broader issues.

Concepts of disease

The practice of medicine predates by thousands of years the science of medicine, and the application of 'therapeutic' procedures by professionals similarly predates any scientific understanding of how the human body works, or what happens when it goes wrong. As discussed in Chapter 1, the ancients defined disease not only in very different terms, but also on a quite different basis from what we would recognize today. The origin of disease and the measures needed to counter it were generally seen as manifestations of divine will and retribution, rather than of physical malfunction. The scientific revolution in medicine, which began in earnest during the 19th century and has been steadily accelerating since, has changed our concept of disease quite drastically, and continues to challenge it, raising new ethical problems and thorny discussions of principle. For the centuries of prescientific medicine, codes of practice based on honesty, integrity and professional relationships were quite sufficient: as therapeutic interventions were ineffective anyway, it mattered little to what situations they were applied. Now, quite suddenly, the language of disease has changed and interventions have become effective; not surprisingly, we have to revise our ideas about what constitutes disease, and how medical intervention should be used. In this chapter, we will try to define the scope and purpose of therapeutics in the context of modern biology. In reality, however, those in the science-based drug discovery business have to recognize the strong atavistic leanings of many healthcare professions[1], whose roots go back much further than the age of science.

Therapeutic intervention, including the medical use of drugs, aims to prevent, cure or alleviate disease states. The question of exactly what we mean by disease, and how we distinguish disease from other kinds of human affliction and dysfunction, is of more than academic importance, because policy and practice with respect to healthcare provision depend on where we draw the line between what is an appropriate target for therapeutic intervention and what is not. The issue concerns not only doctors, who have to decide every day what kind of complaints warrant treatment, but all those involved in the healthcare business – including, of course, the pharmaceutical industry. Much has been written on the difficult question of how to define health and disease, and what demarcates a proper target for therapeutic intervention (Reznek, 1987; Caplan, 1993; Caplan et al., 2004); nevertheless, the waters remain distinctly murky.

One approach is to define what we mean by health, and to declare the attainment of health as the goal of all healthcare measures, including therapeutics.

What is health?

In everyday parlance we use the words 'health', 'fitness', 'wellbeing' on the one hand, and 'disease', 'illness', 'sickness', 'ill-health' etc. on the other, more or less interchangeably, but these words become slippery and evasive when we try to define them. The World Health Organization (WHO), for example, defines health as 'a state of complete physical, mental and social wellbeing and not merely the absence of sickness or infirmity'. On this basis, few humans could claim to possess health, although the majority may not be in the grip of obvious sickness or infirmity. Who is to say what constitutes 'complete physical, mental and social well-being' in a human being? Does physical well being imply an ability to run a marathon? Does a shy and self-effacing person lack social well-being?

We also find health defined in functional terms, less idealistically than in the WHO's formulation: '...health consists in our functioning in conformity with our

natural design with respect to survival and reproduction, as determined by natural selection...' (Caplan, 1993). Here the implication is that evolution has brought us to an optimal – or at least an acceptable – compromise with our environment, with the corollary that healthcare measures should properly be directed at restoring this level of functionality in individuals who have lost some important element of it. This has a fashionably 'greenish' tinge, and seems more realistic than the WHO's chillingly utopian vision, but there are still difficulties in trying to use it as a guide to the proper application of therapeutics. Environments differ. A black-skinned person is at a disadvantage in sunless climates, where he may suffer from vitamin D deficiency, whereas a white-skinned person is liable to develop skin cancer in the tropics. The possession of a genetic abnormality of haemoglobin, known as sickle-cell trait, is advantageous in its heterozygous form in the tropics, as it confers resistance to malaria, whereas homozygous individuals suffer from a severe form of haemolytic anaemia (sickle-cell disease). Hyperactivity in children could have survival value in primitive societies, whereas in western countries it disrupts families and compromises education. Obsessionality and compulsive behaviour are quite normal in early motherhood, and may serve a good biological purpose, but in other walks of life can be a severe handicap, warranting medical treatment.

Health cannot therefore be regarded as a definable state – a fixed point on the map, representing a destination which all are seeking to reach. Rather, it seems to be a continuum, through which we can move in either direction, becoming more or less well adapted for survival in our particular environment. Although we could argue that the aim of healthcare measures is simply to improve our state of adaptation to our present environment, this is obviously too broad. Other factors than health – for example wealth, education, peace, and the avoidance of famine – are at least as important, but lie outside the domain of medicine. What actually demarcates the work of doctors and healthcare workers from that of other caring professionals – all of whom may contribute to health in different ways – is that the former focus on *disease*.

What is disease?

Consider the following definitions of disease:

● A condition which alters or interferes with the normal state of an organism and is usually characterized by the abnormal functioning of one or more of the host's systems, parts or organs (*Churchill's Medical Dictionary*, 1989).
● A morbid entity characterized usually by at least two of these criteria: recognized aetiologic agents,

---

[1]The upsurge of 'alternative' therapies, many of which owe nothing to science – and indeed reject the relevance of science to what its practitioners do – perhaps reflects an urge to return to the prescientific era of medical history.

identifiable groups of signs and symptoms, or consistent anatomical alterations (elsewhere, 'morbid' is defined as diseased or pathologic) (*Stedman's Medical Dictionary*, 1990).

We sense the difficulty that these thoughtful authorities found in pinning down the concept. The first definition emphasizes two aspects, namely *deviation from normality*, and *dysfunction*; the second emphasizes *aetiology* (i.e. causative factors) and *phenomenology* (signs, symptoms etc.), which is essentially the manifestation of dysfunction.

Deviation from normality does not define disease

The criterion of deviation from normality begs many questions. It implies that we know what the 'normal state' is, and can define what constitutes an alteration of it. It suggests that if our observations were searching enough, we could unfailingly distinguish disease from normality. But we know, for example, that the majority of 50-year-olds will have atherosclerotic lesions in their arteries, that some degree of osteoporosis is normal in postmenopausal women. These are not deviations from normality, nor do they in themselves cause dysfunction, and so they do not fall within these definitions of disease, yet both are seen as pathological and as legitimate — indeed important — targets for therapeutic intervention. Furthermore, as discussed below, deviations from normality are often beneficial and much prized.

Phenomenology and aetiology are important factors – the naturalistic view

Setting aside the normality criterion, the definitions quoted above are examples of the *naturalistic*, or observation-based, view of disease, defined by phenomenology and backed up in many cases by an understanding of aetiology; it is now generally agreed that this by itself is insufficient, for there is no *general* set of observable characteristics that distinguishes disease from health. Although individual diseases of course have their defining characteristics, which may be structural, biochemical or physiological, there is no common feature. Further, there are many conditions, particularly in psychiatry, but also in other branches of medicine, where such physical manifestations are absent, even though their existence as diseases is not questioned. Examples would include obsessive–compulsive disorder, schizophrenia, chronic fatigue syndrome, and low back pain. In such cases, of which there are many examples, the disease is defined by symptoms, of which only the patient is aware, or altered behaviour, of which he and those around him are aware: defining features at the physical, biochemical or physiological level are absent, or at least not yet recognized.

Harm and disvalue – the normative view

The shortcomings of the naturalistic view of disease, which is in principle value free, have led some authors to take the opposite view, to the extent of denying the relevance of any kind of objective criteria to the definition of disease. Crudely stated, this value-based (or *normative*) view holds that disease is simply any condition the individual or society finds disagreeable or harmful (i.e. *disvalues*). Taken to extremes by authors such as Szasz and Illich, this view denies the relevance of the physical manifestations of illness, and focuses instead on illness only as a manifestation of *social* intolerance or malfunction. Although few would go this far – and certainly modern biologists would not be among them – it is clear that value-laden judgements play a significant role in determining what we choose to view as disease. In the mid-19th century masturbation was regarded as a serious disease, to be treated if necessary by surgery, and this view persisted well into the 20th century. 'Drapetomania', defined as a disease of American slaves, was characterized by an obsessional desire for freedom. Homosexuality was seen as pathological, and determined attempts were made to treat it.

A definition of disease which tries to combine the concepts of biological malfunction and harm (or disvalue) was proposed by Caplan et al. (1981):

'States of affairs are called diseases when they are due to physiological or psychological processes that typically cause states of disability, pain or deformity, and are generally held to be below acceptable physiological or psychological norms'.

What is still lacking is any reference to aetiology, yet this can be important in recognizing disease, and indeed is increasingly so as we understand more about the underlying biological mechanisms. A patient who complains of feeling depressed may be reacting quite normally to a bereavement, or may come from a suicide-prone family, suggestive of an inherited tendency to depressive illness. The symptoms might be very similar, but the implications, based on aetiology, would be different.

In conclusion, disease proves extremely difficult to define (Scully, 2004). The closest we can get at present to an operational definition of disease rests on a combination of three factors: phenomenology, aetiology and disvalue, as summarized in Figure 2.1.

Labelling human afflictions as diseases (i.e. 'medicalizing' them) has various beneficial and adverse consequences, both for the affected individuals and for healthcare providers. It is of particular relevance to the pharmaceutical industry, which stands to benefit from the labelling of borderline conditions as diseases meriting therapeutic intervention. Strong criticism has been levelled at the industry for the way in which it uses its resources to promote the recognition of questionable

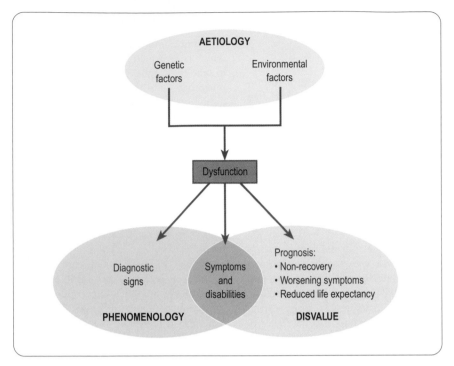

Fig. 2.1
Three components of disease.

disorders, such as female sexual dysfunction or social phobia, as diseases, and to elevate identified risk factors – asymptomatic in themselves but increasing the likelihood of disease occurring later – to the level of diseases in their own right. A recent polemic (Moynihan et al., 2004) starts with the sentence: 'there's a lot of money to be made from telling healthy people they're sick', and emphasizes the thin line that divides medical education from marketing.

The aims of therapeutics

Components of disvalue

The discussion so far leads us to the proposition that the proper aim of therapeutic intervention is to minimize

the disvalue associated with disease. The concept of disvalue is therefore central, and we need to consider what comprises it. The disvalue experienced by a sick individual has two distinct components[2] (Figure 2.1), namely *present symptoms and disabilities* (collectively termed *morbidity*), and future *prognosis* (namely the likelihood of increasing morbidity, or premature death). An individual who is suffering no abnormal symptoms or disabilities, and whose prognosis is that of an average individual of the same age, we call 'healthy'. An individual with a bad cold or a sprained ankle has symptoms and disabilities, but probably has a normal prognosis. An individual with asymptomatic lung cancer or hypertension has no symptoms but a poor prognosis. Either case constitutes disease, and warrants therapeutic intervention. Very commonly, both components of disvalue are present and both need to be addressed with therapeutic measures – different measures may be needed to alleviate morbidity and to im-

---

[2]These concepts apply in a straightforward way to many real-life situations, but there are exceptions and difficulties. For example, in certain psychiatric disorders the patient's judgement of his or her state of morbidity is itself affected by the disease. Patients suffering from mania, paranoid delusions or severe depression may pursue an extremely disordered and self-destructive lifestyle, while denying that they are ill and resisting any intervention. In such cases, society often imposes its own judgement of the individual's morbidity, and may use legal instruments such as the Mental Health Act

to apply therapeutic measures against the patient's will.

Vaccination represents another special case. Here, the disvalue being addressed is the theoretical risk that a healthy individual will later contract an infectious disease such as diphtheria or measles. This risk can be regarded as an adverse factor in the prognosis of a perfectly normal individual.

Similarly, a healthy person visiting the tropics will, if he is wise, take antimalarial drugs to avoid infection – in other words, to improve his prognosis.

prove prognosis. Of course, such measures need not be confined to physical and pharmacological approaches.

The proposition at the beginning of this section sets clear limits to the aims of therapeutic intervention, which encompass the great majority of non-controversial applications. Real life is, of course, not so simple, and in the next section we consider some of the important exceptions and controversies that healthcare professionals and policy-makers are increasingly having to confront.

Therapeutic intervention is not restricted to treatment or prevention of disease

The term 'lifestyle drugs' is a recent invention, but the concept of using drugs, and other types of intervention in a medical setting for purposes unrelated to the treatment of disease is by no means new.

Pregnancy is not by any definition a disease, nor are skin wrinkles, yet contraception, abortion and plastic surgery are well established practices in the medical domain. Why are we prepared to use drugs as contraceptives or abortifacients, but condemn using them to enhance sporting performance? The basic reason seems to be that we attach disvalue to unwanted pregnancy (i.e. we consider it harmful). We also attach disvalue to alternative means of avoiding unwanted pregnancy, such as sexual abstinence or using condoms. Other examples, however, such as cosmetic surgery to remove wrinkles or reshape breasts, seem to refute the disvalue principle: minor cosmetic imperfections are in no sense harmful, but society none the less concedes to the demand of individuals that medical technology should be deployed to enhance their beauty. In other cases, such as the use of sildenafil (Viagra) to improve male sexual performance, there is ambivalence about whether its use should be confined to those with evidence for erectile dysfunction (i.e. in whom disvalue exists) or whether it should also be used in normal men.

It is obvious that departures from normality can bring benefit as well as disadvantage. Individuals with above-average IQs, physical fitness, ball-game skills, artistic talents, physical beauty or charming personalities have an advantage in life. Is it, then, a proper role of the healthcare system to try to enhance these qualities in the average person? Our instinct says not, because the average person cannot be said to be diseased or suffering. There may be value in being a talented footballer, but there is no harm in not being one. Indeed, the value of the special talent lies precisely in the fact that most of us do not possess it. Nevertheless, a magical drug that would turn anyone into a brilliant footballer would certainly sell extremely well, at least until footballing skills

became so commonplace that they no longer had any value[3].

Football skills may be a fanciful example; longevity is another matter. The 'normal' human lifespan varies enormously in different countries, and in the west it has increased dramatically during our own lifetime (Figure 2.2). Is lifespan prolongation a legitimate therapeutic aim? Our instinct – and certainly medical tradition – suggests that delaying premature death from disease is one of the most important functions of healthcare, but we are very ambivalent when it comes to prolonging life in the aged. Our ambivalence stems from the fact that the aged are often irremediably infirm, not merely chronologically old. In the future we may understand better why humans become infirm, and hence more vulnerable to the environmental and genetic circumstances that cause them to become ill and die. And beyond that we may discover how to retard or prevent aging, so that the 'normal' lifespan will be much prolonged. Opinions will differ as to whether this will be the ultimate triumph of medical science or the ultimate social disaster[4].

Conclusions

We have argued that that disease can best be defined in terms of three components, aetiology, phenomenology and disvalue, and that the element of disvalue is the

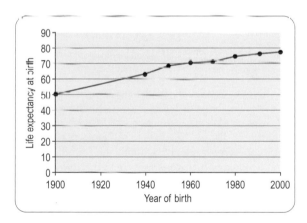

Fig. 2.2
Human lifespan in the USA. (Data from National Centre for Health Statistics, 1998.)

[3]The use of drugs to improve sporting performance is one of many examples of 'therapeutic' practices that find favour among individuals, yet are strongly condemned by society. We do not, as a society, attach disvalue to the possession of merely average sporting ability, even though the individual athlete may take a different view.
[4]Jonathan Swift, in *Gulliver's Travels*, writes of the misery of the Struldbrugs, rare beings with a mark on their forehead who, as they grew older, lost their youth but never died, and who were declared 'dead in law' at the age of 80.

most important determinant of what is considered appropriate to treat. In the end, though, medical practice evolves in a more pragmatic fashion, and such arguments prove to be of limited relevance to the way in which medicine is actually practised, and hence to the therapeutic goals the drug industry sees as commercially attractive. Politics, economics, and above all, social pressures are the determinants, and the limits are in practice set more by our technical capabilities than by issues of theoretical propriety.

Although the drug industry has so far been able to take a pragmatic view in selecting targets for therapeutic intervention, things are changing as technology advances. The increasing cost and sophistication of what therapeutics can offer mean that healthcare systems the world over are being forced to set limits, and are having to go back to the issue of what constitutes disease. Furthermore, by invoking the concept of disease, governments control access to many other social resources (e.g. disability benefits, entry into the armed services, insurance pay-outs, access to life insurance, exemption from legal penalties etc.).

So far, we have concentrated mainly on the impact of disease on individuals and societies. We now need to adopt a more biological perspective, and attempt to put the concept of disease into the framework of contemporary ideas about how biological systems work.

Function and dysfunction: the biological perspective

The dramatic revelations of the last few decades about the molecular basis of living systems have provided a new way of looking at function and dysfunction, and the nature of disease. Needless to say, molecular biology could not have developed without the foundations of scientific biology that were built up in the 19th century. As we saw in Chapter 1, this was the period in which science came to be accepted as the basis on which medical practice had to be built. Particularly significant was cell theory, which established the cell as the basic building block of living organisms. In the words of the pioneering molecular biologist, François Jacob: 'With the cell, biology discovered its atom'. It is by focusing on the instruction sets that define the form and function of cells, and the ways in which these instructions are translated in the process of generating the structural and functional phenotypes of cells, that molecular biology has come to occupy centre stage in modern biology. Genes specify proteins, and the proteins a cell produces determine its structure and function.

From this perspective, deviations from the norm, in terms of structure and function at the cellular level, arise through deviations in the pattern of protein expression by individual cells, and they may arise either through faults in the instruction set itself (genetic mutations) or through environmental factors that alter the way in which the instruction set is translated (i.e. that affect gene expression). We come back to the age-old distinction between inherited and environmental factors (nature and nurture) in the causation of disease, but with a sharper focus: altered gene expression, resulting in altered protein synthesis, is the mechanism through which all these factors operate. Conversely, it can be argued[5] that all therapeutic measures (other than physical procedures, such as surgery) also work at the cellular level, by influencing the same fundamental processes (gene expression and protein synthesis), although the link between a drug's primary target and the relevant effect(s) on gene expression that account for its therapeutic effect may be very indirect. We can see how it has come about that molecular biology, and in particular genomics, has come to figure so largely in the modern drug discovery environment.

Levels of biological organization

Figure 2.3 shows schematically the way in which the genetic constitution of a human being interacts with his or her environment to control function at many different levels, ranging from protein molecules, through single cells, tissues and integrated physiological systems, to the individual, the family and the population at large. For simplicity, we will call this the *bioaxis* . 'Disease', as we have discussed, consists of alterations of function sufficient to cause disability or impaired prognosis at the level of the individual. It should be noted that the arrows along the bioaxis in Figure 2.3 are bidirectional – that is, disturbances at higher levels of organization will in general affect function at lower levels, and vice versa. Whereas it is obvious that genetic mutations can affect function further up the bioaxis (as in many inherited diseases, such as muscular dystrophy, cystic fibrosis or thalassaemia), we should not forget that environmental influences also affect gene function. Indeed, we can state that any long-term phenotypic change (such as weight gain, muscle weakness or depressed mood) *necessarily* involves alterations of gene expression. For example:

---

[5]This represents the ultimate reductionist view of how living organisms work, and how they respond to external influences. Many still hold out against it, believing that the 'humanity' of man demands a less concrete explanation, and that 'alternative' systems of medicine, not based on our scientific understanding of biological function, have equal validity. Many doctors apparently feel most comfortable somewhere on the middle ground, and society at large tends to fall in behind doctors rather than scientists.

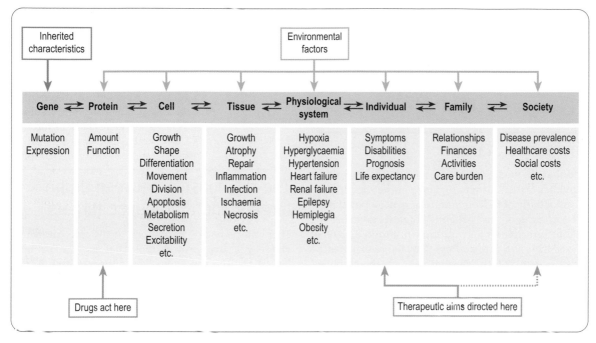

Fig. 2.3
The nature of disease.

- Exposure to a stressful environment will activate the hypothalamopituitary system and thereby increase adrenal steroid secretion, which in turn affects gene transcription in many different cells and tissues, affecting salt metabolism, immune responses and many other functions.
- Smoking, initiated as result of social factors such as peer pressure or advertising, becomes addictive as a result of changes in brain function, phenotypic changes which are in turn secondary to altered gene expression.
- Exposure to smoke carcinogens then increases the probability of cancer-causing mutations in the DNA of the cells of the lung. The mutations, in turn, result in altered protein synthesis and malignant transformation, eventually producing a localized tumour and later, disseminated cancer, with damage to the function of tissues and organs leading to symptoms and premature death.

The pathogenesis of any disease state reveals a similar level of complexity of such interactions between different levels of the bioaxis.

There are two important conclusions to be drawn from the bidirectionality of influence between events at different levels of the bioaxis. One is that it is difficult to pinpoint the *cause* of a given disease. Do we regard the cause of lung cancer in an individual patient as the lack of control over tobacco advertising, the individual's susceptibility to advertising and peer pressure, the state of addiction to nicotine, the act of smoking, the muta-

tional event in the lung epithelial cell, or the individual's inherited tendency to lung cancer? There is no single answer, and the uncertainty should make us wary of the stated claim of many pharmaceutical companies that their aim is to correct the causes rather than the symptoms of disease. The truth, more often than not, is that we cannot distinguish them. Rather, the aim should be to intervene in the disease process in such a way as to minimize the disvalue (disability and impaired prognosis) experienced by the patient.

The second conclusion is that altered gene expression plays a crucial role in pathogenesis and the production of any long-term phenotypic change. If we are thinking of timescales beyond, at maximum, a few hours, any change in the structure and function of cells and tissues will be associated with changes in gene expression. These changes will include those responsible for the phenotypic change (e.g. upregulation of cytokine genes in inflammation, leading to leukocyte accumulation), and those that are consequences of it (e.g. loss of bone matrix following muscle paralysis); some of the latter will, in turn, lead to secondary phenotypic changes, and so on. The pattern of genes expressed in a cell or tissue (sometimes called the 'transcriptome', as distinct from the 'genome', which represents all of the genes present, whether expressed or not), together with the 'proteome' (which describes the array of proteins present in a cell or tissue), provides a uniquely detailed description of how the cell or tissue is behaving. Molecular biology is providing us with powerful methods for mapping the changes in gene and protein expression associated with different functional states – including disease states and therapeutic responses – and we discuss in more detail in Chapters 6 and 7 the way these new windows on function are influencing the drug discovery process (see Debouck and Goodfellow, 1999).

Therapeutic targets

Traditionally, medicine has regarded the interests of the individual patient as paramount, putting them clearly ahead of those of the community or general population. The primacy of the patient's interests remains the guiding principle for the healthcare professions; in other words, their aim is to address disvalue as experienced by the patient, not to correct biochemical abnormalities, nor to put right the wrongs of society. The principal aim of therapeutic intervention, as shown in Figure 2.3, is therefore to alleviate the condition of the individual patient. Genetic, biochemical or physiological deviations which are not associated with any disvalue for the patient (e.g. possession of a rare blood group, an unusually low heart rate or blood pressure, or blood cholesterol concentration) are not treated as diseases because they neither cause symptoms nor carry an unfavourable prognosis. High blood pressure, or high blood cholesterol, on the other hand, do confer disvalue because they carry a poor prognosis, and are targets for treatment – surrogate targets, in the sense that the actual aim is to remedy the unfavourable prognosis, rather than to correct the physiological abnormality per se.

Although the present and future wellbeing of the individual patient remains the overriding priority for medical care, the impact of disease is felt not only by individuals, but also by society in general, partly for economic reasons, but also for ideological reasons. Reducing the overall burden of disease, as measured by rates of infant mortality, heart disease or AIDS, for example, is a goal for governments throughout the civilized world, akin to the improvement of educational standards. The disease-related disvalue addressed in this case, as shown by the secondary arrow in Figure 2.3, is experienced at the national, rather than the individual level, for individuals will in general be unaware of whether or not they have benefited personally from disease prevention measures. As the therapeutic target has come to embrace the population as a whole, so the financial burden of healthcare has shifted increasingly from individuals to institutional providers of various kinds, mainly national agencies or large-scale commercial healthcare organizations. Associated with this change, there has been a much more systematic focus on assessment in economic terms of the burden of disease (disvalue, to return to our previous terminology) in the

community, and the economic cost of healthcare measures. The new and closely related disciplines of *pharmacoeconomics* and *pharmacoepidemiology,* discussed later, reflect the wish (a) to quantify disease-related disvalue and therapeutic benefit in economic terms, and (b) to assess the impact of disease and therapy for the population as a whole, and not just for the individual patient.

The relationship between drug targets and therapeutic targets

There are very few exceptions to the rule, shown in Figure 2.3, that protein molecules are the primary targets of drug molecules. We will come back to this theme repeatedly later, because of its prime importance for the drug discovery process. We should note here that many complex biological steps intervene between the primary drug target and the therapeutic target. Predicting, on the one hand, whether a drug that acts specifically on a particular protein will produce a worthwhile therapeutic effect, and in what disease state, or, on the other hand, what protein we should choose to target in order to elicit a therapeutic effect in a given disease state, are among the thorniest problems for drug discoverers. Molecular biology is providing new insights into the nature of genes and proteins and the relationship between them, whereas time-honoured biochemical and physiological approaches can show how disease affects function at the level of cells, tissues, organs and individuals. The links between the two nevertheless remain tenuous, a fact which greatly limits our ability to relate drug targets to therapeutic effects. Not surprisingly, attempts to bridge this Grand Canyon form a major part of the work of many pharmaceutical and biotechnology companies. Afficionados like to call themselves 'postgenomic' biologists; Luddites argue that they are merely coming down from a genomic 'high' to face once more the daunting complexities of living organisms. We patient realists recognize that a biological revolution has happened, but do not underestimate the time and money needed to bridge the canyon. More of this later.

Therapeutic interventions

Therapeutics in its broadest sense covers all types of intervention aimed at alleviating the effects of disease. The term 'therapeutics' generally relates to procedures based on accepted principles of medical science, that is, on 'conventional' rather than 'alternative' medical practice[6]. The account of drug discovery presented in this book relates exclusively to conventional medicine – and for this we make no apology – but it needs to be realized that the therapeutic landscape is actually much broader, and includes many non-pharmacological procedures in the domain of conventional medicine, as well as quasi-pharmacological practices (e.g. homeopathy and herbalism) in the 'alternative' domain.

As discussed above, the desired effect of any therapeutic interventions is to improve *symptoms* or *prognosis* or both. From a pathological point of view, therapeutic interventions may be directed at *disease prevention, alleviation* of the effects of existing disease, or permanent *cure* (i.e. restoration to a state of function and prognosis equivalent to those of a healthy individual of the same age, without the need for continuing therapeutic intervention). In practice, there are relatively few truly curative interventions, and they are mainly confined to certain surgical procedures (e.g. removal of circumscribed tumours, fixing of broken bones) and chemotherapy of some infectious and malignant disorders. Most therapeutic interventions aim to alleviate symptoms and/or improve prognosis, and there is increasing emphasis on disease prevention as an objective.

It is important to realize that many types of interventions are carried out with therapeutic intent whose efficacy has not been rigorously tested. This includes not only the myriad alternative medical practices, but also many accepted conventional therapies for which a good scientific basis may exist but which have not been subjected to rigorous clinical trials.

Measuring therapeutic outcome

Effect, efficacy, effectiveness and benefit

These terms have acquired particular meanings – more limited than their everyday meanings – in the context of therapeutic trials.

Pharmacological *effects* of drugs (i.e. their effects on cells, organs and systems) are, in principle, simple to

[6]Scientific doctors rail against the term 'alternative', arguing that if a therapeutic practice can be shown to work by properly controlled trials, it belongs in mainstream medicine. If such trials fail to show efficacy, the practice should not be adopted. Paradoxically, whereas 'therapeutics' generally connotes conventional medicine, the term 'therapy' tends to be used most often in the 'alternative' field.

measure in animals, and often also in humans. We can measure effects on blood pressure, plasma cholesterol concentration, cognitive function etc. without difficulty. Such measures enable us to describe quantitatively the pharmacological properties of drugs, but say nothing about their usefulness as therapeutic agents.

Efficacy describes the ability of a drug to produce a desired therapeutic effect in patients under carefully controlled conditions. The gold standard for measurements of efficacy is the randomized controlled clinical trial, described in more detail in Chapter 18. The aim is to discover whether, based on a strictly defined outcome measure, the drug is more or less beneficial than a standard treatment or placebo, in a selected group of patients, under conditions which ensure that the patients actually receive the drug in the specified dose. Proof of efficacy, as well as proof of safety, is required by regulatory authorities as a condition for a new drug to be licensed. Efficacy tests what the drug can do under optimal conditions, which is what the prescriber usually wants to know.

Effectiveness describes how well the drug works in real life, where the patients are heterogeneous, are not randomized, are aware of the treatment they are receiving, are prescribed different doses, which they may or may not take, often in combination with other drugs. The desired outcome is generally less well defined than in efficacy trials, related to general health and freedom from symptoms, rather than focusing on a specific measure. The focus is not on the response of individual patients under controlled conditions, but on the overall usefulness of the drug in the population going about its normal business. Studies of effectiveness are of increasing interest to the pharmaceutical companies themselves, because effectiveness rather than efficacy alone ultimately determines how well the drug will sell, and because effectiveness may depend to a considerable extent on the companies' marketing strategies. Effectiveness measures are also becoming increasingly important to the many agencies that now regulate the provision of healthcare, such as formulary committees, insurance companies, health management organizations, and bodies such as the grandly titled National Institute for Clinical Excellence (NICE), set up by the UK Government in 1999 to advise, on the basis of cost-effectiveness, which drugs and other therapeutic procedures should be paid for under the National Health Service.

Benefit comprises effectiveness expressed in monetary terms. It is popular with economists, as it allows cost and benefit to be compared directly, but treated with deep suspicion by many who find the idea of assigning monetary value to life and wellbeing fundamentally abhorrent.

Returning to the theme of Figure 2.3, we can see that whereas *effect* and *efficacy* are generally measured at the level of cells, tissues, systems and individuals, *effective-*

ness and *benefit* are measures of drug action as it affects populations and society at large. We next consider two growing disciplines that have evolved to meet the need for information at these levels, and some of the methodological problems that they face.

Pharmacoepidemiology and pharmacoeconomics

Pharmacoepidemiology (Strom, 2000) is the study of the use and effects of drugs in human populations, as distinct from individuals, the latter being the focus of clinical pharmacology. The subject was born in the early 1960s, when the problem of adverse drug reactions came into prominence, mainly as a result of the infamous thalidomide disaster. The existence of rare but serious adverse drug reactions which can be detected only by the study of large numbers of subjects, was the initial stimulus for the development of pharmacoepidemiology, and the detection of adverse drug reactions remains an important concern. The identification of Reyes' syndrome as a serious, albeit rare, consequence of using aspirin in children is just one example of a successful pharmacoepidemiological study carried out under the auspices of the US Department of Health and published in 1987. The subject has gradually become broader, however, to cover aspects such as the variability of drug responses between individuals and population groups, the level of compliance of individual patients in taking drugs that are prescribed, and the overall impact of drug therapies on the population as a whole, taking all of these factors into account. The widely used antipsychotic drug *clozapine* provides an interesting example of the importance of pharmacoepidemiological issues in drug evaluation. Clozapine, first introduced in the 1970s, differed from its predecessors, such as haloperidol, in several ways, some good and some bad. On the good side, clozapine has a much lower tendency than haloperidol to cause extrapyramidal motor effects (a serious problem with many antipsychotic drugs), and it appeared to have the ability to improve not only the positive symptoms of schizophrenia (hallucinations, delusions, thought disorder, stereotyped behaviour) but also the negative symptoms (social withdrawal, apathy). Compliance is also better with clozapine, because the patient usually has fewer severe side effects. On the bad side, in about 1% of patients clozapine causes a fall in the blood white cell count (leukopenia), which can progress to an irreversible state of agranulocytosis unless the drug is stopped in time. Furthermore, clozapine does not produce benefit in all schizophrenic patients – roughly one-third fail to show improvement, and there is currently no way of knowing in advance which patients will benefit. Clozapine is also much more expensive than haloperidol. Considered from the perspective of an individual patient, and with hindsight, it is straightforward to balance the pros and cons of using clozapine rather than haloperidol, based on the severity of the extrapyramidal side effects, the balance of positive and negative symptoms which the patient has, whether clozapine is affecting the white cell count, and whether the patient is a responder or a non-responder. From the perspective of the overall population, evaluating the pros and cons of clozapine and haloperidol (or indeed of any two therapies) requires epidemiological data: how frequent are extrapyramidal side effects with haloperidol, what is the relative incidence of positive and negative symptoms, what is the incidence of agranulocytosis with clozapine, what proportion of patients are non-responders, what is the level of patient compliance with haloperidol and clozapine?

In summary, pharmacoepidemiology is a special area of clinical pharmacology which deals with population, rather than individual, aspects of drug action, and provides the means of quantifying *variability* in the response to drugs. Its importance for the drug discovery process is felt mainly at the level of clinical trials and regulatory affairs, for two reasons (Dieck et al., 1994). First, allowing for variability is essential in drawing correct inferences from clinical trials (see Chapter 18). Second, variability in response to a drug is per se disadvantageous, as drug A, whose effects are unpredictable, is less useful than drug B which acts consistently, even though the mean balance between beneficial and unwanted effects may be the same for both. From the population perspective, drug B looks better than drug A, even though for many individual patients the reverse may be true.

Pharmacoeconomics, a branch of health economics, is a subject that grew up around the need for healthcare providers to balance the ever-growing costs of healthcare against limited resources. The arrival of the welfare state, which took on healthcare provision as a national rather than an individual responsibility, was the signal for economists to move in. Good accounts of the basic principles and their application to pharmaceuticals are given by Gold et al. (1996), Johannesson (1996) and McCombs (1998). The aim of pharmacoeconomics is to measure the benefits and costs of drug treatments, and in the end to provide a sound basis for comparing the value for money of different treatments. As might be expected, the subject arouses fierce controversy. Economics in general is often criticized for defining the price of everything but appreciating the value of nothing, and health economics particularly tends to evoke this reaction, as health and quality of life are such ill-defined and subjective, yet highly emotive, concepts. Nevertheless, pharmacoeconomics is a rapidly growing discipline and will undoubtedly have an increasing influence on healthcare provision.

Pharmacoeconomic evaluation of new drugs is often required by regulatory authorities, and is increasingly being used by healthcare providers as a basis for choosing how to spend their money. Consequently, pharmaceutical companies now incorporate such studies into the clinical trials programmes of new drugs. The trend can be seen as a gradual progression towards the right-hand end of the bioaxis in Figure 2.3 in our frame of reference for assessing the usefulness of a new drug. Before 1950, new drugs were often introduced into clinical practice on the basis of studies in animals and a few human volunteers; later, formal randomized controlled clinical trials on carefully selected patient populations, with defined outcome measures, became the accepted standard, along with postmarketing pharmacoepidemiological studies to detect adverse reactions. Pharmacoeconomics represents the further shift of focus to include society in general and its provisions for healthcare. A brief outline of the main approaches used in pharmacoeconomic analysis follows.

Pharmacoeconomics covers four levels of analysis:

- Cost identification
- Cost-effectiveness analysis
- Cost–utility analysis
- Cost–benefit analysis.

Cost identification consists of determining the full cost in monetary units of a particular therapeutic intervention, including hospitalization, working days lost etc., as well as direct drug costs. It pays no attention to outcome, and its purpose is merely to allow the costs of different procedures to be compared. The calculation is straightforward, but deciding exactly where to draw the line (e.g. whether to include indirect costs, such as loss of income by patients and carers) is somewhat arbitrary. Nevertheless, cost identification is the least problematic part of pharmacoeconomics.

Cost-effectiveness analysis aims to quantify outcome as well as cost. This is where the real problems begin. The outcome measure most often used in cost-effectiveness analysis is based on prolongation of life, expressed as *life-years saved per patient treated*. Thus if treatment prolongs the life expectancy of patients, on average, from 3 years to 5 years, the number of life-years gained per patient is 2. Comparing cost and outcome for different treatments then allows the cost per life-year saved to be determined for each. For example, a study of various interventions in coronary heart disease, cited by McCombs (1998), showed that the cost per life-year saved was $5900 for use of a β-adrenoceptor blocker in patients who had suffered a heart attack, the corresponding figure for use of a cholesterol-lowering drug in patients with coronary heart disease was $7200, whereas coronary artery bypass surgery cost $34 000 per life-year saved. Any kind of all-or-nothing event, such as premature births prevented, hospital admissions avoided etc., can be used for this kind of analysis. Its weakness is that it is a very crude measure, making no distinction between years of life spent in a healthy and productive mode and those spent in a state of chronic illness.

Cost–utility analysis is designed to include allowance for quality of life, as well as survival, in the calculation, and is yet more controversial, for it becomes necessary somehow to quantify quality – not an endeavour for the faint-hearted. What the analysis seeks to arrive at is an estimate known as *quality-adjusted life-years (QALYs)*. Thus if the quality of life for a given year, based on the results of the questionnaire, comes out at 70% of the value for an average healthy person of the same age, that year represents 0.7 QALYs, compared with 1 QALY for a year spent in perfect health, the assumption being that 1 year spent at this level of illness is 'worth' 0.7 years spent in perfect health.

Many different questionnaire-based rating scales have been devised to reflect different aspects of an individual's state of health or disability, such as ability to work, mobility, mental state, pain etc. Some relate to specific disease conditions, whereas others aim to provide a general 'quality-of-life' estimate (Jaeschke and Guyatt, 1994), some of the best-known being the *Sickness Impact Profile*, the *Nottingham Health Profile*, the *McMaster Health Index*, and a 36-item questionnaire known as *SF-36*. In addition to these general quality-of-life measures, a range of disease-specific questionnaires have been devised which give greater sensitivity in measuring the specific deficits associated with particular diseases. Standard instruments of this kind are now widely used in pharmacoeconomic studies.

To use such ratings in estimating QALYs it is necessary to position particular levels of disability on a life/death scale, such that 1 represents alive and in perfect health and 0 represents dead. This is where the problems begin in earnest. How can we possibly say what degree of pain is equivalent to what degree of memory loss, for example, or how either compares with premature death? This problem has, of course, received a lot of expert attention (Gold et al., 1996; Drummond et al., 1997; Johannesson, 1996) and various solutions have been proposed, some of which, to the untrained observer, have a distinctly chilling and surreal quality. For example, the standard gamble approach, which is well grounded in the theory of welfare economics, involves asking the individual a question of the following kind:

Imagine you have the choice of remaining in your present state of health for 1 year or taking a gamble between dying now and living in perfect health for 1 year. What odds would you need to persuade you to take the gamble?[7]

---

[7]Imagine being asked this by your doctor! 'But I only wanted something for my sore throat', you protest weakly.

If the subject says 50:50, the implication is that he values a year of life in his present state of health at 0.5 QALYs. An alternative method involves asking the patient how many years of life in their present condition he or she would be prepared to forfeit in exchange for enjoying good health until they die. Although there are subtle ways of posing this sort of question, such an evaluation, which most ordinary people find unreal, is implicit in the QALY concept. Figure 2.4 shows schematically the way in which quality of life, as a function of age, may be affected by disease and treatment, the area between the curves for untreated and treated patients representing the QALYs saved by the treatment. In reality, of course, continuous measurements spanning several decades are not possible, so the actual data on which QALY estimates are based in practice are much less than is implied by the idealized diagram in Figure 2.4. Cost–utility analysis results in an estimate of monetary cost per QALY gained, and is becoming widely accepted as a standard method for pharmacoeconomic analysis. Examples of cost per QALY gained range from £3700 for the use of sildenafil (Viagra) in treating erectile dysfunction (Stolk et al., 2000) to £328 000 for the treatment of multiple sclerosis with β-interferon (Parkin et al., 2000), this high value being accounted for by the high cost and limited therapeutic efficacy of the drug. 'Acceptable' thresholds for cost-effectiveness are suggested to be in the range of £8000–£25 000 per QALY gained. In principle, cost–utility analysis allows comparison of one form of treatment against another, and this explains its appeal to those who must make decisions about the allocation of healthcare resources. It has been adopted as the method of choice for pharmacoeconomic analysis of new medicines by several agencies, such as the US Public Health Service and the Australian Pharmaceutical Benefits Advisory Committee.

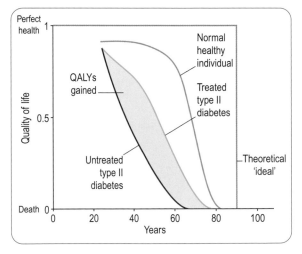

Fig. 2.4
Quality of life affected by disease and treatment.

Hardline economists strive for an absolute scale by which to judge the value of healthcare measures compared with other resource-consuming initiatives that societies choose to support. *Cost–benefit* analysis fulfils this need in principle, by translating healthcare improvements into monetary units that can be directly balanced against costs, to assess whether any given procedure is, on balance, 'profitable'. The science of welfare economics has provided various tools for placing a monetary value on different experiences human beings find agreeable or disagreeable, based generally on the 'willingness-to-pay' principle. Not surprisingly, attempts to value human life and health in cash terms lead rapidly into an ethical and moral minefield, dangerous enough in the context of a single nation and its economy, but much more so in the global context. As a result, cost–benefit analysis has been largely shunned as a practical approach for evaluating medicines.

Summary

In this chapter we have discussed concepts of disease and the aims of therapeutics, the needs newly introduced drugs have to satisfy, and the ways in which their ability to satisfy those needs are judged in practice. There are many uncertainties and ambiguities surrounding the definition of disease, and ideas are constantly shifting, but the two components that most satisfactorily define it are *dysfunction* and *disvalue*. Disvalue, which therapeutic interventions aim to mitigate, in turn has two main components, namely *morbidity* and *prognosis*.

We have described the bioaxis, which represents the various levels in the organizational heirarchy of living systems in general, and human beings in particular, and emphasized that disease inevitably affects all levels on the bioaxis. The drugs that we invent home in very specifically at one level, namely proteins, although the effects we want to produce are at another level, namely individuals. Furthermore, we emphasize that healthcare issues are increasingly being viewed from the perspective of populations and societies, and so the impact of drugs at these levels – even further removed from their primary targets – has to be evaluated. Evaluation of drug effects from these rather lofty perspectives, through the application of the emerging disciplines of pharmacoepidemiology and pharmacoeconomics, although fraught with problems, is an important trend the pharmaceutical industry cannot ignore.

Having taken this rather nervy look at the world about us, we turn in the next chapter to discuss the different therapeutic modalities on which the pharmaceutical and biotechnology industries have focused, before retreating to the safer ground at the left-hand end of the bioaxis, where the modern-day drug discovery business begins.

References

Caplan AL, Engelhardt HT Jr, McCartney JJ (eds) (1981) Concepts of health and disease: interdisciplinary perspectives. London: Addison-Wesley.

Caplan AL (1993) The concepts of health, illness, and disease. In: Bynum WF, Porter R, eds. Companion encyclopedia of the history of medicine. Vol. 1. London: Routledge.

Caplan AL, McCartney JJ, Sisti DA (eds) (2004) Health, disease, and illness: concepts in medicine. Washington, DC: Georgetown University Press.

Debouck C, Goodfellow P N (1999) DNA microarrays in drug discovery and development. Nature Genetics Suppl 21: 48–50.

Dieck G S, Glasser D B, Sachs R M (1994) Pharmacoepidemiology: a view from industry. In: Strom B L, ed. Pharmacoepidemiology. Chichester: John Wiley; 73–85.

Drummond M F, O'Brien B, Stoddart G I, Torrance G W (1997) Methods for the economic evaluation of healthcare programmes. Oxford: Oxford University Press.

Gold M R et al (ed) (1996) Cost-effectiveness in health and medicine. New York: Oxford University Press.

Jaeschke R, Guyatt G H (1994) Using quality-of-life measuremnets in pharmacoepidemiology research. In: Strom BL, ed. Pharmacoepidemiology. Chichester: John Wiley; 495–505.

Johannesson M (1996) Theory and methods of economic evaluation of health care. Dordrecht: Kluwer Academic.

McCombs J S (1998) Pharmacoeconomics: what is it and where is it going? American Journal of Hypertension 11: 112S–119S.

Moynihan R, Heath I, Henry D (2004) Selling sickness: the pharmaceutical industry and disease mongering. British Medical Journal 324: 886–891.

Parkin D, Jacoby A, McNamee P, Miller P, Thomas S, Bates D (2000) Treatment of multiple sclerosis with interferon beta: an appraisal of cost-effectiveness and quality of life. Journal of Neurology, Neurosurgery and Psychiatry 68: 144–149.

Reznek L (1987) The nature of disease. New York: Routledge & Kegan Paul.

Scully JL (2004) What is a disease? EMBO Reports 5: 650–653.

Stolk F.A, Busschbach JJ, Caffa M, Meuleman EJ, Rutten FF (2000) Cost utility analysis of sildenafil compared with papaverine–phentolamine injections. British Medical Journal 320: 1156–1157.

Strom B L (ed) (2000) Pharmacoepidemiology. Chichester: John Wiley.

3 Therapeutic modalities

H P Rang
H LeVine

Introduction

Therapeutics in its broadest sense covers all types of intervention aimed at alleviating the effects of disease. The term 'therapeutics' generally relates to procedures based on accepted principles of medical science, that is, on 'conventional' rather than 'alternative' medical practice.

The account of drug discovery presented in this book relates exclusively to conventional medicine – and for this we make no apology – but it needs to be realized that the therapeutic landscape is actually much broader, and includes many non-pharmacological procedures in the domain of conventional medicine, as well as quasi-pharmacological practices in the 'alternative' domain.

As discussed in Chapter 2, the desired effect of any therapeutic intervention is to improve *symptoms* or *prognosis* or both. From a pathological point of view, therapeutic interventions may be directed at *disease prevention, alleviation* of the effects of existing disease, or *permanent cure* (i.e. restoration to a state of function and prognosis equivalent to those of a healthy individual of the same age, without the need for continuing therapeutic intervention). In practice, there are relatively few truly curative interventions, and they are mainly confined to certain surgical procedures (e.g. removal of circumscribed tumours, fixing of broken bones) and chemotherapy of some infectious and malignant disorders. Most therapeutic interventions aim to alleviate symptoms and/or improve prognosis, and there is increasing emphasis on disease prevention as an objective.

It is important to realize that many types of intervention are carried out with therapeutic intent whose efficacy has not been rigorously tested. This includes not only the myriad alternative medical practices, but also many accepted conventional therapies for which a sound scientific basis may exist but which have not been subjected to rigorous clinical trials.

Therapeutic interventions that lie within the field of conventional medicine can be divided into the following broad categories:

● Advice and counselling (e.g. genetic counselling)
● Psychological treatments (e.g. cognitive therapies for anxiety disorders, depression etc.)

- Dietary and nutritional treatments (e.g. gluten-free diets for celiac disease, diabetic diets etc.)
- Physical treatments, including surgery, radiotherapy
- Pharmacological treatments – encompassing the whole of conventional drug therapy
- Biological and biopharmaceutical treatments, a broad category including vaccination, transplantation, blood transfusion, biopharmaceuticals (see Chapter 12), in vitro fertilization etc.

On the fringe of conventional medicine are preparations that fall into the category of 'nutriceuticals' or 'cosmeceuticals'. Nutriceuticals include a range of dietary preparations, such as slimming diets, and diets supplemented with vitamins, minerals, antioxidants, unsaturated fatty acids, fibre etc. These preparations generally have some scientific rationale, although their efficacy has not, in most cases, been established by controlled trials. They are not subject to formal regulatory approval, so long as they do not contain artificial additives other than those that have been approved for use in foods. Cosmeceuticals is a fancy name for cosmetic products similarly supplemented with substances claimed to reduce skin wrinkles, promote hair growth etc. These products achieve very large sales, and some pharmaceutical companies have expanded their business in this direction. We do not discuss these fringe 'ceuticals' in this book, as most pharmaceutical and biotechnology companies restrict themselves to mainstream therapeutic products.

Within each of the medical categories listed above lies a range of procedures: at one end of the spectrum are procedures that have been fully tried and tested and are recognized by medical authorities; at the other is outright quackery of all kinds. Somewhere between lie widely used 'complementary' procedures, practised in some cases under the auspices of officially recognized bodies, which have no firm scientific foundation. Here we find, among psychological treatments, hypnotherapy and analytical psychotherapy; among nutritional treatments, 'health foods', added vitamins, and diets claimed to avoid ill-defined food allergies; among physical treatments, acupuncture and osteopathy; among chemical treatments, homeopathy, herbalism and aromatherapy. Biological procedures lying in this grey area between scientific medicine and quackery are uncommon (and we should probably be grateful for this) – unless one counts colonic irrigation and swimming with dolphins.

In this book we are concerned with the last two treatment categories on the list, summarized in Table 3.1, and in this chapter we consider the current status and future prospects of the three main fields. namely 'conventional' therapeutic drugs, biopharmaceuticals and various biological therapies.

Conventional therapeutic drugs

Small-molecule drugs, either synthetic compounds or natural products have for long been the mainstay of therapeutics and are likely to remain so, despite the rapid growth of biopharmaceuticals in recent years. For their advantages and disadvantages see Box 3.1.

Although the pre-eminent role of conventional small-molecule drugs may decline as biopharmaceutical products grow in importance, few doubt that they will continue to play a major role in medical treatment. New technologies described in Section 2, particularly combinatorial chemistry, high-throughput screening and genomic approaches to target identification, have already brought about a revolution in drug discovery, the fruits of which are only just beginning to appear. There are also high expectations that more sophisticated drug delivery systems (see Chapter 17) will allow drugs to act much more selectively where they are needed, and thus reduce the burden of side effects.

Biopharmaceuticals

For the purposes of this book, biopharmaceuticals are therapeutic protein or nucleic acid preparations made by techniques involving recombinant DNA technology (Walsh, 2003). Although proteins such as insulin and growth hormone, extracted from human or animal tissues, have long been used therapeutically, the era of biopharmaceuticals began in 1982 with the development by Eli Lilly of recombinant human insulin (Humulin), made by genetically engineered *Escherichia coli*. Recombinant human growth hormone (also produced in *E. coli*), erythropoietin (Epogen) and tissue plasminogen activator (tPA) made by engineered mammalian cells followed during the 1980s. This was the birth of the biopharmaceutical industry, and since then new bioengineered proteins have contributed an increasing proportion of new medicines to be registered (see Table 3.1 for some examples, and Chapters 12 and 22 for more details). The scope of protein biopharmaceuticals includes copies of endogenous mediators, blood clotting factors, enzyme preparations and monoclonal antibodies, as well as vaccines. See Box 3.2 for their advantages and disadvantages.

Immunization against infectious diseases dates from 1796, when Jenner first immunized patients against smallpox by infecting them with the relatively harmless cowpox. Many other immunization procedures were developed in the 19th century, and from the 20th century onwards pharmaceutical companies began producing standardized versions of the antigens, often the attenuated or modified organisms themselves, as well

Table 3.1
The main types of chemical therapeutic agent

Type	Source	Examples	Notes
Conventional small-molecule drugs	Synthetic organic compounds*	Most of the pharmacopoeia	The largest category of drugs in use, and of new registrations
	Natural products	Paclitaxel (Taxol) Many antibiotics and anticancer drugs (e.g. penicillins, aminoglycosides, erythromycin) Opiates (e.g. morphine) Statins (e.g. lovastatin) Ciclosporin, fujimycin	Continues to be an important source of new therapeutic drugs
	Semisynthetic compounds (i.e. compounds made by derivatizing natural products)	Penicillin derivatives (e.g. ampicillin) second-generation statins (e.g. simvastatin)	Strategy for generating improved 'second-generation' drugs from natural products
Peptide and protein mediators	Synthetic	Somatostatin Calcitonin Vasopressin	Peptides up to approximately 20 residues can be reliably made by solid-phase synthesis
	Extracted from natural sources (human, animal, microbial)	Insulin, growth hormone, human γ-globulins, botulinum toxin	At one time the only source of such hormones. Now largely replaced by recombinant biotechnology products. γ-globulins still obtained from human blood
	Recombinant DNA technology	Human insulin, erythropoietin, human growth hormone, GM-CSF TNF-α, hirudin	Many different expression systems in use and in development
Antibodies	Animal antisera, human immunoglobulins	Antisera used to treat infections such as hepatitis A and B, diphtheria, rabies, tetanus. Also poisoning by botulinum, snake and spider venoms etc.	
	Monoclonal antibodies	Trastuzumab (directed against epidermal growth factor receptor) Rituximab (directed against B-cell surface antigen)	A rapidly growing class of biopharmaceuticals, with many products in development.
Enzymes	Recombinant DNA technology	Cerebrosidase Dornase Galactosidase	
Vaccines	Infecting organism (killed, attenuated or non-pathogenic strains)	Smallpox, diphtheria, measles, tuberculosis, tetanus, influenza and many others	The conventional approach, still widely used. Some risk of introducing viable pathogens
	Antigens produced by recombinant DNA technology	Many of the above vaccines now available as recombinant antigens	Advantages are greater consistency and elimination of risk of introducing pathogens
DNA products	Recombinant DNA technology	Antisense oligonucleotides (e.g. Vitravene)	Many products in clinical development. Vitravene (for treating cytomegalovirus infection) is the only marketed product so far.

Table 3.1
The main types of chemical therapeutic agent—cont'd

Type	Source	Examples	Notes
Cells	Human donors Engineered cell lines	Various stem cell therapies in development	
Tissues	Human donors Animal tissues Engineered tissues	Apligraf	Bilayer of human skin cells
Organs	Human donors	Transplant surgery	

*Not considered here are many 'adjunct' therapies, such as oxygen, antiseptic agents, anaesthetic agents, intravenous salts etc., which are beyond the scope of this book.

➤ **Box 3.1 Advantages and disadvantages of small-molecule drugs**

Advantages

- 'Chemical space' is so vast that synthetic chemicals, according to many experts, have the potential to bind specifically to any chosen biological target: the right molecule exists; it is just a matter of finding it.
- Doctors and patients are thoroughly familiar with conventional drugs as medicines, and the many different routes of administration that are available. Clinical pharmacology in its broadest sense has become part of the knowledge base of every practising doctor, and indeed, part of everyday culture. Although sections of the public may remain suspicious of drugs, there are few who will refuse to use them when the need arises.
- Oral administration is often possible, as well as other routes where appropriate.
- From the industry perspective, small-molecule drugs make up more than three-quarters of new products registered over the past decade. Pharmaceutical companies have long experience in developing, registering, producing, packaging and marketing such products.
- Therapeutic peptides are generally straightforward to design (as Nature has done the job), and are usually non-toxic.

Disadvantages

- As emphasized elsewhere in this book, the flow of new small-molecule drugs seems to be diminishing, despite increasing R&D expenditure.
- Side effects and toxicity remain a serious and unpredictable problem, causing failures in late development, or even after registration. One reason for this is that the selectivity of drug molecules with respect to biological targets is by no means perfect, and is in general less good than with biopharmaceuticals.
- Humans and other animals have highly developed mechanisms for eliminating foreign molecules, so drug design often has to contend with pharmacokinetic problems.
- Oral absorption is poor for many compounds. Peptides cannot be given orally.

as antisera which would give immediate passive protection against disease organisms. Vaccines and immune approaches to controlling disease are still a major concern, and increasingly biotechnology-derived vaccines are being developed to improve the efficacy of and reduce the risks associated with preparations made from infectious material.

Overall, biopharmaceuticals offer great promise for the future, and rapid progress is being made in the technologies used to produce them (Scrip Report, 2001). Currently, nearly all approved biopharmaceuticals are proteins, the majority being copies of endogenous mediators, monoclonal antibodies or vaccines. It is possible that most of the clinically useful hormones and mediators that we currently know about have already been produced as biopharmaceuticals, so future advances in this direction are likely to depend on progress in discovering new protein signalling mechanisms. Monoclonal antibodies may offer much broader possibilities, and progress will be greatly facilitated by identifying the genes for important functional proteins, such as key enzymes, transporters etc. Once the DNA sequence of a putative target is known, its amino acid sequence can be inferred and an antibody produced, even if the target protein is of such low abundance that it cannot be isolated biochemically.

Following the wave of successes by the biotechnology industry in producing biopharmaceuticals such as human insulin, erythropoietin and growth hormone during the 1980s and 1990s, medical biotechnology expanded into many other fields, including the development of therapeutic modalities beyond therapeutic proteins and antibodies. Next we briefly discuss two important developments still in the experimental phase, namely gene-based and cell-based therapies, which are under very active investigation.

Gene therapy

Recombinant DNA technology offers the promise of altering the genetic material of cells and thereby correct-

➤ **Box 3.2 Advantages and disadvantages of biopharmaceuticals**

Advantages

- The main benefit offered by biopharmaceutical products is that they open up the scope of protein therapeutics, which was previously limited to proteins that could be extracted from animal or human sources.
- The discovery process for new biopharmaceuticals is often quicker and more straightforward than is the case with synthetic compounds, as screening and lead optimization are not required.
- Unexpected toxicity is less common than with synthetic molecules.
- The risk of immune responses to non-human proteins – a problem with porcine or bovine insulins – is avoided by expressing the human sequence.
- The risk of transmitting virus or prion infections is avoided.

Disadvantages

- Producing biopharmaceuticals on a commercial scale is expensive, requiring complex purification and quality control procedures.
- The products are not orally active and often have short plasma half-lives, so special delivery systems may be required, adding further to costs. Like other proteins, biopharmaceutical products do not cross the blood–brain barrier.
- For the above reasons, development generally costs more and takes longer, than it does for synthetic drugs.
- Many biopharmaceuticals are species specific in their effects, making tests of efficacy in animal models difficult or impossible.

ing the results of genetic defects, whether inherited or acquired. The techniques for manipulating cellular DNA that underpin much of modern molecular biology have great versatility, and can in principle be applied to therapeutic as well as experimental endeavours. Even where the genetic basis of the disease is not well understood, it should be possible to counteract its effects by genetic, as distinct from pharmacological, means. Further technical information about gene therapy is given in Chapter 12, and in reference works such as Meager (1999), Templeton and Lasic (2000), Kresina (2001), and Brooks (2002). Gene therapy has been actively investigated for more than two decades, and many clinical trials have been performed. So far, however, the results have proved disappointing, and there are currently (2004) no gene therapy products approved for clinical use.

The most widely investigated approach involves introducing new genes to replace missing or dysfunctional ones; this is most commonly done by engineering the new gene into a modified virus (the vector), which

has the ability to enter the host cell, causing expression of the artificially introduced gene until the cell dies or expels the foreign DNA. Such non-integrated DNA is usually eliminated quite quickly and is not passed on to the cell's progeny, and so this type of transfection is generally only appropriate in situations where transient expression is all that is required. Retroviral vectors are able to incorporate the new DNA into the host cell's chromosomes, where it will remain and be expressed during the lifetime of the cell and will be passed on to any progeny of that cell. More elaborate gene therapy protocols for treating single-gene disorders are designed actually to correct the disease-producing sequence mutation in the host genome, or to alter gene expression so as to silence dysfunctional genes.

At one time gene therapy directed at germline cells was considered a possibility, the advantage being that an inherited gene defect could be prevented from affecting progeny, and effectively eliminated for good. The serious risks and ethical objections to such human genetic engineering, however, have led to a worldwide ban on germ-cell gene therapy experiments, and efforts are restricted to somatic cell treatments.

How much impact has gene therapy had so far as a therapeutic approach, and what can be expected of it in the future? The first successful trial of gene therapy to be reported was by Anderson and colleagues, who used it in 1990 to replace the dysfunctional gene for the enzyme adenosine deaminase (ADA). ADA deficiency causes *severe combined immunodeficiency syndrome* (SCID), a rare condition which prevents the normal immune response to pathogens, and means that the child can only survive in a germ-free environment. This first gene therapy trial was successful in partly restoring ADA function, but by no means curative. Hundreds of clinical trials were performed during the 1990s, mainly in three clinical areas, namely cancer, AIDS and single-gene inherited disorders such as cystic fibrosis, haemophilia and SCID. Most of these used viral vectors to deliver the DNA, though some used liposome-packaged DNA or other non-viral vectors (see Chapter 17) for this purpose. The genetic material was delivered systemically in some cases, by intravenous or subcutaneous injection; in other cases it was injected directly into solid tumours. An alternative strategy was to harvest bone marrow cells from the patient, transfect these with the necessary DNA construct ex vivo, and return them to the patient so that the genetically modified cells would recolonize the bone marrow and provide the required protein. These techniques had been extensively worked out in laboratory animals, but the clinical results were uniformly disappointing, mainly because transfection rates were too low and expression was too transient. Repeat administration of viral vectors often elicited an immune response which inactivated the vector. So the very high expectation in the early 1990s that gene therapy would revolutionize treatment in many areas of medicine, from arthritis to mental illness, quickly gave way to a much more guarded opti-mism, and in some cases a pessimistic dismissal of the whole concept. There were, however, a few cases in which SCID in children was successfully – and apparently per-manently – cured by gene therapy, and there were other trials in haemophilia and certain cancers where results looked promising. Alarm bells sounded, first in 1999 when a teenager, Jesse Gelsinger, who was participating in a gene therapy trial in Philadelphia, developed an intense immunological reaction and suddenly died 4 days after treatment. Official scrutiny uncovered many other cases of adverse reactions that had not been reported as they should have been. Many ongoing trials were halted, and much tighter controls were imposed. Subsequently, in 2000, immune function was successfully restored in 18 SCID children, 17 of whom are alive 5 years later (the first therapeutic success for human gene therapy), but two later developed leukaemia, thought to be because integra-tion of the retroviral transgene occurred in a way that acti-vated a cancer-promoting gene, raising even more serious concerns about the long-term side effects of gene therapy.

In the much more cautious atmosphere now pre-vailing, some carefully controlled trials are beginning to give positive results, mainly in the treatment of haemophilia, but overall, the general view is that gene therapy, while showing great theoretical potential, has so far proved disappointing in its clinical efficacy, amid con-cerns about its long-term safety and ongoing problems in designing effective delivery systems. (see commentaries by Cavazzana-Calvo et al, 2004 and Relph et al, 2004). Pessimists refer to a decade of failure and note that hun-dreds of trials have failed so far to produce a single approved therapy. A quick survey of the literature, however, shows a profusion of laboratory studies aimed at improving the technology, and exploring many new ideas for using gene therapy in numerous conditions, ranging from transplant rejection to psychiatric disorders.

The main problems to be overcome are (a) to find delivery vectors that are efficient and selective enough to transfect most or all of the target cells without affecting other cells; (b) to produce long-lasting expression of the therapeutic gene; and (c) to avoid serious adverse effects. Additionally, a method for reversing the effect by turning the foreign gene off if things go wrong would be highly desirable, but has not so far been addressed in trials.

Antisense DNA has been investigated as an alternative to the DNA strategies outlined above. Antisense DNA consists of an oligonucleotide sequence complementary to part of a known mRNA sequence. The antisense DNA binds to the mRNA and, by mechanisms that are not fully understood, blocks expression very selectively, though only for as long as the antisense DNA remains in the cell. The practical problems of developing therapeutic anti-sense reagents are considerable, as unmodified oligonu-cleotides are quickly degraded in plasma and do not enter cells readily, so either chemical modification or special delivery systems such as liposomal packaging are re-quired. So far only one antisense preparation has been approved for clinical use, an oligonucleotide used to treat an ocular virus infection in AIDS patients. *Ribozymes*, specific mRNA sequences that inactivate genes by cat-alysing DNA cleavage, are being investigated as an alter-native to antisense DNA, but so far none has been approved for clinical use.

In addition to their chequered clinical trials history, gene therapy products share with other biopharmaceu-ticals many features that cause major pharmaceutical companies to shy away from investing heavily in such products. The reagents are large molecules, or viruses, that have to be delivered to the appropriate sites in tissues, often to particular cells and with high efficiency. Supplying gene therapy reagents via the bloodstream is only effective for luminal vascular targets, and topical administration is usually needed. Viral vectors do not spread far from the site of injection, nor do they infect all cell types. The vectors have their separate toxicology issues. Commercial production, quality control, formu-lation and delivery often present problems.

In summary, the theoretical potential of gene therapy is enormous, and the ingenuity being applied to making it work is very impressive. Still, after 25 years of intense research effort no product has been developed, and many of the fundamental problems in delivering genes effec-tively and controllably still seem far from solution. Most likely, a few effective products for a few specific diseases will be developed and marketed in the next few years, and this trickle will probably grow until gene therapy makes a significant contribution to mainstream therapeu-tics. Whether it will grow eventually to a flood that sup-plants much of conventional therapeutics, or whether it will remain hampered by technical problems, nobody can say at this stage. In the foreseeable future, gene therapy is likely to gain acceptance as a useful adjunct to conven-tional chemotherapy for cancer and viral infections, par-ticularly AIDS. The Holy Grail of a cure for inherited diseases such as cystic fibrosis still seems some way off.

Cell-based therapies

Cell replacement therapies offer the possibility of effec-tive treatment for various kinds of degenerative disease, and much hope currently rests on the potential uses of stem cells, which are undifferentiated progenitor cells that can be maintained in tissue culture and, by the application of appropriate growth factors, be induced to differentiate into functional cells of various kinds. Their ability to divide in culture means that the stock of cells can be expanded as required.

Autologous cell grafts (i.e. returning treated cells to the same individual) are quite widely used for treating leukaemias and similar malignancies of bone marrow cells. A sample of the patient's bone marrow is taken, cleansed of malignant cells, expanded, and returned to colonize the bone marrow after the patient has been treated with high-dose chemotherapy or radiotherapy to eradicate all resident bone marrow cells. Bone marrow is particularly suitable for this kind of therapy because it is rich in stem cells, and can be recolonized with 'clean' cells injected into the bloodstream.

Apart from this established procedure for treating bone marrow malignancies, only two cell-based therapeutic products have so far gained FDA approval: preparations of autologous chondrocytes used to repair cartilage defects, and autologous keratinocytes, used for treating burns. Other potential applications which have been the focus of much experimental work are reviewed by Fodor (2003). They include:

- Neuronal cells injected into the brain (Isaacson, 2003) to treat neurodegenerative diseases such as Parkinson's disease (loss of dopaminergic neurons), amyotrophic lateral sclerosis (loss of cholinergic neurons) and Huntington's disease (loss of GABA neurons);
- Insulin-secreting cells to treat insulin-dependent diabetes mellitus;
- Cardiac muscle cells to restore function after myocardial infarction.

The major obstacle to further development of such cell-based therapies is that the use of embryonic tissues – the preferred source of stem cells – is severely restricted for ethical reasons. Although stem cells can be harvested from adult tissues and organs, they are less satisfactory. Like gene therapy, cell-based therapeutics could in principle have many important applications, and the technical problems that currently stand in the way are the subject of intensive research efforts. Biotechnology companies are active in developing the necessary tools and reagents that are likely to be needed to select and prepare cells for transplantation.

Tissue and organ transplantation

Transplantation of human organs, such as heart, liver, kidneys and corneas, is of course a well established procedure, many of the problems of rejection having been largely solved by the use of immunosuppressant drugs such as ciclosporin and fujimycin. Better techniques for preventing rejection, including procedures based on gene therapy, are likely to be developed, but the main obstacle remains the limited supply of healthy human organs, and there is little reason to think that this will change in the foreseeable future. The possibility of xenotransplantation – the use of non-human organs, usually from pigs – has received much attention. Cross-species transplants are normally rejected within minutes by a

process known as hyperacute rejection. Transgenic pigs whose organs are rendered resistant to hyperacute rejection have been produced, but trials in humans have so far been ruled out because of the risk of introducing pig retroviruses into humans. Despite much discussion and arguments on both sides, there is no sign of this embargo being lifted. Organ transplantation requires such a high degree of organization to get the correct matched organs to the right patients at the right time, as well as advanced surgical and follow-up resources, that it will remain an option only for the privileged minority.

Building two- (e.g. skin) and three-dimensional (e.g. a heart valve) structures that are intended to function mechanically, either from host cells or from banked, certified primordial or stem cell populations, is at the cutting edge of tissue engineering efforts. The aim is to fashion these tissues and organ parts around artificial scaffold materials, and to do this in culture under the control of appropriate growth and differentiation factors. The development of biocompatible scaffolding materials, and achieving the right growth conditions, are problems where much remains to be done. Artificial skin preparations recently became available and others will probably follow.

Also in an early, albeit encouraging, state of development are bionic devices – the integration of mechanical and electronic prostheses with the human body – which will go beyond what has already been accomplished with devices such as cochlear implants and neurally controlled limb prostheses. The role of the major pharmaceutical companies in this highly technological area is likely to be small. The economic realities of the relatively small patient populations will most likely be the limiting factor governing the full implementation of integrated bionics.

Summary

Small organic molecule drugs of molecular weight <500 Da are the preferred therapeutic modality of the major pharmaceutical companies for most disease applications. The advantages summarized above drive this choice. The development over the years of large, chemically diverse small-molecule libraries, many already with 'drug-like' properties (see Chapters 9 and 10) built into their structure, reinforces the commitment. Protein and peptide therapeutics also have their place in the pharmaceutical armamentarium, especially with respect to the immune system and hormonal dysregulation. Many pharmaceutical companies began with immune antisera and vaccines, but the first specialized biotechnology companies took advantage of recombinant DNA methods to produce therapeutic proteins. Although the major pharmaceutical companies have not completely abandoned protein therapeutics, many of the advances in the field have been made by biotechnology companies.

Protein- and DNA-based biopharmaceuticals often face difficult pharmacokinetic problems, in particular poor absorption, rapid degradation, and inability to enter cells or cross the blood–brain barrier. Their successful development therefore often depends on developing suitable delivery systems that help to overcome these problems. For this reason (and also to improve the performance of conventional therapeutic drugs) drug delivery technology (see Chapter 17) is currently receiving a great deal of attention, with many new polymer- and liposome-based formulations being invented and tested. The right delivery system is as necessary as the right drug, and for biopharmaceuticals the two will generally need to be developed in tandem, rather than first developing a compound and then optimizing the delivery system (which is the development strategy usually adopted for small-molecule drugs).

Somatic (non-germline) gene therapy initially was thought to have great promise for curing inborn errors that lead to disease. Thirty years later, although the technology and our understanding have greatly improved, clinical success has proved elusive. Optimizing vectors and delivery systems so as to produce long-lasting gene expression in the tissues where it is needed has proved much more difficult than expected. Nevertheless, there is reason for optimism in the long term. Currently, gene therapy development is being directed mainly at life-threatening disorders such as cancer, AIDs and haemophilia, where the need is greatest and the risks are balanced by the severity of the diseases. It is likely to be another decade or two before gene therapy begins to make a broader clinical impact.

The involvement of pharmaceutical companies in the transplantation field is largely confined to improving the immunosuppressant drugs that are needed to protect transplants from immune rejection. The use of transplants is severely restricted by the availability of human organs, and hopes for improving the situation by the use of xenografts are unlikely to be realized in the foreseeable future. Stem-cell technologies are likely to be used successfully for certain kinds of tissue repair and cell replacement; biotechnology companies, rather than pharmaceutical companies, are likely to make the running in these new fields. Currently, techniques such as bone marrow transplants are being developed and used successfully by clinical teams without any necessary input from commercial research. Probably their use will become more routine, but it seems unlikely that the market size for commercial products in this area will be enough for a large pharmaceutical company.

References

Brooks G (ed) (2002) Gene therapy: the use of DNA as a drug. New York: John Wiley and Sons.

Cavazzano-Calvo M, Thrasher A, Mavilio F (2004) The future of gene therapy. Nature 427: 779–781.

Fodor W L (2003) Tissue engineering and cell based therapies, from the bench to the clinic: the potential to replace, repair and regenerate. Reproductive Biology and Endocrinology 1: 102–107.

Isaacson O (2003) The production and use of cells as therapeutic agents in neurodegenerative diseases. Lancet Neurology 2: 417–424.

Kresina T F (ed) (2001) An introduction to molecular medicine and gene therapy. New York: John Wiley and Sons.

Meager A (1999) Gene therapy technologies: Applications and regulations from laboratory to clinic. Chichester: John Wiley and Sons.

Relph K, Harrington K, Pandha H (2004) Recent developments and current status of gene therapy using viral vectors in the United Kingdom. Br Med J 329: 839–842.

Scrip Report (2001) Biopharmaceuticals: a new era of discovery in the biotechnology revolution.

Templeton N S, Lasic D D (2000) Gene therapy: therapeutic mechanisms and strategies. New York: Marcel Dekker.

Walsh G (2003) Biopharmaceuticals, 2nd edn. Chichester: John Wiley and Sons Ltd.

SECTION 2
DRUG DISCOVERY

The drug discovery process: general principles and some case histories

H P Rang

Introduction

The creation of a new drug can be broadly divided into three main phases (Figure 4.1):

- Drug discovery – from therapeutic concept to molecule
- Drug development – from molecule to registered product
- Commercialization – from product to therapeutic application to sales.

Traditionally, these functions are performed by Research, Development and Marketing, respectively, reflecting the different professional training and expertise required to do the job. Figure 4.1 greatly over-simplifies what is actually a very complex process. For example, development activities, in the form of additional clinical trials, or testing of new formulations, generally continue well beyond the point of registration, with the aim of extending the range of applications of the compound. Often the discovery team, having delivered the first candidate drug, will carry on looking for others, to serve as back-ups in case the lead compound should fail in development, or as follow-up compounds intended to have advantages over the lead compound. The three components of the overall process are not independent and consecutive stages, but have to be closely coordinated at all stages of the project. At the outset of any new project, the criteria against which the plan will be judged include not only its scientific strength and originality but, importantly, development and marketing issues. For example, if the therapeutic target is an ill-defined clinical disorder, such as chronic fatigue syndrome, will it be possible to measure clinical efficacy objectively? Does the project face stiff competition from other companies working in the same area, or from drugs already in clinical use? Is it likely that an esoteric drug delivery system will be required, and if so, can this be developed? If the drug is successfully developed, is the expected market sufficient to justify the cost of development? The answers to questions of this kind are likely to change, for better or for worse, during the course of the project, so it is essential to keep such issues constantly under review, and to adapt the project plan if necessary.

To integrate successfully the different interests – and cultures – of research, development and marketing is

Drug discovery

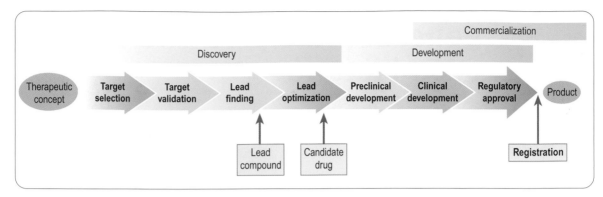

Fig. 4.1
Three main phases of the creation of a new drug: discovery, development and commercialization.

one of the major challenges for a pharmaceutical company, and the need for such integration is a relatively modern development in the industry. As recently as 25–30 years ago in most companies, the process was much more compartmentalized: scientists produced molecules with interesting pharmacological properties, development functions were responsible for checking their safety and turning them into registrable drugs, and the marketing department generated sales and turned them into revenues. At the time this worked well, and many companies prospered. The drop-out rate was not excessive, because regulatory requirements were less stringent, and the failures that did occur were not unduly expensive in terms of time and resources lost. Since then, biomedical science has advanced dramatically, drug discovery and development have become more technology-driven and hence expensive, regulatory requirements much more stringent, and the competition more intense. With bigger teams, and more complex multidisciplinary tasks, effective project management has become much more important than it used to be to keep costs and delays to a minimum.

A more detailed overview of the drug discovery phase of a typical project aimed at producing a new synthetic drug is shown in Figure 4.2. It starts with the choice of a disease area and defining the therapeutic need that is to be met. It proceeds to the identification of the biochemical, cellular or pathophysiological mechanism that will be targeted, and if possible, the identification and validation of a molecular 'drug target'. Next comes the identification of a lead structure, followed by the design, testing and fine-tuning of the drug molecule to the point where it is deemed suitable for development, discussed in more detail in subsequent chapters.

The strong emphasis on defined molecular (normally protein) drug targets as a starting point is too recent to have culminated so far in many actual drugs on the market. The majority of drugs now being registered have their origins in research going back 20 years or more, in the 'premolecular' drug discovery era, when the selected targets were mainly pathophysiological or bio-

chemical mechanisms, such as blood pressure regulation, inflammation or cholesterol metabolism, of which the molecular components were not yet defined. This earlier period, roughly from 1960 to 1980, was actually highly productive in terms of drug discovery, representing a return on R&D investment considerably greater than what can be achieved today, and the discovery approaches used then remain very much alive despite the increasing emphasis on molecular targets. Nevertheless, we now think increasingly in terms of defined molecular targets as the necessary starting point for drug discovery, and turn automatically to molecular technologies to provide the necessary tools. Until about 1980 this was rarely feasible; even when the 'target' was defined, for example as an enzyme or a receptor, it was seldom available in sufficient quantities in a purified functional form to be used as the basis for screening assays. Instead, the functional activity of the target was measured by indirect means in isolated tissue preparations, or even in whole animals, methods which we nowadays regard as too slow, laborious and error prone to place at the front end of a drug discovery project.

The foregoing remarks apply to the discovery of conventional 'small-molecule' therapeutics, but the strategy for developing biopharmaceuticals – an increasing proportion of new drugs appearing on the market – is generally different. Biopharmaceutical agents (see Chapter 3) are very diverse, including endogenous mediators, monoclonal antibodies and vaccines, and in the future, no doubt, products for gene therapy applications. Where endogenous molecules are involved, the concept of targets and lead compounds has much less relevance, as Nature has done the discovery part of the work, so once the therapeutic relevance of the substance has been established, the problems mainly revolve around the production, purification and formulation of the material in a form suitable for the market. With other kinds of biopharmaceuticals, such as therapeutic antibodies, the molecular target will generally be chosen in advance, and the main task is obtain an antibody with the required properties.

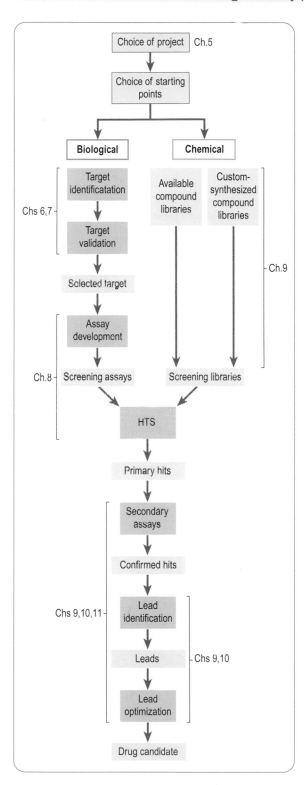

Fig. 4.2
Drug discovery phase of a typical project aimed at producing a new synthetic drug.

A glance at the pharmacopoeia will show that many therapeutic agents, particularly anti-infective and anti-tumour drugs, originate from natural products, rather than synthetic molecules (Table 4.1). Until about 1950, when synthetic chemistry really came into its own as a source of new drugs, most of the pharmacopoeia consisted of natural products, and they continue to be important, as the example of *paclitaxel*, described below, shows. It is reasonable to suppose that such ready-made, highly evolved biomolecules stand a better chance of interacting with selected drug targets than do random synthetic molecules, and the pool from which they come is huge and largely untapped. Exploiting such a ready-made compound library is seen as an attractive strategy which has led to some important therapeutic breakthroughs, such as *ciclosporin* and other immunophilin ligands such as *fujimycin* (FK506) and *rapamycin*, as well as paclitaxel and other potential anti-cancer drugs currently under development, such as *epothilones*. In numerical terms, however, natural products represent only a small proportion of compounds registered recently. In 1999, only one new compound (*sirolimus*, an immunosuppressant used to prevent transplant rejection) out of 40 registered was a natural product, and in 2000 the only example was *galantamine* (a product of the snowdrop, known for many years as an anticholinesterase, used to treat dementia). In practice, the theoretical advantages of natural products are balanced by several practical disadvantages. Access to source material in remote places can be troublesome for geographical reasons, as well as being politically sensitive, and the continuing availability of the active compound, if it cannot be synthesized on a commercial basis, may be uncertain. Microorganisms have an advantage over higher species in this regard, but initial positive test data on microbial samples frequently cannot be replicated, presumably because of inconsistencies in the culture conditions. Purification and structure determination of natural products is now fairly routine, but is often difficult and time-consuming.

Some case histories

It is clear that there are many starting points and routes to success in drug discovery projects (Lednicer, 1993; Drews, 2000). The brief case histories of five successful drugs, *paclitaxel (Taxol)*, *flecainide (Tambocor)*, *omeprazol (Losec)*, *imatinib (Gleevec)* and *trastuzumab (Herceptin)*, are summarized in Figure 4.3 and Table 4.2, and described in more detail below. Each represents a highly innovative 'breakthrough' project rather than an incremental development based on an existing therapy, and they illustrate the variety of different approaches taken by successful projects over the past 30 years. However, for several reasons we should avoid interpreting these as

Table 4.1
Examples of therapeutic drugs derived from natural products

Warfarin	Anticoagulant. Synthetic compound derived from dicoumarol, found in spoiled sweet clover
Heparin	Anticoagulant, occurring naturally in mammalian tissues
Hirudin	Anticoagulant from leech, now produced by genetic engineering
Opiates	Analgesic compounds from poppies
Methylxanthines (caffeine, theophylline)	Phosphodiesterase inhibitors and adenosine receptor antagonists. Produced by tea, coffee and coca plants
Statins	HMG CoA reductase inhibitors used to reduce plasma cholesterol. Lovastatin is a fungal metabolite. Later compounds (mevastatin, pravastatin) synthesized from lovastatin
Cromoglycate	Asthma prohylaxis. Synthetic compound based on khellin, a plant product used as a herbal medicine
Vinca alkaloids (vincristine, vinblastine)	Anticancer drugs produced by plants of the periwinkle family
Paclitaxel	Anticancer drug from yew tree
Etoposide	Anticancer drug synthesized from podophyllotoxin, produced by mandrake plant; used in folk medicine
Artemether	Antimalarial drug, semisynthetic derivative of artemesin, produced by Chinese herb
Ivermectin	Antihelminthic drug, semisynthetic derivative of avermectin, a fungal metabolite
Antibiotics	Too numerous to list. The majority of current antibiotics are derived from fungal metabolites

In earlier times the pharmacopoeia consisted very largely of plant-derived compounds (e.g. opiates, atropine, ephedrine, ergot alkaloids, strychnine, tubocurarine, digoxin, quinine, veratridine, reserpine etc.), many of which remain in therapeutic use or provide valuable research tools.

guidelines for success in the future. For one thing, the approach changes as the underlying technologies advance; furthermore, pharmaceutical companies generally publicize only their successes, and even then the accounts are often somewhat sanitized, and fail to describe the errors that were made, the deadlines missed and the blind alleys that were encountered – the full 'shaggy drug stories' generally remain discreetly hidden.. It must be remembered that, of drug discovery projects begun, only about 1 in 50 is successful in terms of bringing a compound to market. Only at the point when official approval for trials in man is granted does the project become visible to the outside world, so data on success rates, timelines etc. are much more accessible for the minority of projects that progress to Phase I or beyond than for the majority that never get that far. Analysing the success factors for early-stage drug discovery projects is therefore difficult.

Paclitaxel (Taxol)

Paclitaxel is an interesting example of a project based on the development of a natural product (Cragg, 1998). It began in the early 1960s, when the US National Cancer Institute, responding to the Nixon-inspired 'war on cancer', set up one of the first directed screening programmes – still running – to seek new anticancer drugs from plant sources. The sample of bark from the Pacific Yew was collected in 1962 and found to have modest activity against various tumour cell lines. The active substance was isolated in 1969 and joined a collection of moderately active, but not particularly interesting, lead compounds. When this collection was dusted off in 1975 and tested on a new assay, a melanoma cell line, paclitaxel stood out as highly active. Its activity was confirmed in animal models, and it was soon chosen as a development candidate. Interest was further stimulated when its novel mechanism of action, the promotion of microtubule polymerization, was very elegantly demonstrated. Development was difficult, for two main reasons. Paclitaxel is insoluble in water, and the early formulations for injection used in Phase I trials contained a high proportion of the solubilizing agent Cremophor EL, causing frequent severe allergic reactions when given as a bolus intravenous injection. After considerable delay, the problem was overcome by the use of slow infusions and development was resumed. The second problem was the supply of material for

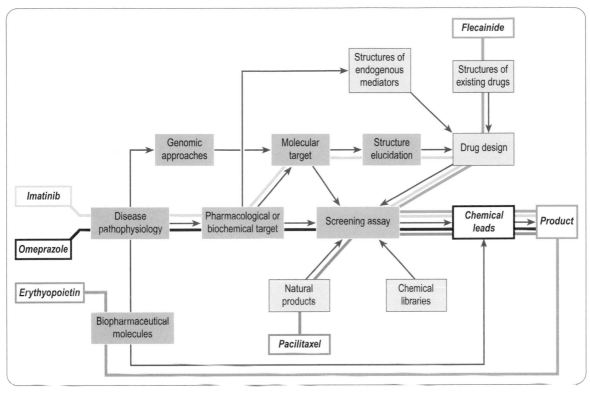

Fig. 4.3
Discovery pathways of some successful projects.

Table 4.2
Timelines for some successful drug discovery projects

Drug	Paclitaxel (Taxol)	Flecainide (Tambocor)	Omeprazol (Losec)	Imatinib (Gleevec)	Trastuzumab (Herceptin)
Mechanism	Natural product inhibitor of tubulin depolymerization	Antidysrhythmic drug. Blocks cardiac Na⁺ channels	Inhibitor of gastric acid secretion. Blocks proton pump	Inhibits Abl kinase	Humanized monoclonal antibody. Blocks Her2 estrogen receptor
Company	US National Cancer Institute/ Bristol Myers Squibb	3M	Astra	Novartis	Genentech/Roche
Indication	Ovarian cancer	Cardiac dyrhythmias	Peptic ulcer	Chronic myeloid leukaemia	Breast cancer
Project start	1964	1965	1966	1983	1988
Compound synthesized or structure determined	1971 (7 years)	1974 (9 years)	1978 (12 years)	1990 (7 years)	1990 (2 years)
Phase I	1983 (19 years)	1976 (11 years)	1981 (15 years)		1991 (3 years)
Registration	1992 (28 years)	1984 (19 years)	1988 (22 years)	2001 (18 years)	1998 (10 years)

clinical trials, and the uncertainty that it could ever be produced on a commercial basis. The Pacific Yew grows slowly and has a restricted habitat, and conservationists were opposed to commercial harvesting. As a result, there was only enough material for limited Phase II studies, on patients with ovarian cancer. The improvement in these patients was dramatic, but continuation of the project, now in collaboration with Bristol Myers Squibb, was seriously hindered by the limited supplies of yew tree bark. The conservation concerns were overcome when a census showed that the tree population was not in fact threatened, and industrial supplies of bark were collected to support the trials programme right through to 1992, when the drug was officially approved.

Commercialization of the material extracted from bark was seen as a major problem, but was solved when it was found that the needles of many yew species contain *baccatin*, from which paclitaxel can be produced. This semisynthetic paclitaxel, made from an abundant and renewable source, was officially approved in 1999 and is a highly successful and clinically valuable form of cancer therapy. The obstacles to progress in this case were (a) the failure of the primary screen to reveal the compound as anything out of the ordinary; (b) the appearance of serious side effects resulting from the properties of the excipient; and (c) the supply problem.

Flecainide (Tambocor)

The story of flecainide (Barritt and Schmid, 1993) represents a completely different route to success, variations of which gave rise to many innovative drugs (e.g. antihypertensive drugs, antidepressants and antipsychotics) during the 1960s. In the early 1960s, the drugs used to treat cardiac dysrhythmias were mainly *quinidine, procainamide, digoxin* (for supraventricular tachycardias) and *lidocaine* (given i.v. for ventricular dysrhythmias). The first three had many troublesome side effects, whereas lidocaine's use was largely confined to intensive care settings. In 1964, the 3M company decided to seek better antidysrhythmic drugs. Their chemists had developed a new synthetic pathway for introducing $-CF_3$ groups, and they started a chemistry programme based on fluorinated derivatives of known local anaesthetic and antidysrythmic drugs. Assays for antidysrhythmic activity at the time involved elaborate studies on anaesthetized dogs, which were quite unsuitable for screening, and so the group developed a simple primary screening assay based on the ability of compounds to prevent ventricular fibrillation induced by chloroform inhalation in mice, which was used to screen hundreds of compounds. Secondary assays on selected compounds were carried out on anaesthetized dogs in the then conventional fashion. Questions of mechanism were not addressed, it being (correctly) assumed that efficacy in these animal models would serve as a good predictor of clinical efficacy irrespective of the cellular mechanisms involved. A potential development com-

pound was synthesized in 1969, but abandoned on account of CNS side effects. After a further 5 years of painstaking chemistry, during which many different structural classes were tested, flecainide was synthesized (1974) and found to have a much improved therapeutic window compared to its predecessors. The first clinical studies were performed in 1976, and development proceeded quite smoothly until the compound was registered in 1984. It was the first deliberate effort to develop an improved antidysrhythmic drug and proved highly successful in the clinic, now accepted as the standard Class 1c antidysrhythmic agent according to the current classification.

With the benefit of hindsight, we can see that the main delaying factor in the flecainide project was simply slow chemistry, guided largely by empiricism. One result of this was that, after encountering side-effect problems with the lead compound, it took 5 years to find the solution (during which, one suspects, the biologists on the team were growing a little bored!). This model of drug discovery research, where chemistry was both the driving force and the rate-limiting factor for the whole project, is typical of many projects around this time (including many that were, like flecainide, ultimately very successful).

Omeprazol (Losec)

Omeprazol, developed by Astra, was the first proton pump inhibitor, which transformed the treatment of peptic ulcers when it was launched in 1988, quickly becoming the company's best-selling drug. The project, however, graphically described by Östholm (1995) had a chequered and death-defying history. In 1966 Astra started a project aimed at developing inhibitors of gastric acid secretion, having previously developed profitable antacid preparations. They started a chemistry programme based on carbamates, and collaborated with an academic group to develop a suitable in vivo screening assay in rats. Compounds with weak activity were quickly identified; initial hepatotoxicity problems were overcome, and a potential development compound was tested in humans in 1968. It had no effect on acid secretion, and the project narrowly escaped termination. In the meantime, good progress was being made by Smith, Kline and French in developing histamine H_2 antagonists for the same indication, thereby adding to the anxiety within Astra. At the same time Searle reported a new class of inhibitory compounds, benzimidazoles, which were active but toxic. Astra began a new chemistry programme based on this series, and in 1973 produced a highly active compound which was proposed for further development. To their dismay, they found that a Hungarian company had a patent on this compound (for a completely different application). However, upon entering licensing negotiations they found that the Hungarian patent had actually lapsed because the company had defaulted on payment of the fees to the patent office! Further studies with this compound revealed problems with thyroid toxicity, however, and more demands to terminate this hapless project were narrowly fought off. The thyroid toxicity was thought to be associated with the thiouracil structure, and further chemistry aimed at eliminating this resulted, in 1976, in the synthesis of *picoprazole*, the forerunner of omeprazole. After yet another toxicological alarm – this time vasculitis in dogs – which turned out to be an artefact, picoprazole was tested in human patients suffering from Zollinger–Ellison syndrome and was found to be highly effective in reducing acid secretion. At around the same time, an academic group showed that acid secretion involved a specific transport mechanism, the proton pump, which was strongly inhibited by the Astra compounds, so their novel mechanism of action was established. Omeprazole, an analogue of picoprazole, was synthesized in 1979, and was chosen for development instead of picoprazole. The chemistry team had by then made over 800 compounds during the 13-year lifetime of the project. The chemical development of omeprazole was complicated by the compound's poor stability and sensitivity to light, requiring special precautions in formulation. Phase II/III clinical trials began in 1981, but were halted for 2 years as a result of yet another toxicology scare – carcinogenicity – which again proved to be a false alarm. Omeprazole was finally registered in 1988.

That omeprazole, one of the most significant new drugs to appear in the early 1990s, should have survived this frightful Odyssey is something of a miracle. One setback after another was faced and overcome, a tribute to the sheer determination and persuasive skills of the discovery team. Nowadays, when research managers pride themselves on their decisiveness and courage in terminating projects at the first hint of trouble, omeprazole would surely stand little chance.

Imatinib (Gleevec)

Imatinib (Druker and Lydon, 2000; Capdeville et al., 2002), registered in 2001, is the most recent example in these brief histories, and exemplifies the shift towards defined molecular targets that has so altered the approach to drug discovery over the last 20 years. In the mid-1980s, it was discovered that a rare form of cancer, chronic myeloid leukaemia (CML), was almost invariably associated with the expression of a specific oncogene product, Bcr-Abl kinase. The enhanced tyrosine kinase activity of this mutated protein was shown to underlie the malignant transformation of the white blood cells. The proven association between the gene mutation[1], the enhanced kinase activity and the distinct

clinical phenotype, provided a particularly clear example of cancer pathogenesis. On this basis, the oncology team of Ciba-Geigy (later Novartis) began a project seeking specific inhibitors of Abl-kinase. It is known that there are many different kinases involved in cellular regulatory mechanisms, all using ATP as a phosphate donor and possessing highly conserved ATP-binding domains. Interest in kinase inhibitors as drugs was, and remains, high (Cohen, 2002), but at the time the known inhibitors were all relatively non-specific and distinctly toxic, and the widely held view was that, as the known compounds all acted at the highly conserved ATP-binding site, specific kinase inhibitors would be difficult to produce. The commercial potential also appeared weak, as CML is a rare disease. Undaunted, the team started by developing routine biochemical assays for this and other kinases, based on purified enzymes produced in quantity by a genetic engineering technique based on the baculovirus expression system. Screening of synthetic compound libraries revealed that compounds of the 2-phenylaminopyrimidine class showed selectivity in blocking Abl and PDGF-receptor kinases, and systematic chemical derivatization led to the synthesis of imatinib in 1992, roughly 8 years after starting the project. Although crystallographic analysis of the kinase structure played no part in guiding the chemistry that produced imatinib, a later structural study (Schindler et al., 2000) provided an explanation for its selectivity for Abl-kinase by showing that its binding site extends beyond the ATP site to other, less conserved domains. Imatinib proved to have no major shortcomings in relation to pharmacokinetics or toxicology, and was highly effective in suppressing the growth of cells engineered to express Bcr-Abl, and of human tumour cells transplanted into mice. Importantly, it also inhibited the growth in culture of peripheral blood or bone marrow cells from CML patients (Druker et al., 1996). The latter result was particularly valuable for the project, as it is rarely possible to carry out such ex vivo tests on material from patients – normally, it is necessary to wait until the compound enters Phase II trials before any evidence relating to clinical efficacy emerges. On that basis the project was given high priority and an accelerated clinical trials programme was devised. The first trials (Druker et al., 2001), beginning in 1998, were performed not on normal subjects, but on 83 CML patients who had failed to respond to treatment with interferon. Different doses were tested in groups of six to eight patients, and the pharmacokinetic parameters, adverse effects and clinical response were measured in parallel. These highly streamlined studies showed an unequivocal clinical effect, with 100% of patients receiving the higher doses showing a good haematological response. As a result, and because the regulatory procedures were dispatched particularly rapidly, the drug was registered in record time, in May 2001, just 3 years after being tested for the

---

[1]Identifiable by a chromosomal staining technique able to detect the translocation of DNA between two chromosomes, producing the characteristic 'Philadelphia chromosome' which gives rise to the abnormal kinase.

first time in humans. Imatinib is the first 'designer' kinase inhibitor to be registered (other drugs, such as *rapamycin*, probably act by kinase inhibition, but this was not known at the time). Imatinib has proved efficacious also in certain gastrointestinal tumours, and is almost certainly the forerunner of further kinase inhibitors developed for the treatment, not only of cancer, but also of inflammatory and immunological disorders (and who knows what else!).

In retrospect, the imatinib project owes its success to several factors, most obviously to the selection of a precisely defined molecular target which was known to be disease relevant, and was amenable to modern assay technologies. Setting up the various kinase assays took 4–5 years, but thereafter screening produced the lead series of compounds rather quickly, and imatinib itself was made within about 4 years of starting the screening programme. Avoiding the pitfalls of pharmacokinetics and toxicology, which so often hinder development, was very fortunate. What was quite exceptional was the speed of clinical development and registration. This was possible partly because CML is resistant to conventional anticancer drugs, and so imatinib did not need to be compared with other treatments. Also, the designation of imatinib as an 'orphan drug' (see Chapter 20), based on the rarity of CML, allowed the trials programme to be simplified and accelerated. Its action is readily monitored by haematological tests, permitting a rapid clinical readout. The therapeutic effect of the drug on circulating white cells is directly related to its plasma level, which is often not the case for drugs acting on solid tumours. It is an example where the choice of indication, initially made on the basis of a solid biological hypothesis, proved highly advantageous in allowing the clinical development to progress rapidly.

Trastuzumab (Herceptin)

Trastuzumab is a humanized monoclonal antibody which selectively blocks the estrogen receptor Her2. This project, which took 8 years from compound discovery to registration, shows the speed with which biopharmaceuticals can, under the right conditions, be developed. The Her2 receptor was first cloned in 1985, and 2 years later it was found to be strongly overexpressed in the most aggressive breast cancers. Genentech used its in-house technology to develop a humanized mouse monoclonal antibody that blocked the function of the receptor and suppressed the proliferation of receptor-bearing cells. Compared with conventional lead-finding and lead optimization of synthetic molecules, this took very little time – only 2 years from the start of the project. Antibodies generally exhibit much simpler and more predictable pharmacological effects than synthetic compounds, and run into fewer problems with chemical development, formulation and toxicology, so that trastuzumab was able to enter Phase

I within 2 years. Clear-cut efficacy was evident in Phase II, and the rest of the clinical development was rapid and straightforward. Trastuzumab represents a significant step forward in the treatment of breast cancer, as well as a commercial success. Given the right circumstances, biopharmaceuticals can be developed more quickly and more cheaply than conventional drugs, a fact reflected in the growing proportion (approximately 35% in 2001) of biopharmaceuticals among new chemical entities being registered.

Comments and conclusions

One common feature that emerges from a survey of the many anecdotal reports of drug discovery projects is that they often have outcomes quite different from what was originally intended. The first tricyclic antidepressant drug, *imipramine*, emerged from a project aimed at developing antihistamines based on the structure of promethazine. *Clonidine* was synthesized in the early 1960s as part of a project intended to develop α-adrenoceptor agonists as vasoconstrictors for use as decongestant nose drops. The physician involved tested the nose drops on his wife, who had a cold, and was surprised by the fact that her blood pressure plummeted. She also slept for 24 hours. It turned out that the dose was about 30 times what was later found effective in humans. The experiment revealed the unexpected hypotensive action of clonidine upon which its subsequent commercial development was based. More recently, it is well known that *sildenafil (Viagra)* was originally intended as a vasodilator for treating angina, and only during clinical testing did its erection-inducing effect become evident.

It might be supposed that the increasing emphasis now being placed on defined molecular targets as starting points for drug discovery projects would reduce the likelihood of such therapeutic surprises. However, the molecular targets used for screening nowadays lie further, in the functional sense, from the therapeutic response that is being sought than do the physiological responses relied on previously (see Chapter 2, Figure 2.3). Thus compounds aimed with precision at well-defined targets commonly fail to produce the desired therapeutic effect, evidently because we do not sufficiently understand the pathophysiological pathway linking the two. Recent examples of such failures include *ondansetron*, a $5HT_3$-receptor antagonist conceived as an antimigraine drug but ineffective in this indication (developed instead as an antiemetic), and substance P receptor antagonists which were expected to have analgesic properties in humans, but which proved ineffective. Lack of efficacy in clinical trials – a measure of our inability to predict therapeutic efficacy on the basis of pharmacological properties – remains one of the commonest

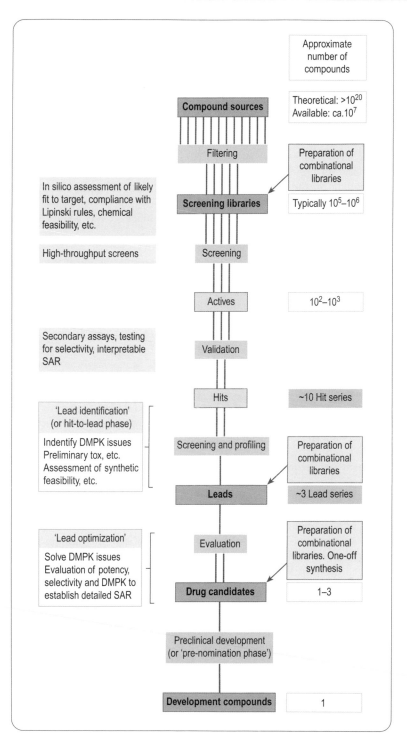

Fig. 4.4
Stages of drug discovery.

The stages of drug discovery

causes of project failure, accounting for 30% of failures (Kennedy, 1997), second only to pharmacokinetic short-comings (39%).

In this section we are concerned with the initial stages of the overall project outlined in Figure 4.1, up to the point at which a molecule makes its solemn rite of passage from research to development. Figure 4.4 summarizes the main stages that make up a 'typical' drug discovery project, from the identification of a target to the production of a candidate drug[2].

A huge number of 'theoretical' compounds (far too many to be physically accessible) is first 'filtered' in silico to reduce it to a practicable number of compounds that are available, or can be synthesized, as screening libraries. High-throughput screening is then used to identify 'hits', which show significant activity in the chosen screen. This may throw up hundreds or thousands of compounds, depending on the nature of the screen and the size and quality of the library. Normally, a significant proportion of these prove to be artefacts of one sort or another, for example results that cannot be repeated when the compound is resynthesized, positives in the assay resulting from non-specific effects, or simply 'noise' in the assay system. 'Validation' of hits is therefore necessary to eliminate artefacts, and this may involve repeating the screening of the hits, confirming the result in a different assay designed to measure activity on the chosen target, as well as resynthesis and retesting of the hit compounds. Validation will also entail assessment of the structure–activity relationships within the screening library, and whether the hit belongs to a family of compounds – a 'hit series' – which represents a reasonable starting point for further chemistry.

In the next stage, lead identification, the validated hits are subjected to further scrutiny, particularly in respect of their pharmacokinetic properties and toxicity, as well as addressing in more detail the feasibility of building a synthetic chemistry programme. In this process, the handful of 'hit series' is further reduced to one or a few 'lead series'. Up to this point, the aim has been to reduce the number of compounds in contention from millions to a few – 'negative chemistry', if you will.

Synthetic chemistry then begins, in the 'lead optimization' stage. This usually involves parallel synthesis to generate derivatives of the lead series, which are screened and profiled with respect to pharmacology, pharmacokinetics and toxicology, to home in on a small number of 'drug candidates' (often a single compound, or if the project is unlucky, none at all) judged suitable for further development, at which point they are taken into preclinical development.

The flow diagram in Figure 4.4 provides a useful basis for the more detailed accounts of the various activities that contribute to the drug discovery process, described in the chapters that follow. It should be realized, though, that many variations on this basic scheme take place in real life. A project may, for example, work

on one lead series and at the same time go back to library screening to find new starting points. New biological discoveries, such as the identification of a new receptor subtype, may cause the project to redefine its objectives midstream.

Increasingly, large companies are tending to centralize the early stages of drug discovery, up to the identification of lead series, and to carry out many screens in parallel with very large compound libraries, focusing on putative drug targets often identified on the basis of genomics, rather than on pharmacology and pathophysiology relating to specific disease indications. In this emerging scenario, the work of the drug discovery team effectively begins from the chemical lead.

Trends in drug discovery

Increasingly, drug discovery has become focused on cloned molecular targets that can be incorporated into high-throughput screens. Target selection, discussed in Chapter 6, has therefore assumed a significance that it rarely had in the past: of the projects described above, three began without any molecular target in mind, which would seldom be the case nowadays.

The examples summarized in Table 4.2 show that it took 7–12 years from the start of the project to identificaton of the compound that was finally developed. That interval has now been substantially reduced, often to 3 years or less once a molecular target has been selected, mainly as a result of (a) high-throughput screening of large compound libraries (including natural product libraries) to identify initial lead compounds; (b) improvements at the lead optimization stage, including the use of combinatorial synthesis to generate large families of related compounds, and increased use of molecular modelling techniques, whereby the results of compound screening are analysed to reveal the molecular configurations that are associated with biological activity.

There is strong motivation to improve not only the speed of lead optimization, but also the 'quality' of the compound selected for development. Quality, in this context, means a low probability that the compound will fail later in development. The main reasons that compounds fail, apart from lack of efficacy or unexpected side effects, are that they show toxicity, or that they have undesirable pharmacokinetic properties (e.g. poor absorption, too long or too short plasma half-life, unpredictable metabolism, accumulation in tissues etc.). In the past, these aspects of a drug's properties were often not investigated until the discovery/development hurdle had been crossed, as investigating them was traditionally regarded as a responsibility of 'development' rather than 'research'. Frequently a compound would fail after several months in preclinical development – too late for the problem to be

---

[2]The process of developing a new biopharmaceutical generally follows a different path, and is described more fully in Chapter 12.

addressed by the drug discovery team, which had by then moved on. This highlighted the need to incorporate pharmacokinetic and toxicological studies, as well as pharmacological ones, at an earlier stage of the project, during the lead optimization phase. As described in Chapter 10, studies of this kind are now routinely included in most drug discovery projects. Inevitably this has a cost in terms of time and money, but this will be more than justified by a reduction in the likelihood of compounds failing during clinical development.

The main trends that have occurred over the last two decades are summarized in Table 4.3, the key ones being, as discussed above:

- A massive expansion of the compound collections used as starting points, from large 'white-powder' libraries of 100 000 or more compounds created during the 1990s, to massive virtual libraries of tens of millions;
- Use of combinatorial synthesis methods to accelerate lead optimization;
- To deal with large, compound libraries, the introduction of high-throughput screens for actual compounds, and in silico screens for virtual compounds;
- Increasing reliance on in silico predictions to generate leads;

Table 4.3
Trends in drug discovery

		Ca 1980	Ca 1990	Ca 2000
Target finding	Sources of targets	Insights from pathophysiology Known pharmacological targets Serendipitous findings	Known pharmacological targets Defined molecular targets	Defined human molecular targets based on genomics
Hit finding	Compound sources	Available natural products 'One-at-a-time' synthesis	Large compound libraries, selected on basis of availability Natural product libraries	Massive virtual libraries, then focused combinatorial libraries
	Screens	In vitro and in vivo pharmacological screens. Radioligand binding assays	High-throughput screen in vitro Hits validated by secondary functional assays in vitro	Virtual library screened in silico for predicted target affinity, 'rule-of-5' compliance, chemical and metabolic stability, toxic groups, etc
			Selection of leads mainly 'in cerebro'*	Combinatorial libraries screened by HTS, several screens in parallel
Validated hits				
Lead finding	Compound sources	Custom synthesis based on medicinal chemistry insights Natural products	Analogues synthesized one at a time or combinatorially	Combinatorial synthesis of analogues
	Screens	Low throughput pharmacological assays in vitro and in vivo	Functional assays in vitro and in vivo	Medium throughput in vitro screens for target affinity, DMPK characteristics Preliminary measurements of DMPK in vivo
Leads				
Lead optimization	Compound sources	Analogues of active compounds synthesized one at a time	Combinatorial or one at a time synthesis of analogues	Combinatorial or one at a time synthesis of analogues
Drug candidate	Screens	Animal models	Efficacy in animal models Simple PK measurements in vivo Safety pharmacology In vitro genotoxicity	Efficacy in animal models Detailed DMPK analysis Safety pharmacology In vitro genotoxicity

*The cerebrum required being that of an experienced medicinal chemist.

- Focus on cloned human targets as starting points;
- Progressive 'front-loading' of assessment of DMPK (drug metabolism and pharmacokinetic) characteristics, including in silico assessment of virtual libraries.

Project planning

When a project moves from the phase of exploratory research to being an approved drug discovery project to which specific resources are assigned under the direction of a project leader, its objectives, expected timelines and resource requirements need to be agreed by the members of the project team and approved by research management.

The early drug discovery phase of the project will typically begin when a target has been selected and the necessary screening methods established, and its aim will be to identify one or a few 'drug candidates' suitable for progressing to the next stage of preclinical development. The properties required for a drug candidate will vary from project to project, but will invariably include chemical, pharmacological, pharmacokinetic and toxicological aspects of the compound. Table 4.4 summarizes the criteria that might apply to a typical drug acting on a target such as an enzyme or receptor, and intended for oral use. Where appropriate (e.g. potency, oral bioavailability), quantitative limits will normally be set. Such a list of necessary or desirable features, based on results from many independent assessments and experimental tests, provides an essential focus for the project. Some of these, such as potency on target, or oral bioavailability, will be absolute requirements, whereas others, such as water solubility or lack of in vitro genotoxicity, may be highly desirable but not essential. There are, in essence, two balancing components of a typical project:

- Designing and synthesizing novel compounds;
- Filtering, to eliminate compounds that fail to satisfy the criteria.

Whereas in an earlier era of drug discovery these two activities took place independently – chemists made compounds and handed over white powders for testing, while pharmacologists tried to find ones that worked – nowadays the process is invariably an iterative and interactive one, whereby the design and synthesis of new compounds continuously takes into account the biological findings and shortcomings that have been revealed to date. Formal project planning, of the kind that would be adopted for the building of a new road, for example, is therefore inappropriate for drug discovery. Experienced managers consequently rely less on detailed advance planning, and more on good communication between the various members of the project team, and frequent meetings to review progress and agree on the best way forward.

An important aspect of project planning is deciding what tests to do when, so as to achieve the objectives as quickly and efficiently as possible. The factors that have to be taken into account for each test are:

- Compound throughput;
- Cost per compound;

Table 4.4
Typical selection criteria for drug candidates intended for oral use*

Chemical	Pharmacological	Pharmacokinetic	Toxicological
Patentable structure	Defined potency on target	Cell-permeable in vitro	In vitro genotoxicity tests negative
Water-soluble	Selectivity for specific target relative to other related targets	Adequate oral bioavailability	Preliminary in vivo toxicology tests showing adequate margin between expected 'therapeutic' dose and maximum No Adverse Effect Dose
Chemically stable	Pharmacodynamic activity in vitro and in vivo	For CNS drugs: penetrates blood–brain barrier	
Large-scale synthesis feasible	No adverse effects in standard safety pharmacology tests	Appropriate plasma half-life	
Non-chiral	Active in disease models	Defined metabolism by human liver microsomes	
No known 'toxophoric' groups		No inhibition or induction of cytochrome P450	

*Criteria such as these, which will vary according to the expected therapeutic application of the compound, would normally be applied to compound selection in the drug discovery stage of a project, culminating in lead optimization and the identification of a drug candidate, when preclinical development begins, focusing mainly on pharmacokinetics, toxicology, chemistry and formulation.

- Amount of compound required in relation to amount available;
- Time required. Some in vivo pharmacodynamic tests (e.g. bone density changes, tumour growth) are inherently slow. Irrespective of compound throughput, they cannot provide rapid feedback;
- 'Salience' of result (i.e. is the criterion an absolute requirement, or desirable but non-essential?);
- Probability that the compound will fail. In a typical high-throughput screen more than 99% of compounds will be eliminated, so it is essential that this is done early. In vitro genotoxicity, in contrast, will be found only occasionally, so it would be wasteful to test for this early in the sequence.

The current emphasis on fast drug discovery, to increase the time window between launch and patent expiry, and on decreasing the rate of failure of compounds during clinical development, is having an important effect on the planning of drug discovery projects. As discussed above, there is increasing emphasis on applying fast-result, high-throughput methods of testing for pharmacokinetic and toxicological properties at an early stage ('front-loading'; see Chapter 10), even though the *salience* (i.e. the ability to predict properties needed in the clinic) of such assays may be limited. The growth of high-throughput test methods has had a major impact on the work of chemists in drug discovery (see Chapter 9), where the emphasis is on preparing 'libraries' of related compounds to feed the hungry assay machines. These changes have undoubtedly improved the performance of the industry in finding new lead compounds of higher quality for new targets. The main bottlenecks now in drug discovery are in lead optimization (see Chapter 9) and animal testing (see Chapter 11), areas so far largely untouched by the high-throughput revolution.

Research in the pharmaceutical industry

Pharmaceutical companies perform research for commercial reasons and seek to ensure that it produces a return on investment. The company owns the data, and is free to publish it or keep it secret as it sees fit. Although most pharmaceutical companies include altruistic as well as commercial aims in their mission statements, the latter necessarily take priority. The company will therefore wish to ensure that the research it supports is in some way relevant to its commercial objectives. Clearly, studies aimed directly at drug discovery present no problems. At the other end of the spectrum lies pure curiosity-driven ('blue-skies') research. Although such work may – and often does –

lead to progress in drug discovery in the long term, the commercial pay-off is highly uncertain and inevitably long delayed. Generally speaking, such long-term research is not performed in a commercial setting. Between the two lies a large territory of 'applied' research, more clearly focused on drug discovery, though still medium-term and somewhat uncertain in its applicability. Many technological projects come into this category, such as novel high-throughput screening methods, imaging technologies etc., as well as research into pathophysiological mechanisms aimed at the identification of new drug targets. The many applications of genomics and molecular biology in drug discovery make up an increasing proportion of work in this applied research category. Small biotechnology companies which started during the 1980s and 1990s moved quickly into this territory, and several large pharmaceutical companies, notably SmithKlineBeecham (now merged with GlaxoWellcome), also made major investments. The extent to which pharmaceutical companies invest in medium-term applied research projects varies greatly. A growing tendency seems to be for larger companies to set up what amounts to an in-house biotechnology facility, often incorporating one or more acquired biotech companies. The technological revolution in drug discovery, referred to frequently in this book, has yet to pay dividends in terms of improved performance, so it is uncertain whether this level of commitment to medium-term applied research can be sustained.

The cultural difference between academic and commercial research is real, but less profound than is often thought. Quality, in the sense of good experimental design, methodology and data interpretation, is equally important to both, as is creativity, the ability to generate new ideas and see them through. Key differences are that, in the industry environment, freedom to choose projects and to publish is undoubtedly more limited, and effective interdisciplinary teamwork is obligatory, rather than a matter of personal choice: there is little room in industry for the lone genius. These differences are, however, becoming narrower as the bodies funding academic research take a more 'corporate' approach to its management. Individual researchers in academia are substantially constrained to work on projects that attract funding support, and are increasingly being required to collaborate in interdisciplinary projects. They are certainly more free to publish, but are also under much more pressure to do so, as, in contrast to the situation in industry, publications are their only measure of research achievement. Pharmaceutical companies also have incentives to publish their work: it gives their scientists visibility in the scientific community and helps them to establish fruitful collaborations, as well as strengthening the company's attractiveness as an employer of good scientists. The main restrictions to publication are the company's need to avoid compromising its future patent position, or giving away information that might help its competitors. Companies vary in their attitude to publication, some being much more liberal than others.

Scientists in industry have to learn to work, and communicate effectively, with the company's management. Managers are likely to ask 'Why do we need this information?' which, to scientists in academia, may seem an irritatingly silly question. To them, the purpose of any research is to add to the edifice of human knowledge, and working towards this aim fully justifies the time, effort and money that supports the work. The long-term benefits to humanity are measured in terms of cultural richness and technological progress. In the short term the value of what has been achieved is measured by peer recognition and grant renewal; the long-term judgment is left to history.

Within a pharmaceutical company, research findings are aimed at a more limited audience and their purpose is more focused. The immediate aim is to provide the data needed for prediction of the potential of a new compound to succeed in the clinic. The internal audiences are the research team itself and research management; the external audiences are the external scientific community and, importantly, the regulatory authorities.

We should, however, resist the tendency to think of drug discovery as a commercial undertaking comparable developing a new sports car, where the outcome is assured provided that operatives with the necessary skill and experience fulfil what is asked of them. They are not likely by chance to invent a new kind of aeroplane or vacuum cleaner.

Like all research, drug discovery is more likely than not to come up with unexpected findings, and these can have a major impact on the plan and its objectives. So, frequent review – and, if necessary, amendment – of the plan is essential, and research managers need to understand (as most do, having their own research experiences to draw on) that unexpected results, and the problems that may follow for the project, reflect the complexity of the problem, rather than the failings of the team. Finding by experiment that a hypothesis is wrong is to be seen as a creditable scientific achievement, not at all the same as designing a car with brakes that do not work.

References

Barritt E H, Schmid J R (1993) In: Lednicer D, ed. Chronicles of drug discovery. Vol. 3. Washington DC: American Chemical Society.

Capdeville R, Buchdunger E, Zimmermann J, Matter A (2002) Glivec (STI571, imatinib), a rationally developed, targeted anticancer drug. Nature Reviews Drug Discovery 1: 493–502.

Cohen P (2002) Protein kinases – the major drug targets of the twenty-first century? Nature Reviews Drug Discovery 1: 309–316.

Cragg G M (1998) Paclitaxel (Taxol): a success story with valuable lessons for natural product drug discovery and development. Medical Research Review 18: 315–331.

Drews J (2000) Drug discovery: a historical perspective. Science 287: 1960–1964.

Druker B J, Lydon N B (2000) Lessons learned from the development of an Abl tyrosine kinase inhibitor for chronic myelognous leukemia. Journal of Clinical Investigation 105: 3–7.

Druker B J, Tamura S, Buchdunger E et al. (1996) Effects of a selective inhibitor of the Abl tyrosine kinase on the growth of Bcr-Abl positive cells. Nature Medicine 2: 561–566.

Druker BJ, Talpaz M, Resta DJ et al. (2001) Efficacy and safety of a specific inhibitor of the Bcr-Abl tyrosine kinase in chronic myeloid leukemia. New England Journal of Medicine 344: 1031–1037.

Kennedy T (1997) Managing the drug discovery/development interface. Drug Discovery Today 2: 436–444.

Lednicer D (1993) Chronicles of drug discovery. Vol. 3. Washington DC: American Chemical Society.

Östholm I 1995 Drug discovery: a pharmacist's view. Stockholm: Swedish Pharmaceutical Press.

Schindler T, Bornmann W, Pellicana P, Miller W T, Clarkson B, Kuriyan J (2000) Structural mechanism for STI-571 inhibition of Abelson tyrosine kinase. Science 289: 1938–1942.

5 Choosing the project

H P Rang

Introduction

In this chapter we discuss the various criteria that are applied when making the initial decision of whether or not to embark on a new drug discovery project. The point at which a project becomes formally recognized as a drug discovery project with a clear-cut aim of delivering a candidate molecule for development, and the amount of managerial control that is exercised before and after this transition, vary considerably from company to company. Some encourage – or at least allow – research scientists to pursue ideas under the general umbrella of 'exploratory research', whereas others control the research portfolio more tightly and discourage their scientists from straying off the straight and narrow path of a specific project. Generally, however, some room is left within the organization for exploratory research in the expectation that it will generate ideas for future drug discovery projects. When successful, this strategy results in research-led project proposals, which generally have the advantage of starting from proprietary knowledge and having a well-motivated and expert in-house team. Historically, such research-led drug discovery projects have produced many successful drugs, including β-blockers, ACE inhibitors, statins, tamoxifen and many others, but also many failures, for example prostanoid receptor ligands, which have found few clinical uses. Facing harder times, managements are now apt to dismiss such projects as 'drugs in search of a disease', so it is incumbent upon research teams to align their work, even in the early exploratory stage, as closely as possible with the business objectives of the company, and to frame project proposals accordingly.

Making the decision

The first, and perhaps the most important, decision in the life history of a drug discovery project is the decision to start. Imagine a group considering whether or not to climb a mountain. *Strategically*, they decide whether or not they want to get to the top of that particular mountain; *technically*, they decide whether there is a feasible route; and *operationally* they decide whether or not they

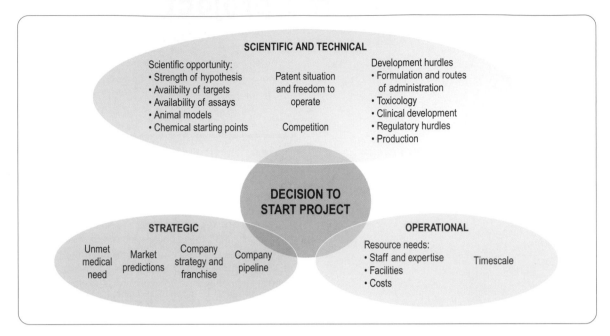

Fig. 5.1
Criteria for project selection.

have the wherewithal to accomplish the climb. In the context of a drug discovery project, the questions are:

● *Should we do it?* (strategic issues)
● *Could we do it?* (scientific and technical issues)
● *Can we do it?* (operational issues).

The main factors that need to be considered are summarized in Figure 5.1.

Strategic issues

Strategic issues relate to the *desirability* of the project from the company's perspective, reflecting its mission (a) to make a significant contribution to healthcare, and (b) to make a profit for its shareholders. These translate into assessments respectively of medical need and market potential.

Unmet medical need

Unmet medical need represents what many would regard as the most fundamental criterion to be satisfied when evaluating any drug discovery project, though defining and evaluating it objectively is far from straightforward. Of course there are common and serious diseases, such as many cancers, viral infections, neurodegenerative diseases, certain developmental abnormalities etc., for

which current treatments are non-existent or far from ideal, and these would be generally accepted as areas of high unmet need. Nevertheless, trying to rank potential drug discovery projects on this basis is full of difficulties, because it assumes that we can assess disease severity objectively, and somehow balance it against disease prevalence. Does a rare but catastrophic disease represent a greater or a lesser medical need than a common minor one? Is severity best measured in terms of reduced life expectancy, or level of disability and suffering? Does reducing the serious side effects of existing widely used and efficacious drugs (e.g. gastric bleeding with conventional non-steroidal anti-inflammatory drugs) meet a need that is more important than finding a therapy for a condition that was previously untreatable? Does public demand for baldness cures, antiwrinkle creams and other 'lifestyle' remedies constitute a medical need?

Assessing medical need is not simply a matter of asking customers what they would regard as ideal; this usually results in a product description which falls into the category of 'a free drug, given once orally with no side effects, that cures the condition'. Nevertheless, this trite response can serve a useful purpose when determining the medical need for a new product: how closely do existing and future competitors approach this ideal? How big is the gap between the reality and the ideal, and would it be profitable to try and fill it? Using this type of 'gap analysis' we can ask ourselves the following questions:

- How close do we come to 'free'? In other words, can we be more cost-effective?
- Compliance is important: a drug that is not taken cannot work. Once-daily oral dosing is convenient, but would a long-lasting injection be a better choice for some patients?
- If an oral drug exists, can it be improved, for example by changing the formulation?
- The reduction of side effects is an area where there is often a medical need. Do we have a strategy for improving the side-effect profile of existing drugs?
- Curing a condition or retarding disease progression is preferable to alleviating symptoms. Do we have a strategy for achieving this?

Market considerations

These overlap to some extent with unmet medical need, but focus particularly on assessing the likelihood that the revenue from sales will succeed in recouping the investment. Disease prevalence and severity, as discussed above, obviously affect sales volume and price. Other important factors include the extent to which the proposed compound is likely to be superior to drugs already on the market, and the marketing experience and reputation of the company in the particular disease area. The more innovative the project, the greater is the degree of uncertainty of such assessments. The market for *ciclosporin*, for example, was initially thought to be too small to justify its development – as transplant surgery was regarded as a highly specialized type of intervention that would never become commonplace – but in the end the drug itself gave a large boost to organ transplantation, and proved to be a blockbuster. There are also many examples of innovative and well-researched drugs that fail in development, or perform poorly in the marketplace, so creativity is not an infallible passport to success. Recognizing the uncertainty of market predictions in the early stages of an innovative project, companies generally avoid attaching much weight to these evaluations when judging which projects to support at the research stage.

Company strategy and franchise

The current and planned franchise of a pharmaceutical company plays a large part in determining the broad disease areas, such as cancer, mental illness, cardiovascular disease, gastroenterology etc., addressed by new projects, but will not influence the particular scientific approach that is taken. All companies specialize to a greater or lesser extent on particular disease areas, and this is reflected in their research organization and scientific recruitment policies. Biotechnology companies are more commonly focused on particular technologies and scientific approaches, such as drug delivery, genomics, growth factors, monoclonal antibodies etc., rather than on particular disease areas. They are therefore more pragmatic about the potential therapeutic application of their discoveries, which will generally be licensed out at an appropriate stage for development by companies within whose franchise the application falls. In the biotech environment, strategic issues therefore tend to be involved more with science and technology than may be the case in larger pharmaceutical companies – a characteristic that is often appealing to research scientists.

The state of a company's development pipeline, and its need to sustain a steady flow of new compounds entering the market, sometimes influences the selection of drug discovery projects. The company may, for example, need a product to replace one that is nearing the end of its patent life, or is losing out to competition, and it may endeavour to direct research to that end. In general, though, in the absence of an innovative scientific strategy such top-down commercially driven priorities often fail. A better, and quicker, solution to the commercial problem will often be to license in a partly developed compound with the required specification.

In general, the management of a pharmaceutical company needs to choose and explain which therapeutic areas it wishes to cover, and to communicate this effectively to the drug discovery research organization, but most will avoid placing too much emphasis on market analysis and commercial factors when it comes to selecting specific projects. This is partly because market analysis is at best a very imprecise business and the commercial environment can change rapidly, but also because success in the past has often come from exploiting unexpected scientific opportunities and building a marketing and commercial strategy on the basis of what is discovered, rather than the other way round.. The interface between science and commerce is always somewhat turbulent.

Legislation, government policy, reimbursement and pricing

Unlike the products of many other industries, pharmaceuticals are subject to controls on their pricing, their promotional activities, and their registration as 'safe and effective' products that can be put on the market, and so their commercial environment is significantly altered by government intervention. The socialized medicine that is a feature of European and Canadian healthcare means that the government is not only the major provider of healthcare, but also a monopoly purchaser of drugs for use in the healthcare system. The USA is the only major market where the government does not exert price controls, except as a feature of Medicare, where it acts as a major buyer and expects discounts commensurate with its purchasing power. Governments have great influence on the marketing of drugs, and they have an interest in limiting the prescription of newer, generally more expensive products, and this affects where the industry can sell premium-priced products. Governments and their associated regulatory bodies have gradually extended their power from a position of regulation for public safety to one of guardians of the public purse. Products deemed to be 'clinically essential or life-saving' now may be fast-tracked, whereas those that are thought to be inessential may take twice as long to obtain approval. Many countries, such as Canada, Australia and the UK, have additional reimbursement hurdles, based on the need for cost–efficacy data. As a consequence, the choice of drug development candidate will have to reflect not only the clinical need of the patient, but also government healthcare policies in different countries. The choice of indications for a new drug is thus increasingly affected by the willingness of national healthcare systems to offer accelerated approval and reimbursement for that drug.

Scientific and technical issues

These issues relate to the *feasibility* of the project, and several aspects need to be considered:

- The scientific and technological basis on which the success of the drug discovery phase of the project will depend;
- The nature of the development and regulatory hurdles that will have to be overcome if the development phase of the project is to succeed;
- The state of the competition;
- The patent situation.

The scientific and technological basis

Evaluation of the *scientific opportunity* should be the main factor on which the decision as to whether or not to embark on a project rests once its general alignment with corporate strategy, as described above, is accepted. Some of the key elements are listed in Figure 5.1. In this context it is important to distinguish between public knowledge and proprietary knowledge, as a secure but well known scientific hypothesis or technology may provide a less attractive starting point than a shakier scientific platform based on proprietary information. Regardless of the strength of the underlying scientific hypothesis, the other items listed in Figure 5.1 – availability of targets, assays, animal models and chemical starting points – need to be evaluated carefully, as weaknesses in any of these areas are likely to block progress, or at best require significant time and resources to overcome. They are discussed more fully in Chapters 6–9.

Competition

Strictly speaking, competition in drug discovery is unimportant, as the research activities of one company do not impede those of another, except to the limited extent that patents on research tools may restrict a company's 'freedom to operate', as discussed below. What matters greatly is competition in the marketplace. Market success depends in part on being early (not necessarily first) to register a drug of a new type, but more importantly on having a product which is better. Analysis of the external competition faced by a new project therefore involves assessing the chances that it will lead to earlier registration, and/or a better product, than other companies will achieve. Making such an assessment involves long-range predictions based on fragmentary and unreliable information. The earliest solid information comes from patent applications, generally submitted around the time a compound is chosen for preclinical development, and made public soon thereafter (see Chapter 19), and from official clinical trial approvals. Companies are under no obligation to divulge information about their research projects. Information can be gleaned from gossip, publications, scientific meetings and unguarded remarks, and scientists are expected to keep their antennae well tuned to these signals – a process referred to euphemistically as 'competitive intelligence'. There are also professional agencies that specialize in obtaining commercially sensitive information and providing it to subscribers in database form. Such sources may reveal which companies are active in the area, and often which targets they are focusing on, but will rarely indicate how close they are to producing development compounds, and they are often significantly out of date.

At the drug discovery stage of a project overlap with work in other companies is a normal state of affairs and should not, per se, be a deterrent to new initiatives. The fact that 80–90% of compounds entering clinical development are unsuccessful should be borne in mind. So, a single competitor compound in early clinical development theoretically reduces the probability of our new project winning the race to registration by only 10–20%, say from about 2% to 1.7%. In practice, nervousness tends to influence us more than statistical reasoning, and there may be reluctance to start a project if several companies are working along the same lines with drug discovery projects, or if a competitor is well ahead with a compound in development. The incentive to identify novel proprietary drug targets (Chapter 6) stems as much from scientific curiosity and the excitement of breaking new ground as from the potential therapeutic benefits of the new target.

Development and regulatory hurdles

Although many of the problems encountered in developing and registering a new drug relate specifically to the compound and its properties, others are inherent to the therapeutic area and the clinical need being addressed, and can be anticipated at the outset before any candidate compound has been identified. Because development consumes a large proportion of the time and money spent on a project, likely problems need to be assessed at an early stage and taken into account in deciding whether or not to embark on the discovery phase.

The various stages of drug development and registration are described in more detail in Section 3. Here we give some examples of the kinds of issue that need to be considered in the planning phase.

- *Will the drug be given as a short course to relieve an acute illness, or indefinitely to relieve chronic symptoms or prevent recurrence?* Many anti-infective drugs come into the former category, and it is notable that development times for such drugs are much shorter than for, say, drugs used in psychiatry. The need for longer clinical trials and more exhaustive toxicity testing mainly accounts for the difference.
- *Is the intended disease indication rare or common?* Definitive trials of efficacy in rare diseases may be slow because of problems in recruiting patients. (For recognized 'orphan indications' (see Chapter 20), the clinical trials requirements may be less stringent.)
- *What clinical models and clinical end-points are available for assessing efficacy?* Testing whether a drug relieves an acute symptom, such as pain or nausea, is much simpler and quicker than, for example, testing whether it reduces the incidence of stroke or increases the life expectancy of patients with a rare cancer. Where accepted surrogate markers exist (e.g. lowering of LDL cholesterol as an indicator of cardiovascular risk, or improved bone density on X-ray as a marker of fracture risk in osteoporosis), this enables trials to be carried out more quickly and simply, but there remain many conditions where symptoms and/or life expectancy provide the only available measures of efficacy.
- *How serious is the disease, and what is the status of existing therapies?* Where no effective treatment of a condition exists, comparison of the drug with placebo will generally suffice to provide evidence of efficacy. Where standard therapies exist several comparative trials will be needed, and the new drug will have to show clear evidence of superiority before being accepted by regulatory authorities. For serious disabling or life-threatening conditions the regulatory hurdles are generally lower, and the review process is conducted more quickly.
- *What kind of product is envisaged (synthetic compound, biopharmaceutical, cell or gene-based therapy etc.), and what route of administration?* The development track and the main obstacles that are likely to be encountered depend very much on the type of product and the route of administration. With protein biopharmaceuticals, for example, toxicology is rarely a major problem, but production may be, whereas the reverse is generally true for synthetic compounds. With proteins, the route of administration is often a difficult issue, whereas with synthetic compounds the expectation is that they will be developed for oral or topical use. Cell- or gene-based products are likely to face serious safety and ethical questions before clinical trials can be started. The development of a special delivery system, such as a skin patch, nasal spray or slow-release injectable formulation, will add to the time and cost of development.

The patent situation

As described in Chapter 19, patent protection in the pharmaceutical industry relates mainly to specific chemical substances, their manufacture and their uses. Nevertheless, at the start of a project, before the drug substance has been identified, it is important to evaluate the extent to which existing patents on compounds or research tools may limit the company's 'freedom to operate' in the research phase. Existing patents on compounds of a particular class (see Chapter 19) will obviously rule out using such compounds as the starting point for a new project.

By 'research tool' is meant anything that contributes to the discovery or development of a drug, without being part of the final product. Examples include genes, cell lines, reagents, markers, assays, screening methods, animal models etc.

A company whose business it is to sell drugs is not usually interested in patenting research tools, but it is the business of many biotech companies to develop and commercialize such tools, and these companies will naturally wish to obtain patent protection for them. For pharmaceutical companies, such research tool patents and applications raise issues of freedom to operate, particularly if they contain 'reach-through' claims purporting to cover drugs found by using the patented tools.

Some scientists may believe that research activities, in contrast to manufacture and sale of a product, cannot be patent infringement. This is not the case. If I have invented a process that is useful in research and have a valid patent for it, I can enforce that patent against anyone using the process without my permission. I can make money from my patent by granting licenses for a flat fee, or a fee based on the extent to which the process is used; or by selling kits to carry out the process or reagents for use in the process (for example the enzymes used in the PCR process). What I am not entitled to do is to charge a royalty on the sale of drugs developed with the help of my process. I can patent an electric drill, but I should not expect a royalty on everything it bores a hole in!

Nevertheless, some patents have already been granted containing claims that would be infringed, for example, by the sales of a drug active in a patented assay, and although it is hoped that such claims would be held invalid if challenged in court, the risk that such claims might be enforceable cannot be dismissed.

Should research tool patents be the subject of a freedom to operate search at an early stage of project planning? Probably not. There are simply too many of them, and if no research project could be started without clearance on the basis of such a search, nothing would ever get done. At least for a large company, it is an acceptable business risk to go ahead and assume that if problems arise they can be dealt with at a later stage.

Operational issues

It might seem that it would be a straightforward management task to assess what resources are likely to be needed to carry through a project, and whether they can be made available when required. Almost invariably, however, attempts to analyse the project piece by piece, and to estimate the likely manpower and time required for each phase of the work, end up with a highly over-optimistic prediction, as they start with the assumption that everything will run smoothly according to plan: targets will be established, leads will be found and 'optimized', animal models will work as expected, and the project will most likely be successful in identifying a development compound. In practice, of course, diversionary or delaying events almost invariably occur. The gene that needs to be cloned and expressed proves difficult; obtaining an engineered cell line and devising a workable assay runs into problems; new data are pub-lished which necessitate revision of the underlying hypothesis, and possibly a switch to an alternative target; a key member of the team leaves or falls ill; or an essential piece of equipment fails to be delivered on time. However, project champions seeking management support for their ideas do their case no good if they say: 'We plan to set up this animal model and validate it within 3 months, but I have allowed 6 months just in case...'. Happy accidents do occur, of course, but unplanned events are far more likely to slow down a project than to speed it up, so the end result is almost invariably an overrun in terms of time, money and manpower.

Experienced managers understand this and make due allowance for it, but the temptation to approve more projects than the organization can actually cope with is hard for most to resist.

A final word

To summarize the key message in a sentence: The drug discovery scientist needs to be aware that many factors other than inherent scientific novelty and quality affect the decision whether or not to embark on a new project. And the subtext: The more the drug discovery scientist understands about the realities of development, patenting, registration and marketing in the pharmaceutical industry, the more effective he or she will be in adapting research plans to the company's needs, and the better at defending them.

6 Choosing the target

H P Rang

Introduction: the scope for new drug targets

The word 'target' in the context of drug discovery has several common meanings, including the market niche that the drug is intended to occupy, therapeutic indications for the drug, the biological mechanism that it will modify, the pharmacokinetic properties that it will possess, and – the definition addressed in this chapter – the molecular recognition site to which the drug will bind. For the great majority of existing drugs the target is a protein molecule, most commonly a receptor, an enzyme, a transport molecule or an ion channel, although other proteins such as tubulin and immunophilins are also represented. Some drugs, such as alkylating agents, bind to DNA, and others, such as bisphosphonates, to inorganic bone matrix constituents, but these are exceptions, and the search for new drug targets is nowadays directed mainly at finding new proteins.

Since the 1950s, when the principle of drug discovery based on identified (then pharmacological or biochemical) targets became established, the pharmaceutical industry has recognized the importance of identifying new targets as the key to successful innovation. As the industry has become more confident in its ability to invent or discover candidate molecules once the target has been defined – a confidence, some would say, based more on hubris than history – the selection of novel targets, preferably exclusive and patentable ones, has assumed increasing importance in the quest for competitive advantage.

In this chapter we look at drug targets in more detail, and discuss old and new strategies for seeking out and validating them.

How many drug targets are there?

Even when we restrict our definition to defined protein targets, counting them is not simple. An obvious starting point is to estimate the number of targets addressed by existing therapeutic drugs, but even this is difficult. For many drugs, we are ignorant of the precise molecular target. For example, several antiepileptic drugs apparently work by blocking voltage-gated sodium channels, but there are many molecular subtypes of

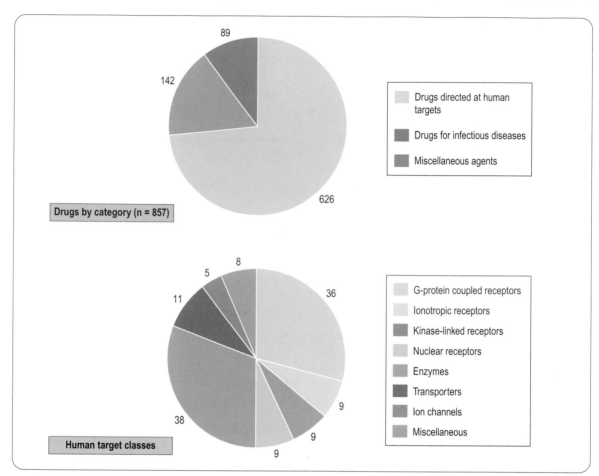

Fig. 6.1
Therapeutic drug targets.

these, and we do not know which are relevant to the therapeutic effect. Similarly, antipsychotic drugs block receptors for several amine mediators (dopamine, serotonin, norepinephrine, acetylcholine), for each of which there are several molecular subtypes expressed in the brain. Again, we cannot pinpoint the relevant one or ones that represent the critical targets.

A recent compendium of therapeutic drugs licensed in the UK and/or US (Dollery, 1999) lists a total of 857 compounds (Figure 6.1), of which 626 are directed at human targets. Of the remainder, 142 are drugs used to treat infectious diseases, and are directed mainly at targets expressed by the infecting organism, and 89 are miscellaneous agents such as vitamins, oxygen, inorganic salts, plasma substitutes etc., which are not target-directed in the conventional sense.

Drews and Ryser (1997) estimated that these drugs addressed approximately 500 distinct human targets, but this figure includes all of the molecular subtypes of the generic target (e.g. 14 serotonin receptor subtypes and seven opioid receptor subtypes, most of which are not known to be therapeutically relevant, or to be specifically targeted by existing drugs), as well as other pu-

tative targets such as calcineurin, whose therapeutic relevance is unclear. A more conservative analysis (Figure 6.1) suggests that the 626 drugs address about 125 known human targets (disregarding their molecular heterogeneity, whose therapeutic relevance is unclear). Drews and Ryser estimated that the number of potential targets might be as high as 5000–10 000. Adopting a similar but more restrictive approach, Hopkins and Groom (2002) found that 120 drug targets accounted for the activities of compounds used therapeutically, and estimated that 600–1500 'druggable' targets exist in the human genome. From an analysis of all prescribed drugs produced by the 10 largest pharmaceutical companies, Zambrowicz and Sands (2003) identified fewer than 100 targets; when this analysis was restricted to the 100 best-selling drugs on the market, the number of targets was only 43, reflecting the fact that more than half of the successful targets (i.e. those leading to therapeutically effective and safe drugs) failed to achieve a significant commercial impact. Their analysis also revealed that during the 1990s only two or three new targets were exploited by the 30 or so new drugs registered each year, most of which addressed targets that were already well known. The small target base of existing drugs, and the low rate of emergence of new targets, suggests that the number yet to be discovered may be considerably smaller than some optimistic forecasters have predicted. Based on an analysis of gene deletion mutations in transgenic mice, Zambrowicz and Sands (2003) estimate that 100–150 high-quality targets in the human genome may remain to be discovered, roughly doubling the number currently represented in the pharmacopoeia. In the earlier analysis by Drews and Ryser (1997), about one-quarter of the targets identified were associated with drugs used to treat infectious diseases, and belonged to the parasite, rather than the human, genome. Their number is even harder to estimate. Most anti-infective drugs have come from natural products, reflecting the fact that organisms in the natural world have faced strong evolutionary pressure, operating over millions of years, to develop protection against parasites. It is likely, therefore, that the 'druggable genome' of parasitic microorganisms has already been heavily trawled – more so than that of humans, in whom many of the diseases of current concern are too recent for evolutionary countermeasures to have developed.

In summary, estimates of the number of useful drug targets that remain to be discovered are highly speculative. The fact that, over the last decade, roughly three new targets have emerged each year as a basis for 'first-in-class' drugs (Zambrowicz and Sands, 2003), whereas the previous century of drug discovery revealed about 120 targets, suggests that adequate scope remains.

The nature of existing drug targets

The human targets of the 626 drugs, where they are known, are summarized in Figure 6.1. Of the 125 known targets, the largest groups are enzymes and G-protein-coupled receptors, each accounting for about 30%, the remainder being transporters, other receptor classes, and ion channels. This analysis gives only a crude idea of present-day therapeutics, and underestimates the number of molecular targets currently addressed, since it fails to take into account the many subtypes of these targets that have been identified by molecular cloning. In most cases we do not know which particular subtypes are responsible for the therapeutic effect, and the number of distinct targets will certainly increase as these details become known. Also there are many drugs whose targets we do not yet know. There is a growing number of examples where drug targets consist, not of a single protein, but of an oligomeric assembly of different proteins. This is well established for ion channels, most of which are hetero-oligomers, and recent studies show that G-protein-coupled receptors (GPCRs) may form functional dimers (Bouvier, 2001) or may associate with accessory proteins known as RAMPs (McLatchie

et al., 1998; Morphis et al., 2003), which strongly influence their pharmacological characteristics. The human genome is thought to contain about 1000 genes in the GPCR family, of which about one-third could be odorant receptors. Excluding the latter, and without taking into account the possible diversity factors mentioned, the 40 or so GPCR targets for existing drugs represent only about 10% of those cloned so far, and perhaps about 6% of the total. Roughly one-third of cloned GPCRs are classed as 'orphan' receptors, for which no endogenous ligand has yet been identified, and these could certainly emerge as attractive drug targets when more is known about their physiological role. Broadly similar conclusions apply to other major classes of drug target, such as nuclear receptors, ion channels and kinases.

The above discussion relates to drug targets expressed by human cells, and similar arguments apply to those of infective organisms. The therapy of infectious diseases, ranging from viruses to multicellular parasites, is one of medicine's greatest challenges. Current antibacterial drugs – the largest class – originate mainly from natural products (with a few, e.g. sulfonamides and oxazolidinediones, coming from synthetic compounds) first identified through screening on bacterial cultures, and analysis of their biochemical mechanism and site of action came later. In many cases this knowledge remains incomplete, and the molecular targets are still unclear. Since the pioneering work of Hitchings and Elion (see Chapter 1), the strategy of target-directed drug discovery has rarely been applied in this field[1]; instead, the 'antibiotic' approach, originating with the discovery of penicillin, has held sway. For the 142 current anti-infective drugs (Figure 6.1), which include antiviral and antiparasitic as well as antibacterial drugs, we can identify approximately 40 targets (mainly enzymes and structural proteins) at the biochemical level, only about half of which have been cloned. The urgent need for drugs that act on new targets arises because of the major problem of drug resistance, with which the traditional chemistry-led strategies are failing to keep up. Consequently, as with other therapeutic classes, genomic technologies are being increasingly applied to the problem of finding new antimicrobial drug targets (Rosamond and Allsop, 2000; Buysse, 2001). In some ways the problem appears simpler than finding human drug targets. Microbial genomes are being sequenced at a high rate, and identifying prokaryotic genes

---

[1]A notable exception is the recent discovery (Wengelnik et al., 2002) of a new class of antimalarial drug designed on biochemical principles to interfere with choline metabolism, which is essential for membrane synthesis during the multiplicatory phase of the malaria organism within the host's red blood cells. Hitchings and Elion would have approved.

that are essential for survival, replication or pathogenicity is generally easier than identifying genes that are involved in specific regulatory mechanisms in eukaryotes.

Conventional strategies for finding new drug targets

Two main routes have been followed so far:

- Analysis of pathophysiology
- Analysis of mechanism of action of existing therapeutic drugs.

There are numerous examples where the elucidation of pathophysiological pathways has pointed to the existence of novel targets that have subsequently resulted in successful drugs, and this strategy is still adopted by most pharmaceutical companies. To many scientists it seems the safe and logical way to proceed – first understand the pathway leading from the primary disturbance to the appearance of the disease phenotype, then identify particular biochemical steps amenable to therapeutic intervention, then select key molecules as targets. The pioneers in developing this approach were undoubtedly Hitchings and Elion (see Chapter 1), who unravelled the

steps in purine and pyrimidine biosynthesis and selected the enzyme dihydrofolate reductase as a suitable target. This biochemical approach led to a remarkable series of therapeutic breakthroughs in antibacterial, anticancer and immunosuppressant drugs. The work of Black and his colleagues, based on mediators and receptors, also described in Chapter 1, was another early and highly successful example of this approach, and there have been many others (Table 6.1a). In some cases the target has emerged from pharmacological rather than pathophysiological studies. The 5HT$_3$ receptor was identified from pharmacological studies and chosen as a potential drug target for the development of antagonists, but its role in pathophysiology was at the time far from clear. Eventually animal and clinical studies revealed the antiemetic effect of drugs such as *ondansetron*, and such drugs were developed mainly to control the nausea and vomiting associated with cancer chemotherapy. Similarly, the GABA$_B$ receptor (target for relaxant drugs such as *baclofen*) was discovered by analysis of the pharmacological effects of GABA, and only later exploited therapeutically to treat muscle spasm.

The identification of drug targets by the 'backwards' approach – involving analysis of the mechanism of action of empirically discovered therapeutic agents – has produced some major breakthroughs in the past (see examples in Table 6.1b). Its relevance is likely to decline

Table 6.1
Examples of drug targets identified, (a) by analysis of pathophysiology, and (b) by analysis of existing drugs

(a) Targets identified via pathophysiology

Disease indication	Target identified	Drugs developed
AIDS	Reverse transcriptase HIV protease	Zidovudine Saquinavir
Asthma	Cysteinyl leukotriene receptor	Zafirlukast
Bacterial infections	Dihydrofolate reductase	Trimethoprim
Malignant disease	Dihydrofolate reductase	6-mercaptopurine Methotrexate
Depression	5HT transporter	Fluoxetine
Hypertension	Angiotensin-converting enzyme Type 4 phosphodiesterase Angiotensin-2 receptor	Captopril Sildenafil Losartan
Inflammatory disease	COX-2	Celecoxib
Alzheimer's disease	Acetylcholinesterase	Donepezil
Breast cancer	Oestrogen receptor	Tamoxifen Herceptin
Chronic myeloid leukemia	Abl-kinase	Imatinib
Parkinson's disease	Dopamine synthesis MAO-B	Levodopa Selegiline
Depression	MAO-A	Moclobemide

Table 6.1 (b) Targets identified via drug effects

Drug	Disease	Target
Benzodiazepines	Anxiety, sleep disorders	BDZ binding site on $GABA_A$ receptor
Aspirin-like drugs	Inflammation, pain	COX enzymes
Ciclosporin, FK506	Transplant rejection	Immunophilins
Vinca alkaloids	Cancers	Tubulin
Dihydropyridines	Cardiovascular disease	L-type calcium channels
Sulfonylureas	Diabetes	K_{ATP} channels
Classic antipsychotic drugs	Schizophrenia	Dopamine D_2 receptor
Tricyclic antidepressants	Depression	Monoamine transporters
Fibrates	Raised blood cholesterol	$PPAR\alpha$

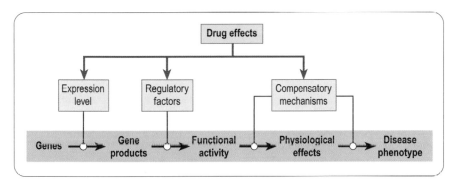

Fig. 6.2
Drug effects in relation to disease aetiology.

as drug discovery becomes more target focused, though natural product pharmacology will probably continue to reveal novel drug targets.

It is worth reminding ourselves that there remain several important drug classes whose mechanism of action we still do not understand in detail (e.g. acetaminophen (paracetamol)[2], gabapentin, valproate). Whether their targets remain elusive because their effects depend on a cocktail of interactions at several different sites, or whether novel targets will emerge for such drugs, remains uncertain.

---

[2]Recently, COX-3, a novel splice variant of cyclooxygenase-1, has been identified as the likely target underlying the analgesic action of acetaminophen (Chandrasekharan et al., 2002), spurring several companies to set up screens for new acetaminophen-like drugs.

New strategies for identifying drug targets

Figure 6.2 summarizes the main points at which drugs may intervene along the pathway from genotype to phenotype, namely by altering gene expression, by altering the functional activity of gene products, or by activating compensatory mechanisms. This is of course an oversimplification, as changes in gene expression or the activation of compensatory mechanisms are themselves indirect effects, following pathways similar to that represented by the primary track in Figure 6.2. Nevertheless, it provides a useful framework for discussing some of the newer genomics-based approaches. A useful account of the various genetic models that have been developed in different organisms for the identification of new drug targets, and elucidating the mechanisms of action of existing drugs, is given by Carroll and Fitzgerald (2003).

Trawling the genome

The conventional route to new drug targets, starting from pathophysiology, will undoubtedly remain as a standard approach. Understanding of the disease mechanisms in the major areas of therapeutic challenge, such as Alzheimer's disease, atherosclerosis, cancer, stroke, obesity etc., is advancing rapidly, and new targets are continually emerging. But this is generally slow, painstaking, hypothesis-driven work, and there is a strong incentive to seek shortcuts based on the use of new technologies to select and validate novel targets, starting from the genome. In principle, it is argued, nearly all drug targets are proteins, and are therefore represented in the proteome, and also as corresponding genes in the genome. There are, however, some significant caveats, the main ones being:

- Splice variants may result in more than one pharmacologically distinct type of receptor being encoded in a single gene. These are generally predictable from the genome, and represented as distinct species in the transcriptome and proteome.
- There are many examples of multimeric receptors, made up of non-identical subunits encoded by different genes. This is true of the majority of ligand-gated ion channels, whose pharmacological characteristics depend critically on the subunit composition (Hille, 2001). Recent work also shows that G-protein-coupled receptors often exist as heteromeric dimers, with pharmacological properties distinct from those of the individual units (Bouvier, 2001). Moreover, association between receptors and non-receptor proteins can determine the pharmacological characteristics of certain G-protein-coupled receptors (McLatchie et al., 1998).

Despite these complications, studies based on the appealingly simple dogma:

one gene → one protein → one drug target

have been extremely productive in advancing our knowledge of receptors and other drug targets in recent years, and it is expected that genome trawling will reveal more 'single-protein' targets, even though multiunit complexes are likely to escape detection by this approach.

How might potential drug targets be recognized among the 30 000 or so genes in the human genome?

Several approaches have been described for homing in on genes that may encode novel drug targets, starting with the identification of certain gene categories:

- 'Disease genes', i.e. genes, mutations of which cause or predispose to the development of human disease.
- 'Disease-modifying' genes. These comprise (a) genes whose altered expression is thought to be involved in the development of the disease state; and (b) genes that encode functional proteins, whose activity is altered (even if their expression level is not) in the disease state, and which play a part in inducing the disease state.
- 'Druggable genes', i.e. genes encoding proteins likely to possess binding domains that recognize drug-like small molecules. Included in this group are genes encoding targets for existing therapeutic and experimental drugs. These genes and their paralogues (i.e. closely related but non-identical genes occurring elsewhere in the genome) comprise the group of druggable genes.

On this basis (Hopkins and Groom, 2002), novel targets are represented by the intersection of disease-modifying and druggable gene classes, excluding those already targeted by therapeutic drugs. Next, we consider these categories in more detail.

Disease genes

The identification of genes in which mutations are associated with particular diseases has a long history in medicine (Weatherall, 1991), starting with the concept of 'inborn errors of metabolism' such as phenylketonuria. The strategies used to identify disease-associated genes, described in Chapter 7, have been very successful. Examples of common diseases associated with mutations of a single gene are summarized in Table 7.3. There are many more examples of rare inherited disorders of this type. Information of this kind, important though it is for the diagnosis, management and counselling of these patients, has so far had little impact on the selection of drug targets. None of the gene products identified appears to be directly 'targetable'. Much more common than single-gene disorders are conditions such as diabetes, hypertension, schizophrenia, bipolar depressive illness and many cancers, in which there is a clear genetic component, but, together with environmental factors, several different genes contribute as risk factors for the appearance of the disease phenotype. The methods for identifying the particular genes involved (see Chapter 7) were until recently difficult and laborious, but are becoming much easier as the sequencing and annotation of the human genome progresses. The Human Genome Consortium (2001) found 971 'disease genes' already listed in public databases, and identified 286 paralogues of these in the sequenced genome.

The value of information about disease genes in better understanding the pathophysiology is unquestionable, but how useful is it as a pointer to novel drug targets? Many years after being identified, the genes involved in several important single-gene disorders, such as thalassaemia, muscular dystrophy and cystic fibrosis, have not so far proved useful as drug targets. On the other hand, the example of Abl-kinase, the molecular target for the recently introduced anticancer drug *imatinib (Gleevec*; see Chapter 4*)*, shows that the proteins encoded by mutated genes can themselves constitute drug targets, but so far there are few instances where this has proved successful. The finding that rare forms of familial Alzheimer's disease were associated with mutations in the gene encoding the amyloid precursor protein (APP) or the secretase enzyme responsible for formation of the β-amyloid fragment present in amyloid plaques, were strong pointers that confirmed the validity of secretase as a drug target (although it had already been singled out on the basis of biochemical studies). Secretase inhibitors reached late-stage clinical development as potential anti-Alzheimer's drugs in 2001. Similar approaches have been successful in identifying disease-associated genes in defined subgroups of patients with conditions such as diabetes, hypertension and hypercholesterolaemia, and there is reason to hope that novel drug targets will emerge in these areas. However, in other fields, such as schizophrenia and asthma, progress in pinning down disease-related genes has been very limited. The most promising field for identifying novel drug targets among disease-associated mutations is likely to be in cancer therapies, as mutations are the basic cause of malignant transformation. In general, one can say that identifying disease genes may provide valuable pointers to possible drug targets further down the pathophysiological pathway, even though their immediate gene products will rarely be targetable. The identification of a new disease gene often hits the popular headlines on the basis that an effective therapy will quickly follow, though this rarely happens, and never quickly.

In summary, the class of disease genes does not seem to include many drug targets.

Disease-modifying genes

In this class lie many non-mutated genes that are directly involved in the pathophysiological pathway leading to the disease phenotype. The phenotype may be associated with over- or underexpression of the genes, detectable by expression profiling (see below), or by the over- or underactivity of the gene product – for example, an enzyme – independently of changes in its expression level.

This is the most important category in relation to drug targets, as therapeutic drug action generally occurs by changing the activity of functional proteins, whether or not the disease alters their expression level. Finding new ones, however, is not easy, and there is as yet no shortcut screening strategy for locating them in the genome.

Two main approaches are currently being used, namely gene expression profiling and comprehensive gene knockout studies.

Gene expression profiling

The principle underlying gene expression profiling as a guide to new drug targets is that the development of any disease phenotype necessarily involves changes in gene expression in the cells and tissues involved. Long-term changes in the structure or function of cells cannot occur without altered gene expression, and so a catalogue of all the genes whose expression is up- or down-regulated in the disease state will include genes where such regulation is actually required for the development of the disease phenotype. As well as these 'critical path' genes, which may represent potential drug targets, others are likely to be affected as genes involved in sec-

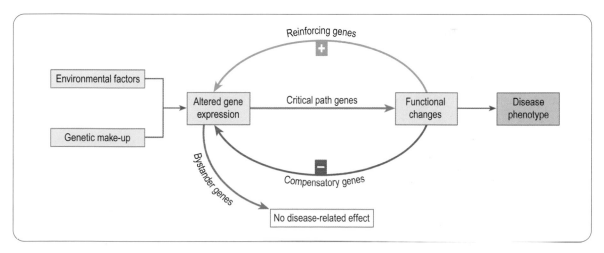

Fig. 6.3
Gene expression in disease.

ondary reinforcing of compensatory mechanisms following the development of the disease phenotype (which may also represent potential drug targets), but many will be irrelevant 'bystander genes' (Figure 6.3). The important problem, to which there is no simple answer, is how to eliminate the bystanders, and how to identify potential drug targets among the rest. Zanders (2000), in a thoughtful review, emphasizes the importance of focusing on signal transduction pathways as the most likely source of novel targets identifiable by gene expression profiling.

The methods available for gene expression profiling are described in Chapter 7. DNA microarrays ('gene chips') are most commonly used, their advantage being that they are quick and easy to use. They have the disadvantage that the DNA sequences screened are selected in advance, but this is becoming less of a limitation as more genomic information accumulates. They also have limited sensitivity, which (see Chapter 7) means that genes expressed at low levels – including, possibly, a significant proportion of potential drug targets – can be missed. Methods based on the polymerase chain reaction (PCR), such as serial analysis of gene expression (SAGE; Velculescu et al., 1995), are, in principle, capable of detecting all transcribed RNAs without preselection, with higher sensitivity than microarrays, but are more laborious and technically demanding. Both technologies produce the same kind of data, namely a list of genes whose expression is significantly altered as a result of a defined experimental intervention. A large body of gene expression data has been collected over the last few years, showing the effects of many kinds of disturbance, including human disease, animal models of disease and drug effects, some examples being listed in Table 6.2. In most cases, several thousand genes have been probed with microarrays, covering perhaps 20% of the entire genome, so the coverage is by no means complete. Commonly, it is found that some 2–10% of the genes studied show significant changes in response to such disturbances. Thus, assuming a total of 25–35 000 genes in man, with perhaps 20% expressed in a given tissue, we can expect several hundred to be affected in a typical disease state. Much effort has gone into (a) methods of analysis and pattern recognition within these large data sets, and (b) defining the principles for identifying possible drug targets within such a group of regulated genes. Techniques for analysis and pattern recognition fall within the field of bioinformatics (Chapter 7), and the specific problem of analysing transcription data is discussed by Quackenbush (2001) and Butte (2002). Because altered mRNA levels do not always correlate with changes in protein expression, protein changes should be confirmed independently where possible. This normally entails the production and validation of an antibody-based assay or staining procedure.

Identifying potential drug targets among the array of differentially expressed genes that are revealed by ex-pression profiling is neither straightforward nor exact. Possible approaches are:

- On the basis of prior biological knowledge, genes that might plausibly be critical in the pathogenesis of the disease can be distinguished from those (e.g. housekeeping genes, or genes involved in intermediary metabolism) that are unlikely to be critical. This, the plausibility criterion, is in practice the most important factor in identifying likely drug targets. As genomic analysis proceeds, it is becoming possible to group genes into functional classes, e.g. tissue growth and repair, inflammation, myelin formation, neurotransmission, etc. and changes in expression are often concentrated in one or more of these functional groups, giving a useful pointer to the biological pathways involved in pathogenesis.
- Anatomical studies can be used to identify whether candidate genes are regulated in the cells and tissues affected by the disease.
- Timecourse measurements reveal the relationship between gene expression changes and the development of the disease phenotype. With many acute interventions, several distinct temporal patterns are detectable in the expression of different genes. 'Clustering' algorithms (see Chapter 7; Quackenbush, 2001) are useful to identify genes which are co-regulated and whose function might point to a particular biochemical or signalling pathway relevant to the pathogenesis.
- The study of several different clinical and animal models with similar disease phenotypes can reveal genes whose expression is consistently affected and hence representative of the phenotype.
- The effects of drug or other treatments can be studied in order to reveal genes whose expression is normalized in parallel with the 'therapeutic' effect.

Gene knockout screening

Another screening approach for identifying potential drug target genes is based on generating transgenic 'gene knockout' strains of mice, as performed by biotechnology company Lexicon Genetics (Walke et al., 2001; Zambrowicz and Sands, 2003), who are aiming to study 5000 genes within 5 years. The 5000 genes are selected on several criteria, including existing evidence of association with disease and membership of families of known drug targets (GPCRs, transporters, kinases etc.). The group has developed an efficient procedure for generating transgenic knockout mice, and a standardized set of tests to detect phenotypic effects relevant to a range of disease states. In a recent review, Zambrowicz and Sands (2003) present many examples where the effects of gene knockouts in mice produce effects consistent with the known actions and side effects of therapeutic drugs. For example, inactivation of the genes for angiotensin con-

Table 6.2
Examples of gene expression profiling studies, showing numbers of mRNAs affected under various conditions

Test system	Method	Number of genes analysed	Number of genes affected (threshold)	Number up	Number down	Ref
Activated vs quiescent human fibroblasts	Microarray	8600	517 (2.2-fold)) (Some genes showed both up- and down regulation at different times)	148	242	Iyer V R et al (1999) Science 283: 83–87
Differentiated vs undifferentiated mouse neural stem cells	Microarray	8700	156 (twofold)	94	62	Somogyi R (1999) Pharma Informatics Trends Supplement 17—24
Small diameter vs large diameter rat sensory neurons	Microarray	477	40 (1.5-fold)	26	14	Luo L et al. (1999) Nature Medicine 5: 117–122
Ischaemic vs control rat brain	Microarray	1179	20 (1.8-fold)	6	14	Keyvani K et al. (2002) J Cerebral Blood Flow Metab. 22: 153–160
Inflamed vs normal mouse lung	Microarray	6000	470 (twofold) (Many genes showed both up- and down regulation at different times)			Kaminski N et al. (2000) Proc Nat Acad Sci USA 97: 1778–1783
Old vs young mouse brain (cortex)	Microarray	6347	110 (1.7-fold)	63	47	Lee C-K et al. (2000) Nature Genetics 25: 294–297
Old vs young mouse skeletal muscle	Microarray	6300	113 (twofold)	58	55	Lee C-K et al. (1999) Science 285: 1390–1393
Human colorectal cancer vs normal tissue	SAGE	~49 000	289 (difference significant at $p < 0.01$)	108	181	Zhang L et al. (1997) Science 276: 1268–1272
Human MS plaques vs normal brain	Microarray	>5000	(~twofold)	29	ND	Whitney L W et al. (1999) Ann Neurol 46: 425–428
Human ovarian cancer vs normal ovary	Microarray	5766	726 (threefold)	295	431	Wang K et al. (1999) Gene 229: 101–108
Human Alzheimer's disease plaques vs non-plaque regions	Microarray	6800	18 (1.8-fold)	–	18	Ho L et al. (2001) Neuroscience Letters 298: 191–194
Mouse liver, thyroid treated vs hypothyroid	Microarray	2225	55 (twofold)	14	41	Feng X et al. (2000) Mol Endocrinol 14: 947–955
Mouse, hypertophied vs normal heart muscle	Microarray	>4000	47 (~1.8-fold)	21	26	Friddle C J (2000) Proc Natl Acad Sci USA 97: 5745–5750
Human post-mortem prefrontal cortex, schizophrenia vs control	Microarray	~7000	179 (1.9-fold)	97	82	Mimic K et al. (2000) Neuron 28: 53–67

Table 6.2
Examples of gene expression profiling studies, showing numbers of mRNAs affected under various conditions—cont'd

Test system	Method	Number of genes analysed	Number of genes affected (threshold)	Number up	Number down	Ref
Human post-mortem prefrontal cortex, schizophrenia vs control	Microarray	~6000	88 (1.4-fold)	71	17	Hakak Y et al. (2001) Proc Natn Acad Sci 98: 4746–4751
Single neurons from human post-mortem entorhinal cortex, schizophrenia vs control	Microarray	>18 000	4139 (2-fold)	1574	1565	Hemby S E el al. (2002) Arch Gen Psychiat 59: 631–640

verting enzyme (ACE) or the angiotensin receptor results in lowering of blood pressure, reflecting the clinical effect of drugs acting on these targets. Similarly, elimination of the gene encoding one of the subunits of the $GABA_A$ receptor produces a state of irritability and hyperactivity in mice, the opposite of the effect of benzodiazepine tranquillizers, which enhance $GABA_A$ receptor function. However, using transgenic gene knockout technology (sometimes dubbed 'reverse genetics') to confirm the validity of previously well established drug targets is not the same as using it to discover new targets. Success in the latter context will depend greatly on the ability of the phenotypic tests that are applied to detect therapeutically relevant changes in the knockout strains. Some new targets have already been identified in this way, and deployed in drug discovery programmes; they include *cathepsin K*, a protease involved in the genesis of osteoporosis, and *melanocortin receptors*, which may play a role in obesity. The Lexicon group has developed a systems-based panel of primary screens to look for relevant effects on the main physiological systems (cardiovascular, CNS, immune system etc.). On the basis of their experience with the first 750 of the planned 5000 gene knockouts, they predict that about 100 new high-quality targets could be revealed in this way. Programmes such as this, based on mouse models, are time-consuming and costly, but have the great advantage that mouse physiology is fairly similar to human. The use of species such as flatworm (*C. elegans)* and zebrafish (*Danio rerio*) is being explored as a means of speeding up the process (Shin and Fishman, 2002).

'Druggable' genes

For a gene product to serve as a drug target, it must possess a recognition site capable of binding small molecules. Hopkins and Groom (2002) found a total of 399 protein targets for registered and experimental drug molecules. The 399 targets belong to 130 distinct protein families, and the authors suggest that other members of these families – a total of 3051 proteins – are also likely to possess similar binding domains, even though specific ligands have not yet been described, and propose that this total represents the current limit of the druggable genome. Of course, it is likely that new targets, belonging to different protein families, will emerge in the future, so this number may well expand. 'Druggable' in this context implies only that the protein is likely to possess a binding site for a small molecule, irrespective of whether such an interaction is likely be of any therapeutic value. To be useful as a starting point for drug discovery, a potential target needs to combine 'druggability' with disease-modifying properties.

Target validation

The techniques discussed so far are aimed at identifying potential drug targets within the diversity warehouse represented by the genome, the key word being 'potential'.

Few companies will be willing to invest the considerable resources needed to mount a target-directed drug discovery project without more direct evidence that the target is an appropriate one for the disease indication. Target validation refers to the experimental approaches by which a potential drug target can be tested and given further credibility. It is an open-ended term, which can be taken to embrace virtually the whole of biology, but for practical purposes the main approaches are *pharmacological* and *genetic*.

Although these experimental approaches can go a long way towards supporting the validity of a chosen target, the ultimate test is in the clinic, where efficacy is or is not confirmed. Lack of clinical efficacy causes the abandonment of roughly one-third of drugs in Phase II, reflecting the unreliability of the earlier surrogate evidence for target validity.

Pharmacological approaches

The underlying question to be addressed is whether drugs that influence the potential drug target actually produce the expected effects on cells, tissues or whole animals. Where a known receptor, for example the metabotropic glutamate receptor (mGluR), was identified as a potential target for a new indication (e.g. pain) its validity could be tested by measuring the analgesic effect of known mGluR antagonists in relevant animal models. For novel targets, of course, no panel of active compounds will normally be available, and so it will be necessary to set up a screening assay to identify them. Where a company is already active in a particular line of research – as was the case with Ciba Geigy in the kinase field – it may be straightforward to refine its assay methods in order to identify selective inhibitors. Ciba Geigy was able to identify active Abl-kinase inhibitors within its existing compound collection, and hence to show that these were effective in cell proliferation assays.

A variant of the pharmacological approach is to use antibodies raised against the putative target protein, rather than small-molecule inhibitors.

Many experts predict that, as high-throughput screening and combinatorial chemistry develop (see Chapters 8 and 9), allowing the rapid identification of families of selective compounds, these technologies will be increasingly used as tools for target validation, in parallel with lead finding. 'Hits' from screening that show a reasonable degree of target selectivity, whether or not they represent viable lead compounds, can be used in pharmacological studies designed to test their efficacy in a selection of in vitro and in vivo models. Showing that such prototype compounds, regardless of their suitability as leads, do in fact produce the desired effect greatly strengthens the argument for target validity. Although contemporary examples are generally shrouded in confidentiality, it is clear that this approach is becoming more common, so that target validation and lead finding are carried out simultaneously.

Genetic approaches

These approaches involve various techniques for suppressing the expression of specific genes to determine whether they are critical to the disease process. This can be done acutely in genetically normal cells or animals by the use of antisense oligonucleotides or RNA interference, or constitutively by generating transgenic animals in which the genes of interest are either overactive or suppressed.

Antisense oligonucleotides

Antisense oligonucleotides (Phillips, 2000; Dean, 2001) are stretches of RNA complementary to the gene of interest, which bind to cellular mRNA and prevent its translation. In principle this allows the expression of specific genes to be inhibited, so that their role in the development of a disease phenotype can be determined. Although simple in principle, the technology is subject to many pitfalls and artefacts in practice, and attempts to use it, without very careful controls, to assess genes as potential drug targets are likely to give misleading results. As an alternative to using synthetic oligonucleotides, antisense sequences can be introduced into cells by genetic engineering. Examples where this approach has been used to validate putative drug targets include a range of recent studies on the novel cell surface receptor uPAR (urokinase plasminogen-activator receptor; see review by Wang, 2001). This receptor is expressed by certain malignant tumour cells, particularly gliomas, and antisense studies have shown it to be important in controlling the tendency of these tumours to metastasize, and therefore to be a potential drug target. In a different field, antisense studies have supported the role of a recently cloned sodium channel subtype, PN3 (Porreca et al., 1999) and of the metabotropic glutamate receptor mGluR1 (Fundytus et al., 2001) in the pathogenesis of neuropathic pain in animal models. Antisense oligonucleotides have the advantage that their effects on gene expression are acute and reversible, and so mimic drug effects more closely than, for example, the changes seen in transgenic animals (see below), where in most cases the genetic disturbance is present throughout life. It is likely that, as more experience is gained, antisense methods based on synthetic oligonucleotides will play an increasingly important role in drug target validation.

RNA interference (RNAi)

This technique depends on the fact that short lengths of double-stranded RNA (*short interfering RNAs, or siRNAs*) activate a sequence-specific *RNA-induced silencing complex (RISC)*, which destroys by cleavage the corresponding functional mRNA within the cell (Hannon, 2000; Kim, 2003). Thus specific mRNAs or whole gene families can be inactivated by choosing appropriate siRNA sequences. Gene silencing by this method is highly efficient, particularly in invertebrates such as *Caenorhabditis elegans* and *Drosophila*, and can also be used in mammalian cells and whole animals. Its use for studying gene function and validating potential drug targets is increasing rapidly, and it also has potential for therapeutic applications.

Transgenic animals

The use of the gene knockout principle as a screening approach to identify new targets is described above. The same technology is also valuable, and increasingly being used, as a means of validating putative targets. In principle, deletion or overexpression of a specific gene in vivo can provide a direct test of whether or not it plays a role in the sequence of events that gives rise to a disease phenotype. The generation of transgenic animal – mainly mouse – strains is, however, a demanding and time-consuming process (Houdebine, 1997; Jackson and Abbott, 2000). Therefore, although this technology has an increasingly important role to play in the later stages of drug discovery and development, it is currently too cumbersome to be used routinely at the stage of target selection, though Harris and Foord (2000) predict that high-throughput 'transgenic factories' may soon come to be used in this way. One problem relates to the genetic background of the transgenic colony. It is well known that different mouse strains differ in many significant ways, for example in their behaviour, susceptibility to tumour development, body weight etc. For technical reasons, the strain into which the transgene is introduced is normally different from that used to establish the breeding colony, so a protocol of back-crossing the transgenic 'founders' into the breeding strain has to proceed for several generations before a genetically homogeneous transgenic colony is obtained. Limited by the breeding cycle of mice, this normally takes about 2 years. It is mainly for this reason that the generation of transgenic animals for the purposes of target validation is not usually included as a stage on the critical path of the project. Sometimes, studies on transgenic animals tip the balance of opinion in such a way as to encourage work on a novel drug target. For example, the vanilloid receptor, TRPV1, which is expressed by nociceptive sensory neurons, was confirmed as a potential drug target when the knockout mouse proved to have a marked deficit in the development of inflammatory hyperalgesia (Davis et al., 2000), thereby confirming the likely involvement of this receptor in a significant clinical condition. Most target-directed projects, however, start on the basis of other evidence for (or simply faith in) the relevance of the target, and work on developing transgenic animals begins at the same time, in anticipation of a need for them later in the project. In many cases, transgenic animals have provided the most useful (sometimes the only available) disease models for drug testing in vivo. Thus, cancer models based on deletion of the p53 tumour suppressor gene are widely used, as are atherosclerosis models based on deletion of the ApoE or LDL-receptor genes. Alzheimer's disease models involving mutation of the gene for amyloid precursor protein, or the presenilin genes, have also proved extremely valuable, as there was hitherto no model that replicated the amyloid deposits typical of this disease. In summary, transgenic animal models are often helpful for post hoc target validation, but their main – and increasing – use in drug discovery comes at later stages of the project (see Chapter 11).

Summary and conclusions

In the present drug discovery environment most projects begin with the identification of a molecular target, usually one that can be incorporated into a high-throughput screening assay. Drugs currently in therapeutic use cover about 100–120 distinct human molecular targets, and the great majority of new compounds registered in the last decade are directed at targets that were already well known; on average, about three novel targets are covered by drugs registered each year. The discovery and exploitation of new targets is considered essential for therapeutic progress and commercial success in the long term. Estimates from genome sequence data of the number of potential drug targets, defined by disease relevance and 'druggability', suggest that from about 100 to several thousand 'druggable' new targets remain to be discovered. The uncertainty reflects two main problems: the difficulty of recognizing 'druggability' in gene sequence data, and the difficulty of determining the relevance of a particular gene product in the development of a disease phenotype. Much effort is currently being applied to these problems, often taking the form of new 'omic' disciplines whose role and status are not yet defined. Proteomics and structural genomics are expected to improve our ability to distinguish druggable proteins from the rest, and 'transcriptomics' (another name for gene expression profiling) and the study of transgenic animals will throw light on gene function, thus improving our ability to recognize the disease-modifying mechanisms wherein novel drug targets are expected to reside.

References

Bouvier M (2001) Oligomerization of G-protein-coupled transmitter receptors. Nature Reviews Neuroscience 2: 274–286.

Butte A (2002) The use and analysis of microarray data. Nature Reviews Drug Discovery 1: 951–960.

Buysse J M (2001) The role of genomics in antibacterial drug discovery. Current Medicinal Chemistry 8: 1713–1726.

Carroll P M, Fitzgerald K (eds) (2003) Model organisms in drug discovery. Chichester: John Wiley.

Chandrasekharan NV, Dai H, Roos KL et al. (2002) COX-3, a cyclooxygenase-1 variant inhibited by acetaminophen and other analgesic/antipyretic drugs: cloning, structure, and expression. Proceeding of the National Academy of Sciences 99: 13926–13931.

Davis JB, Gray J, Gunthorpe MJ et al. (2000) Vanilloid receptor-1 is essential for inflammatory thermal hyperalgesia. Nature 405: 183–187.

Dean NM (2001) Functional genomics and target validation approaches using antisense oligonucleotide technology. Current Opinion in Biotechnology 12: 622–625.

Dollery C T (ed) (1999) Therapeutic drugs. Edinburgh: Churchill Livingstone.

Drews J, Ryser S (1997) Classic drug targets. Nature Biotechnology 15: 1318–1319.

Fundytus M E, Yashpal K, Chabot JG et al. (2001) Knockdown of spinal metabotropic receptor 1 (mGluR1) alleviates pain and restores opioid efficacy after nerve injury in rats. British Journal of Pharmacology 132: 354–367.

Hannon G J (2000) RNA interference. Nature 418: 244–251.

Harris S, Foord SM. (2000) Transgenic gene knock-outs: functional genomics and therapeutic target selection. Pharmacogenomics 1: 433–443

Hille B (2001) Ion channels of excitable membranes, 3rd edn. Sunderland, Mass: Sinauer.

Hopkins AL, Groom CR (2002) The druggable genome. Nature Reviews Drug Discovery 1: 727–730.

Houdebine L M (1997) Transgenic animals – generation and use. Amsterdam: Harwood Academic.

Jackson I J, Abbott C M (2000) Mouse genetics and transgenics. Oxford: Oxford University Press.

Kim V N (2003) RNA interference in functional genomics and medicine. Journal of Korean Medical Science 18: 309–318

McLatchie L M, Fraser N J, Main M J et al. (1998) RAMPs regulate the transport and ligand specificity of the calcitonin-receptor-like receptor. Nature 393: 333–339.

Morphis M, Christopoulos A, Sexton P M (2003) RAMPs: 5 years on, where to now? Trends in Pharmacological Sciences 24: 596–601.

Phillips M I (2000) Antisense technology, Parts A and B. San Diego: Academic Press.

Porreca F, Lai J, Bian D et al. (1999) A comparison of the potential role of the tetrodotoxin-insensitive sodium channels, PN3/SNS and NaN/SNS2, in rat models of chronic pain. Proceedings of the National Academy of Sciences of the USA 96: 7640–7644.

Quackenbush J (2001) Computational analysis of microarray data. Nature Reviews Genetics 2: 418–427.

Rosamond J, Allsop A (2000) Harnessing the power of the genome in the search for new antibiotics. Science 287: 1973–1976.

Shin JT, Fishman MC (2002) From zebrafish to human: molecular medical models. Annual Review of Genomics and Human Genetics 3: 311–340.

Velculescu VE, Zhang L, Vogelstein B, Kinzler KW (1995) Serial analysis of gene expression. Science 270: 484–487.

Walke DW, Han C, Shaw J, Wann E, Zambrowicz B, Sands A (2001) In vivo drug target discovery: identifying the best targets from the genome. Currrent Opinion in Biotechnology 12: 626–631.

Wang Y (2001) The role and regulation of urokinase-type plasminogen activator receptor gene expression in cancer invasion and metastasis. Medicinal Research Reviews 21: 146–170.

Weatherall D J (1991) The new genetica and clinical practice, 3rd edn. Oxford: Oxford University Press.

Wengelnik K et al. (2002) A class of potent antimalarials and their specific accumulation in infected erythrocytes. Science 295. 1311–1314.

Zambrowicz BP, Sands AT (2003) Knockouts model the 100 best-selling drugs – will they model the next 100? Nature Reviews Drug Discovery 2: 38–51.

Zanders ED (2000) Gene expression profiling as an aid to the identification of drug targets. Pharmacogenomics 1: 375–384.

The role of genomics and bioinformatics

H LeVine

H P Rang

Introduction to '-OMICS'

The genome is defined as 'the full complement of genetic information, both coding and non-coding, in the organism', an idea first conceived in 1932. Pharmaceutical utility inherent in this vast array of information lies in understanding how information translates into function at the organism level. This is true both for the human genome and for the genomes of pathogenic organisms in which the search is going on for new therapeutic targets. The availability of the nucleic acid sequence for the entire complement of human genes, and all of the code specifying the regulation of expression of those genes, will signal a major shift in the way we approach life science, a revolution already well under way. We will soon have the lexicon, but are left with the questions of when, how, and why life patterns unfold.

Biotechnology companies which promoted the methodologies that made the Human Genome Project a reality are positioning themselves to be the leaders in managing and tapping this vast new information resource. Companies specializing in genomic technology, bioinformatics, and related fields were the fastest expanding sector of the biotechnology industry during the 1990s, aspiring to lead the pharmaceutical industry into an era of rapid identification and exploitation of novel targets (Chandra and Caldwell, 2003). Despite the perceived failure of the genomic revolution so far to deliver the goods in terms of drug discovery (Drews, 2003), there is consensus that the Genome Project will be worth the investment of billions of dollars and millions of man-hours, though exactly how the information can be translated into drugs is much less certain. Just how prominent should genome-based strategies be in the research portfolio of pharmaceutical companies?

The answer to that question has become clearer the more we learn about the genome. First, only about 2% of the human genome is sequence that codes for protein or RNA. What are we missing in the other 98%? Initially considered to be 'junk' DNA, fossil relics of evolution, the role of intergenic sequences in gene regulation, chromatin structure, recombination templating, and sponsoring heterogeneity in polymorphic loci is only now emerging. On the other hand, 75–85% of bacterial genomes are coding sequence. Although it is important to know all of the possible gene products that a species is capable of producing, understanding which ones are altered in disease and how that affects pathology is more pharmaceutically relevant.

The genome is the basic instruction set from which various subsets of gene products are derived (Greenbaum et al., 2001). The resulting hierarchy of '-omes' is shown in Table 7.1. Whereas the genome is a static compilation of the sequence of the four DNA bases, the other groupings are dynamic and much more complex. It is these shifting, adapting pools of cellular components that determine health and pathology. Each of them is a mini genome project, with ground rules that are much less well defined. Some worry that '-omics' will prove to be a spiral of knowing less and less about more and more.

Genomes

By mid-2004 the genomes of more than 180 organisms had been completely sequenced. Most are bacteria, but about 32 eukaryote genomes have been sequenced, including plants, fungi, yeasts, invertebrates such as the fruit fly *Drosophila melanogaster*, the flatworm *Chaenorhabditis elegans*, the malaria-carrying mosquito *Anopheles gambiae*, the malaria parasite, a number of higher plants, and seven vertebrates – mouse, rat, dog, chicken, puffer fish, chimpanzee and, notably, human (Lander et al., 2001; Venter et al., 2001). The list (see www.genomenewsnetwork.org) grows monthly. The massive amount of information generated in the various genome projects and gene mapping studies has to be stored, disseminated and analysed electronically, relying heavily on bioinformatics software systems and the Internet (see later section). Here we may note that defining the nucleotide sequence is only the starting point of the genomic approach. Although identifying genes within the genome sequence is not straightforward, earlier estimates of about 100 000 genes in the human genome came down, rather startlingly, to about 35 000 when the sequence was determined, and later (International Human Genome Sequencing Consortium, 2004) to about 25 000. Even more difficult is to elucidate the likely functions of the encoded proteins, how their expression is controlled, and how disease states can arise, all of which we need to understand in order to apply genomic principles effectively to the business of drug discovery.

Genetic approaches to drug target identification

The principle of using genomic information as the starting point for identifying novel drug targets is described in Chapter 6. Here we discuss two main approaches in more detail: chromosomal mapping and identification of 'disease genes', and the analysis of gene expression in diseased and normal tissue.

Table 7.1
Gene to function is paved with 'omes'

Commonly used terms		
Genome	Full complement of genetic information (i.e. DNA sequence, including coding and non-coding regions)	Static
Transcriptome	Population of mRNA molecules in a cell under defined conditions at a given time	Dynamic
Proteome	Either: the complement of proteins (including post-translational modifications) encoded by the genome	Static
	or: the set of proteins and their post-translational modifications expressed in a cell or tissue under defined conditions at a specific time (also sometimes referred to as the translatome)	Dynamic
Terms occasionally encountered (to be interpreted with caution)		
Secretome	Population of secreted proteins produced by a cell	Dynamic
Metabolome	Small molecule content of a cell	Dynamic
Interactome	Grouping of interactions between proteins in a cell	Dynamic
Glycome	Population of carbohydrate molecules in a cell	Dynamic
Foldome	Population of gene products classified by tertiary structure	Dynamic
Phenome	Population of observable phenotypes describing variations of form and function in a given species.	Dynamic

Genes and disease

The tendency of certain illnesses to run in families has been recognized for centuries, and human gene mapping efforts predate the discovery of DNA or even knowledge of the number of human chromosomes. Following Mendel's description of the transmission and independent assortment of hereditary factors in 1865, Hardy and Weinberg in 1908 used a mathematical approach to predict the behaviour of alleles and to calculate allele frequencies in a large population. For two allele systems, carrier frequencies of diseases, disease prevalence, and approximate degree of penetrance could be calculated from the Hardy–Weinberg Equilibrium theory. Linkage analysis (see below) rests on the principle that two genes that lie close together on a chromosome will only rarely be separated by a recombination event (chromosome crossover) at the time of conception, and so will tend to remain linked through many generations. By measuring the frequency with which a particular allele of an identified marker gene occurs in affected individuals, the proximity of the marker gene to the putative disease gene can be estimated.

Monogenic diseases

Over 7000 inherited human diseases have been described, and by mid-2003 about 8500 disease-associated genes had been identified (see http://www.ncbi.nlm.nih.gov/Omim/searchomim.html for a regularly updated compilation). Most of these are rare single-gene metabolic disorders, whose genetics follow relatively straightforward models of inheritance within families (Scriver, 2001). For more than 1000 of these diseases the responsible gene has been mapped to a chromosomal region by genetic linkage analysis. An increasing number are being defined at a molecular level, and our knowledge of the complete human genome sequence will greatly speed up this endeavour. Table 7.2 lists a few of the more common diseases for which the responsible gene has been mapped and cloned. Of course, as discussed in Chapter 6, knowing the responsible component and the exact defect does not guarantee that improved treatments can be found.

Nucleotide changes that occur naturally in DNA can be *point mutations*, where a single nucleotide base is changed; *deletions/insertions*, where stretches of nucleotides can be deleted/inserted/duplicated; *inversions*, where a portion of the nucleotide sequence is reversed; and *translocations*, where a piece of DNA on one chromosome is moved and incorporated into another chromosome. Point mutations within exons (protein coding sequence) can be *silent* (no observable effect) because of the degeneracy of the genetic protein code; *missense*, where the wrong amino acid is incorporated; and *nonsense*, where a stop codon is introduced, leading to a truncated protein product. Mutations within introns can disrupt splicing of mRNAs and may affect other forms of regulation that are controlled by intronic sequences. Mutations also occur in regulatory regions of genes such as control elements up- and downstream of the protein coding sequence, or in more distant regulatory elements involved in enhancement or repression of transcriptional activity.

At its simplest (see Griffiths et al, 2000, for details of genetic analysis), transmission of a trait, mutation or polymorphism is characterized as *dominant* (one copy of the gene needed for expression of the trait) or *recessive* (two copies needed for expression), and as *autosomal* (gene present on a chromosome other than X) or *sex-linked* (gene present on X chromosome). These characteristics determine the pattern of transmission of the trait and, for recessive genes, the carrier state, from parents to offspring. Table 7.2 shows the classification on this basis of some of the major genetic disorders.

Complications in interpreting genetic data

Variations on straightforward unitary inheritance cloud the interpretation of many genetic data (see Griffiths et al, 2000). '*Pseudodominant*' transmission of a recessive mutation occurs in situations where the disease allele is relatively common in the population and can be brought into a pedigree even if the mates are not related. Mutations occurring in the zygote yield mosaicism – expression in some tissues or cells but not others – which can skew phenotypic expression. Germline mosaicism can result in apparent *pseudorecessive* transmission of a dominant trait whereby unaffected parents produce affected offspring.

Frequently, the inheritance is difficult to follow if the phenotype or observable trait is not visible to the same degree in different individuals. Because the inheritance of the mutation itself is more constant than the expression of the trait, non-uniformity of phenotype and hence assignment of the pedigree is attributed to a variety of causes, described as variations of gene *penetrance* of various sorts, or *expressivity*. With autosomal dominant transmission this can mean that a heterozygous individual, though strictly 'affected', actually shows little or no sign of disease, yet still passes on the gene to offspring, so that the expected vertical transmission can appear to skip a generation. The genetic modelling of the disease needs to be adjusted for this and to take into account the difficulty in making the phenotype assignment. Such corrections can be critical in the interpretation of linkage studies.

A common problem in epidemiological and genetic studies is that disease classification may be uncertain and sometimes controversial, and does not necessarily reflect the underlying cause. The clinical syndromes recognized as heart failure or epilepsy, for example, can have many different causes, which need to be distinguished if genetic analysis is to have any meaning.

Table 7.2
Examples of common single gene disorders

Disease	Inheritance pattern	Gene	Notes
Achrondroplasia	Autosomal recessive	Fibroblast growth factor receptor	Involved in growth of long bones
Cystic fibrosis	Autosomal recessive	Cystic fibrosis transporter regulator	Causes deficient NaCl transport, affecting secretory epithelia, especially in lungs
Duchenne muscular dystrophy	Sex-linked recessive	Dystrophin	Muscle-specific protein involved in contractile function
Fragile X syndrome	Sex-linked dominant	Fragile X mental retardation (FMR-1) gene	Triplet repeat in untranslated region of gene, affecting stability of X chromosome
Gaucher's disease	Autosomal recessive	β-Glucosidase	One of several similar lipid storage diseases. Enzyme replacement therapy developed
Hemophilia A	Sex-linked recessive	Factor VIII	Treated with blood-derived or recombinant factor VIII
Huntington's chorea	Autosomal dominant	Huntingtin	Triplet repeat disorder. Function of huntingtin not known
Marfan's syndrome	Autosomal dominant	Fibrillin	Involved in elastin deposition
Myotonic muscular dystrophy	Autosomal dominant	Myotonin protein kinase	Triplet repeat disorder
Neurofibromatosis	Autosomal dominant	Neurofibromin	Involved in regulation of G-protein signalling, affecting cell growth and division
Phenylketonuria	Autosomal recessive	Phenylalanine hydroxylase	One of many 'inborn errors of metabolism' associated with lack of a single enzyme
Sickle cell anemia	Autosomal recessive	β-Globin	Affects conformational state of haemoglobin in red cells

Complex diseases

Most common diseases are not due to a single defective gene, but nevertheless show varying degrees of heritability. Such diseases – like most human traits – arise from the interaction of many different genes with each other, and with the environment (Schafer and Hawkins, 1998). Nucleotide changes that tend to occur in a sizeable fraction of the population, and whose effects, if any, lie within the normal range of individual variation are known as *polymorphisms*. These changes can contribute to complex genetic diseases in which multiple genes, interacting with environmental factors, contribute to the disease phenotype. Many human diseases, for example diabetes, schizophrenia, hypertension and most cancers, fall into this category.

Schizophrenia is an example of a complex genetic disease. Its incidence in the population at large is approximately 0.8%, whereas its incidence in first-degree relatives of individuals with the disease is 8–12%, a difference not due to environmental factors. The fact that in schizophrenia, as in many other diseases, such as type 1 diabetes, multiple sclerosis and many cancers, the concordance rate for the condition among monozygotic (genetically identical) twins is 50% or less, shows clearly that the cause is not exclusively genetic – rather, we have to look for *susceptibility* genes, the possession of which increases the chance of developing the disease. In the case of schizophrenia there have been many false leads, but recently a number of susceptibility genes have been identified (Harrison and Owen, 2003). The class of polymorphic leukocyte antigens known as HLA was one of the first to be identified as susceptibility genes for a variety of autoimmune diseases, including rheumatoid arthritis, type 1 diabetes and multiple sclerosis, as well as certain drug hypersensitivity reactions. More recently, variation in the gene encoding apolipoprotein E (ApoE) has been associated with an increased risk of developing Alzheimer's disease (Rocchi et al., 2003); new examples are flooding in.

Genetic associations of this kind, on which the identification of disease susceptibility genes rests, are revealed by epidemiological studies in human populations, the reliability of which depends critically on:

- The need for accurate diagnosis
- Avoidance of sampling bias
- Ensuring sample sizes large enough to give the required statistical power.

That the task is a difficult one is reflected in the large number of published studies purporting to have identified genes associated with disorders such a schizophrenia and bipolar depression, but whose conclusions have not stood up to further investigation. The pace of discovery is, however, increasing rapidly.

Gene mapping

The tendency of alleles of two loci to segregate together across generations if they are physically close on the same chromosome is known as genetic linkage. The closer the loci are to one another, the less likely is it that crossing-over will occur between them. The LOD (logarithm of the odds of linkage) score is used to express this: the higher the LOD score for a pair of genes, the closer they are on the chromosome.

Recombination between loci is caused by crossing-over between chromatids during meiosis. In fruit flies, generations of genetics students have performed crosses and noted the coincidence of phenotypic markers such as eye colour and the presence of wing veins to map the unknown gene relative to the marker traits. For medical genetic studies, the co-occurrence of anonymous chromosomal markers that have a defined chromosome position, in association with the phenotypic trait, is used to measure co-segregation. The Human Genome Project used a series of physical and genetic marker maps to verify the ordering of these markers. The paucity of genetic markers suitably spread over the human genome to use for linkage analysis, and the need for computerized algorithms for data analysis, were obstacles to linkage

analysis until the 1980s, when the use of *restriction fragment length polymorphisms* (RFLP; Box 7.1) opened up most of the rest of the genome to analysis. Further refinement of linkage analysis has been achieved by the mapping of increasingly dense sets of anonymous nucleotide sequence markers – *minisatellites, sequence-tagged sites* (STSs), *microsatellites* and single nucleotide polymorphisms (SNPs) (Box 7.1). The more closely spaced markers of linkage are, given adequate patient population sizes, the better the resolution of the technique and the smaller the region of DNA sequence that must be searched through to identify the altered gene responsible for the observed trait. Conventional linkage studies, as used, for example, in locating the cystic fibrosis gene (Riordan et al., 1989), are able to locate the gene within a few megabases – often called a 'hotspot'. Before the genome sequence was known it was still a laborious task to pin the gene down precisely, but this is becoming much easier as the location of all the genes is being worked out.

A problem in the past has been that markers equally spaced at convenient intervals were not available. The advent of polymerase chain reaction (PCR) amplification of short tandem repeats of two, three or four bases defined by unique flanking sequences and their physical ordering on chromosomes has alleviated this as an issue. Dinucleotide repeats occur on average every 0.4 cM (roughly 400 kb). Single nucleotide polymorphisms, estimated to be about 5 million in number, occur much more frequently – every 600 bp. These substitutions account for the bulk of the DNA sequence variation between individuals. Each is likely to have

> **Box 7.1 Anonymous nucleotide marker sequences used in gene mapping**

Restriction length polymorphism
Cutting DNA containing a probe sequence gives different length fragments after cleavage by the particular endonuclease because of a polymorphism in the site that either creates or removes a cleavage site.

Minisatellites
Stretches of DNA that contain tandem arrangements of repeats of a short (12 or more bp) core sequence.

Sequence-tagged sites
Short (60–1000 bp) sequences that can be detected by PCR with primers to defined sequences. If the length of the amplified fragment varies polymorphically then the sequence-tagged site is useful for genetic mapping.

Microsatellites
Short (2–4 bp) tandem repeats that can be detected by PCR with primers to defined sequences. These markers are highly polymorphic and uniformly dispersed throughout the genome.

occurred once in the history of humankind. A subset of these markers can be used for mapping studies. A consortium has been established to collect informative SNPs to be used in genomic mapping studies (see SNP website).

The details of sample mapping and the statistical analysis of the data are beyond the scope of this chapter. The reader is referred to Liu (1998) and Griffiths et al. (2000) for entry into that subject. Technology has improved greatly over the past decade, and mapping projects that were inconceivable a few years ago are well within the reach of many groups. Patient collection and clinical evaluation remain a stumbling block. The more complex the disease process under investigation, the more patients of the appropriate kind are required and the harder they are to find. Diseases such as schizophrenia and bipolar disorder can require up to several thousand patients. In addition, a mapping study must be replicated, usually in a smaller number of patients, but in a separate population. Many studies initially focus on geographically isolated areas where certain diseases are common and genetic variation is low due to inbreeding.

The next slow and expensive segment of the process comes at the end of the initial mapping – transforming a chromosomal localization to an identified gene. Chromosome-level mapping studies have tended to localize genes to a 5–20 cM (roughly 5–20 million base pairs) region, which can contain hundreds of genes. However, based on knowledge of the entire genome sequence, it is now possible to use much more efficient screening paradigms to detect the nucleotide changes responsible for the altered trait. Identifying the mutational allelic change by completely sequencing the candidate region for each of the patients is unrealistic. Instead, candidate genes in the region are identified that fit in with what is known about the disease biology, and these are chosen for sequencing. Still, depending on what other genes are in the region, this could be a large undertaking. This information may be sufficient to identify an interesting therapeutic target. Sometimes candidate genes are selected early on and evaluated as targets while the linkage project continues. With the completion of the human genome sequencing project and the improving annotation of the sequence, this approach may become more fruitful.

Animal models of human disease

Hereditary diseases are common in domestic animals, partly as a result of inbreeding and selection. Hip dysplasia, progressive retinal atrophy and corneal cataract are examples of hereditary diseases affecting particular dog breeds. Inbred strains of laboratory mice and rats differ in their susceptibility to pathogens and drugs, and in some cases, such as the spontaneously hypertensive rat (SHR) strain, and the Brattleborough rat, whose pathology resembles human diabetes insipidus (see Chapter 11), such animals are widely used for drug testing.

Several single- and polygenic models of human disease have been defined in the laboratory mouse, often with symptoms similar to that of the human disease counterpart (Bedell et al., 1997a,b). The Jackson Laboratory maintains a collection of characterized mouse mutants for study (see JAXMICE database), in addition to transgenic and knockout mouse strains created by genetic engineering (see TBASE database). The mouse genome sequence was completed in 2002 and proved to be closely related to the human genome, with a very similar gene order and relative positioning of large chromosomal regions. This *synteny* is a great advantage for the localization and identification of genes. For monogenic disorders there are numerous examples of single-gene mutations in the mouse resulting in phenotypic expression indistinguishable from the human condition. Mapping the synteny of several polygenic disorders in mice and in humans suggests that mice will be useful models, although it is not certain whether the same genes control the same trait in both organisms. Numerous inbred strains of mice with complex polygenic diseases such as epilepsy, obesity, hypertension, asthma, and diabetes have been developed, along with outbred strains selected for their phenotype. The production of congenic strains of mice that contain defined regions of single chromosomes from inbred strains with a particular trait will help in the analysis of polygenic disorders.

Model organisms

Although mice are one of the closest accessible mammalian models for the genetic analysis of human disease, other less closely related organisms possess significant advantages for the study of gene–phenotype relationships. The fruit fly *Drosophila melanogaster* and the flatworm *Caenorhabditis elegans* are particularly useful, because a great deal is known about their genetics and large collections of phenotypically characterized mutants are available. They are anatomically and physiologically fairly simple, yet have quite complex behavioural repertoires that are easily observed. These features have made them the multicellular organisms of choice for genetic analysis. RNA interference (RNAi; see Chapter 6), a technique for specifically silencing individual genes or families of genes, is being used in these species for systematic 'gene screening' in order to elucidate the functional role of particular genes and to generate potential animal models for drug testing. (Kim, 2003; Lee et al., 2004).

Saccharomyces cerevisiae, a yeast, is particularly suitable for genetic manipulations, and human proteins often substitute for their yeast homologues, which makes the organism also a useful tool for mechanistic studies at the cellular level (Munder and Hinnen, 1999). Although the relevance of such distantly related species to the mammalian – and especially the human – situation is often questioned in pharmaceutical circles, the fact is that genes are remarkably well conserved across the large species gap, even though their functions may differ. At the molecular level eukaryotes all look much the same, despite their amazing biological diversity. The utility and ease of genetic manipulations in organisms such as yeasts, fruit flies and flatworms constitute a big advantage over higher organisms. Currently, the mouse is the only mammalian species suitable for routine generation of transgenic strains, and it takes months or years of breeding to produce a new pure strain, a task that can be finished in days or weeks – and much more cheaply – with lower organisms.

Gene expression profiling

The principle of using gene expression profiling as an approach to identifying novel drug targets was described in Chapter 6. In practice, what is measured is the number of individual mRNA species present in cells or tissues, and it is important to realize that the result is a snapshot of a kinetic process. Messenger RNAs have different stabilities regulated by their composition, by sequestered proteins, and by subcellular compartmentalization. The balance between synthesis and degradation determines the net amount of an mRNA present at any particular time. The relationship between the amount of mRNA and the rate of translation into protein is also uncertain. Nevertheless, the population of mRNAs present at any time (the transcriptome; see Table 7.1), provides a highly detailed picture of cell function – a new window through which to observe what is going on. Like the genome itself, the transcriptome is readily codified, stored and analysed by bioinformatics software. It represents the first step on the trail linking genes to function, and transcriptome data sets are proving increasingly useful in a wide range of pathological, physiological, pharmacological and toxicological studies (see Chapter 6). This approach holds great promise, but the compiling of reliable databases is hampered by the varying experimental protocols and analytical procedures used in different experiments.

The most commonly used technique for transcription profiling is the use of DNA *microarrays* (Marshall and Hodgson, 1998; Ramsay, 1998; Friend and Stoughton,

2002), the principle of which is illustrated in Figure 7.1. The microarray consists of a square of plastic on to which is spotted, in a tightly packed rectangular array, a series of DNA sequences representing genes of interest. With modern robotic techniques, several thousand known sequences can be spotted on to an area of a few square centimetres. A typical experiment, designed to measure, for example, changes in gene expression associated with inflammation, would be carried out as follows. mRNA is extracted from normal (control) and inflamed (test) tissues and converted to cDNA, which is much more stable than RNA. Test and control cDNAs, representing all of the different gene transcripts, are labelled with fluorescent dyes (green for control, say, and red for test), and then mixed together and applied to the DNA microarray under controlled conditions for several hours. During this time the various cDNA species will hybridize with the corresponding arrayed DNAs, so that the arrayed spots become fluorescent. The fluorescence will be red or green if a particular cDNA is more strongly represented in either test or control tissue, or red/green (=orange) if it is the same in both. A robotic laser-scanning and imaging procedure is used to record the fluorescence signal from each spot of the array, allowing differentially expressed genes to be rapidly identified. Microarrays ('gene chips') representing many different collections of genes of different species are now commercially available, and the technique is very widely used for transcription profiling – the first step in the chain of

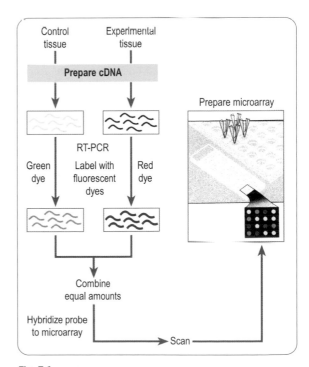

Fig. 7.1
Microarray experiment: technology for analysing mRNA expression.

events linking genes with functions. Current microarray methods are somewhat limited in sensitivity, and are unable to detect transcripts representing fewer than about 1 in 100 000 mRNA molecules. Low-abundance transcripts can be present at levels below this detection limit. As it happens, many of the well known pharmacological targets, such as G-protein-coupled receptors (GPCRs), ion channels and transporters, fall into this class, and so highly sensitive techniques are needed to capture the information likely to be most relevant to drug discovery.

mRNA profiles can also be monitored with subtractive libraries of various sorts and differential display of cDNAs (Hunt and Livesey, 2000) without a great deal of expensive technology, particularly if only a few genes are being followed. These older techniques lack the sensitivity and accuracy needed to detect relatively small changes in the abundance of rare transcripts, and have largely been supplanted by microarray-based methods. Other techniques, such as SAGE (Serial Analysis of Gene Expression; Velculescu et al., 1995), its less extravagant cousin SADE (SAGE Adaptation for Downsized Extracts; Virlon et al., 1999) and DEPD (Digital Expression Pattern Display; Maelicke and Lubbert, 2002) , rely on using several restriction enzymes to cut DNA strands at specific sites and separating the resulting fragments by gel or capillary electrophoresis, giving several thousand peaks of different magnitudes, each representing the expression of a particular gene. Such methods (Powell, 2000) generally have high sensitivity and resolving power, and (in contrast to array-based methods), do not require the experimenter to decide in advance which genes are likely to be of interest. Though generally slower and more technically demanding than microarray methods, and therefore less widely used, such methods are useful where the need is for a more comprehensive picture, covering unknown and low-abundance genes, than microarrays can provide.

The simultaneous analysis of large numbers of different mRNAs can give a uniquely detailed view of how cells and tissues react to different challenges, such as infection, physical stimuli or chemicals. Interpreting these large data sets poses two types of problem. One is the need for careful statistical analysis to reduce the likelihood of being misled by chance or artefactual variations. It is usually necessary to 'normalize' results obtained with replica microarrays, as experimental variation in the efficiency of hybridization is common. Signals from a range of common 'housekeeping' genes can be used for this purpose, it being assumed that their expression levels will be the same in all experiments. Alternatively, the sum of signals from all the genes in the microarray can be used. Either procedure involves assumptions that are not necessarily correct. It is essential to replicate the measurements so that due allowance for experimental variation can be included, and an estimate made of the likely proportion of false negatives

and false positives. When large numbers of transcripts are being compared across a number of different experimental conditions, a small degree of experimental variation can substantially degrade the confidence that can be placed on conclusions about which transcripts show significant up- or down-regulation. Failure to replicate experiments sufficiently and to apply rigorous statistical analysis can easily lead to false interpretations. The second, more fundamental, problem is to link the observed changes in gene expression to changes in function – the broad and ill-defined field of functional genomics, discussed briefly below and in Chapter 6.

Analysis of gene expression data

The end result of an expression profiling study, whether based on microarrays or other technologies, is a list of genes whose expression levels changed, either up or down, in one or more of the experimental groups, and the associated estimates of their expression levels. Imagine an experiment in which groups of animals were treated with five different drugs, each at three different doses, and mRNA was extracted from three different tissues – a total of 45 experimental groups. Suppose that 2000 genes were studied, of which 100 were identified as showing substantial changes in expression, giving a total of 90 000 data points, 4500 of which are of potential interest. What can we expect to learn from this daunting pile of numbers? Reasonable questions to ask might be:

- Do all the drugs produce much the same changes in gene expression?
- Are the effects of the five drugs all quite different, or can they be grouped?
- Similarly, do all three tissues behave similarly, or are they all different?
- Do the effects seen resemble the results obtained in published studies, say with another set of drugs?
- Are there particular groups of genes that behave in a similar way, for example showing upregulation in one of the three tissues in response to the same four drugs?
- Do the gene expression changes correlate with the pharmacological effects and dose–response relationships of the drugs studied?

None of these answers is likely to leap out at us spontaneously as we browse through the data pile: special ways of quantifying the 'similarity' of multidimensional (genes, drugs, doses, tissues in the example above) gene expression patterns are required. Many approaches have been tried to address this problem (Quackenbush, 2001; Dopazo et al., 2001; European Bioinformatics Institute website, www.ebi.ac.uk). If we consider the expression levels of two genes in several experimental groups, their overall behaviour can be

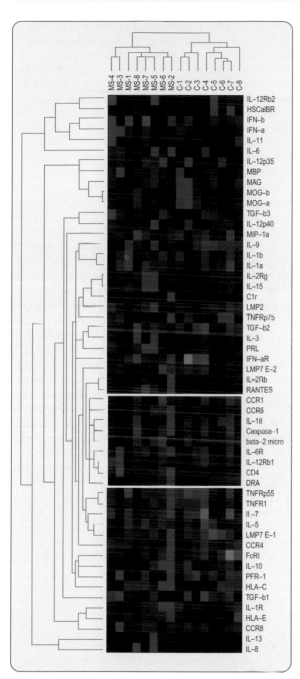

Fig. 7.2
Cluster analysis of gene expression experiment. Expression
levels of 54 genes (listed on right) in eight control and eight multiple
sclerosis brain samples (listed above). Relative expression levels are
indicated in shades of red for high values and green for low values.
A computer algorithm was used to calculate similarity between the
expression pattern of each gene for all subjects, and the expression
pattern for each subject for all genes, and to display the results as a
dendrogram. The top dendrogram shows that MS and control
samples are clearly distinguishable, the intragroup distance being
much greater than the intersample difference within each group. The
left-hand dendrogram shows the grouping of genes into clusters that
behave similarly. A group of genes with highly similar expression
patterns is outlined in yellow. (Reproduced with permission from
Baranzini et al., 2000.)

compared by calculating a *correlation coefficient*, which
will be large and positive if the two are affected in the
same way in all of the experimental groups, large and
negative if they are consistently affected in opposite
directions, and close to zero if they behave independently of each other. A correlation matrix is generated
by calculating correlation coefficients for every pair of
genes. Other metrics for estimating the 'distance' between the expression profiles of genes under different
experimental conditions can also be used (Quackenbusch, 2001), and one needs to be aware that the choice
of algorithm can have a large effect on the conclusions.
Whatever the method used, once the distance matrix
has been calculated, various pattern recognition algorithms (see Valafar, 2002 for details) can be used to classify
genes into groups with similar behaviours, or alternatively to classify the experimental groups according
to their overall effect on gene expression. Figure 7.2
shows an example in which the expression of 56 selected
genes was compared between normal post-mortem brain
tissue and the characteristic 'plaques' in post-mortem
brain tissue from multiple sclerosis (MS) patients
(Baranzini et al., 2000). The dendrograms obtained by
cluster analysis show that MS lesions form a cluster that
is quite distinct from the cluster of controls, and that
groups of genes that behave similarly can be identified.
In Figure 7.2, the group highlighted includes a number
of cytokines believed to be involved in MS pathology.
The groupings shown, even in this simple example, could
not have been picked out by merely inspecting the data.

Proteomics

Proteins are a great deal more complicated than genes or
mRNA transcripts. Although their amino acid sequence
can be determined experimentally, or inferred from the
gene sequence, they often undergo post-translational
modification, and – most importantly – adopt distinct
three-dimensional structures that are critical to their function. Neither of these characteristics is easy to address by
the kind of screening procedure used in genomics. It is
thought that splice variants and post-translational
modifications mean that ~25 000 genes in the human
genome may give rise to 200 000 or more functional proteins. The demands on resolution and sensitivity are
therefore much harder to meet in proteomics than in
genomics. Unlike DNA sequences, proteins cannot be
amplified, nor can powerful methods based on hybridization of complementary sequences – which form the basis
of much nucleic acid technology – be applied to proteins.

The main tools used in proteomics are large-scale two-
dimensional gel electrophoresis and mass spectrometry
(Burbaum and Tobel, 2002; Michaud and Snyder, 2002).
Two-dimensional electrophoresis, separating proteins by

charge in one direction and by mass in the other, is capable of resolving hundreds or even thousands of distinct proteins spots on a single gel. About 100 µg of protein can be loaded on to the gel, and the detection sensitivity of the separated spots is about 3 ng, so that proteins accounting for fewer than about 1 in 30 000 molecules will escape detection – one of the main limitations of the technique. The spots, once located, can be sequenced and further analysed to reveal post-translational modifications by a variety of mass spectroscopic techniques – a rapidly advancing field. Information about 3D structure is obtained mainly by nuclear magnetic resonance (NMR) studies of the protein in solution, or X-ray analysis of crystals, techniques that require relatively large amounts of pure protein.

Many public domain databases have been set up to store the very large amount of data on protein sequence, structure and function (see later section). The main sequence database (SwissProt, www.expasy.ch/swissprot) currently (mid-2004) contains about 160 000 proteins, including about 11 000 human proteins. Proteomic approaches involving the analysis of proteins expressed by human tumours is becoming widely used as a diagnostic tool to distinguish subtypes of cancers, and many other clinical applications are also being developed.

Protein microarrays (Mitchell, 2002; Cutler, 2003), analogous to DNA microarrays, are becoming available and can be used in screening for compounds that bind to specific proteins (Jeffrey and Bogyo, 2003), or for obtaining a broad 'binding profile' for novel compounds whose biochemical mechanism of action is uncertain. This application is proving valuable as a screen for likely toxicity, based on arrays of proteins known to be targets for toxic chemicals (Bandara and Kennedy, 2002).

In summary, proteomics embraces a broad range of technologies for detecting, isolating and characterizing the proteins present in cells and tissues. The technologies are evolving rapidly and improving in sensitivity. The major problem remains the use of the cumbersome technique of 2D gel electrophoresis as the main method of separating proteins, and the relatively low sensitivity of methods for detecting individual spots. The role of proteomics in drug discovery is not yet clearly defined, but is likely to increase as the technology improves. Its application to clinical diagnosis, particularly in the field of cancer (Dwek and Rawlings, 2002; Wulfkuhle et al., 2003), is already well established, and its use for toxicological screening is also advancing rapidly (Kennedy, 2002).

Functional genomics

Functional genomics in its broadest interpretation seeks to assign all of the genes of an organism to their place in a functional framework. This includes understanding both the activity of the encoded protein and the overall role of the gene in the biology of particular cell types as well as in the life of the organism. Knowing the primary amino acid sequence of the protein, or the nucleic acid sequence of the gene's regulatory regions, is just the beginning of this process. Fortunately, genetic engineering technology provides several tools to manipulate cells and whole organisms to obtain answers to at least some of these questions, if investigators are clever enough to ask the right questions and interpret the answers.

When applied to drug discovery (see review by Kramer & Cohen, 2004), the primary role is to identify and validate possible drug targets (see Chapter 6). Once a putative target is implicated in a disease-related phenotype, it can be manipulated in a variety of ways to assess its role in the pathologic state. Mutating or deleting the gene for the protein of interest either in cells or in whole organisms allows the assessment of what an inhibitor would do in a biological system. Many cell types can readily be manipulated by transfection, resulting in overexpression or deletion of the genes of interest, or introducing mutations of selected residues or regions of the protein by homologous recombination. Postmitotic cells such as differentiated neurons or cardiocytes, though, are notoriously difficult to transfect.

Transgenic animals, into which an abnormal gene is introduced or a normal gene is overexpressed or suppressed, do not always give a clear picture of gene function. Some genes code for multifunctional proteins that fulfil different roles (e.g. structural, enzymatic, or ligand recognition) in different tissues or at different stages of development. Disruption of developmentally important genes may be lethal or cause major developmental abnormalities. To overcome some of these problems, techniques to control the expression of particular genes have been developed. Two widely used techniques are the *Tet-on/Tet-off* system, which allows the experimenter to determine when the transgene will be switched on or off, and the *Cre/Lox* system, which allows for tissue-specific expression of the transgene. Both are commercially available.

The *Tet-on/Tet-off* system involves introducing a bacterial tetracycline-responsive (TetR) gene into the promoter region of a particular target gene. Depending on the nature of the TetR, introduction of the tetracycline analogue *doxycycline* reversibly switches the targeted gene either on or off.

Cre is a recombinase enzyme which excises stretches of DNA lying between two *Lox* sites, and reunites the ends. *Lox* sites are specific 34-residue DNA sequences not normally found in eukaryotes. Transgenic mice are produced which possess two *Lox* sites introduced on either side of a particular target gene. They function normally. This strain is then crossed with transgenic mice possessing the *Cre* gene linked to a tissue-specific promoter. In offspring that possess both transgenes, tissue-specific *Cre* expression results in excision of the target gene restricted to those tissues. By a simple modification, the same principle can be used to induce tissue-specific expression of an abnormal transgene.

Temporary or regulatable manipulations of specific genes can also be accomplished by antisense nucleotide or ribozyme-catalysed lowering of cellular mRNA levels for specific gene products, or by RNA interference (RNAi, see Chapter 6). For further details of these and other procedures for controlling gene expression, see Latchman (2002).

These are now standard ways of defining the role of proteins in cells. Complete or partial phenocopies of the pathological condition produced by the gene manipulation provide support – though not iron-clad proof – for the involvement of the target gene in the disease state.

The next step – animal models

For most diseases pathology is not manifest – or at least not recognized – at the cellular level, but at a tissue, organ, or whole organism level. Fortunately, technology is rapidly being developed which allows much of the spectrum of manipulations performed in cell culture to be carried out in whole animals. Animal models are useful for proof of concept experiments as well as the later testing of putative drug candidates (see Chapter 11). Natural or induced mutations, or strain-dependent susceptibilities derived from inbreeding that result in a phenocopy of a disease of interest, have been used for decades for drug discovery.

The ability to engineer specific genetic modifications as fine as a single nucleotide and as much as an entire gene (or more) in animals, and to do so rapidly, provides an unprecedented degree of control. The use of bacterial artificial chromosome (BAC) and yeast artificial chromosome (YAC) constructs allows large pieces of genomic DNA, or even complete genes, together with endogenous promoters and other regulatory elements, to be incorporated, which allows normal tissue-specific expression of the correct mRNA splice products from the gene. It should be noted that models derived from simple overexpression or deletion of genes do not necessarily model defects due to altered post-translational modifications, unless such defects are suspected and specific mutations made to test that hypothesis. The role of post-translational reactions such as phosphorylation, sulfation or glycosylation in producing the pathological phenotype can be investigated by mutating the amino acids involved and thus preventing the reaction.

Transgenic manipulation of animals for research applications is almost always done using mice, though simpler organisms such as the flatworm (*C. elegans*), the fruitfly (*Drosophila*) and the zebrafish (*Danio*) are being increasingly used in drug discovery applications (See Kramer & Cohen, 2004). Mice, because of their size and relatively rapid generation time, together with our advanced understanding of their genetics and genome sequence, are the mammalian transgenic animal of choice. Other mammalian species are generally much more difficult to engineer transgenically. Even if the transgene can be successfully introduced, it is important for experimental purposes to work with animals with a defined genetic background, which requires several generations of selective breeding to accomplish once the first transgenic animals have been born. This takes about 2 years even with mice, and longer for other mammalian species. With transgenic animals, as well as in cultured cells, the human forms of proteins can be introduced ('humanization'), which is important in systems where there is species specificity of the target, provided that the human protein substitutes well for the cognate protein. Deletion or knockout of candidate genes that reproduce a pathological phenotype can provide support for involvement of that gene. Similarly, manipulation of pathways designed to alleviate a defect can mimic the effect of an inhibitory drug on a putative target. Knockouts can also be used to show that the effect of a drug requires the presence of a particular target protein, giving valuable evidence of the drug's mechanism of action. Similar principles apply to assigning mechanisms of toxicity. Technical aspects and applications of transgenic animals are described in detail by Pinkert (2002) and Offermanns and Hein (2004).

Pharmacogenetics and pharmacogenomics

Variation of drug effects, including therapeutic efficacy, side effects and toxicity, between individuals is a major clinical problem. Apart from environmental factors, what causes individuals to differ is their genetic make-up, the differences being reflected mainly in the pattern of minisatellites, microsatellites and SNPs (see Table 7.2). It was realized many years ago that genetic factors have a strong influence on drug responses. The rate of acetylation of the antituberculosis drug *isoniazid* shows a clear bimodal distribution in the population, roughly half being *fast acetylators* in whom isoniazid has relatively few side effects, and half *slow acetylators* who suffer side effects unless the dose is reduced, this being an inherited trait. Several similar examples are known (Weinshilboum, 2003), many of which are due to polymorphism of the gene for cytochrome P450 (see Chapter 10). The rate of metabolic degradation of the anticoagulant drug *coumarin* is some 20 times more variable between fraternal twins than between identical twins, a clear indication of a predominantly genetic cause of the variation.

Pharmacodynamic, as well as pharmacokinetic, variability is also genetically determined in some instances. Polymorphisms affecting the gene for the β_2-adrenoceptor affects the clinical response to β_2-adrenoceptor antagonists such as *salbutamol*, used in the treatment of asthma (Liggett, 2000). Mutations affecting cardiac K^+ channels can increase the incidence of dangerous cardiac dysrhythmias in response to a range of drugs (see Chapter 10), and new examples are rapidly emerging (Tribut et al., 2002). The application of genetic analysis to our understanding of the variation of human response to therapeutic efficacy and the side effects of drugs and differences in metabolism will undoubtedly increase. Besides providing insight into the reasons why drugs work for some people and not for others, genotyping also holds promise for assessing drug risks and benefits for prospective patients. A number of biotechnology companies have been founded on the basis of this potential clinical application.

Both pharmaceutical companies and regulatory authorities such as the FDA are beginning to assess the possible impact of reducing patient variability on the costs of clinical trials, and on improving safety by reducing the potential for adverse events during testing of new drugs. Companies are searching for the most effective way of integrating pharmacogenomics into their drug development systems (Lindpaintner, 2002; Frank and Hargreaves, 2003). They have traditionally been cautious about developments that might segment the market for a drug. On the other hand, they have readily embraced applications of the technology that might identify individuals susceptible to drug-induced toxicity. The possible savings in time and cost if proof-of-efficacy clinical trials are performed in smaller groups of patients, genetically selected as responders with a reduced likelihood of adverse reaction, are considerable. In the future, it is likely that routine genetic testing will substantially reduce response variability, and hence improve the safety margin, of therapeutic drugs by enabling responders and adverse reactors to be identified in advance, and that pharmacogenomic evaluation of new compounds will become a regulatory requirement for some classes of drug.

An important initiative that is expected to provide a sound basis for – among other things – correlating human genotypes with variations in drug effects, is the creation of a detailed map of human single nucleotide polymorphisms (SNPs; see above). Correlating SNP haplotypes with drug response phenotypes will be a long and complex task. The first part of the project, involving the identification and mapping of human SNPs, is already under way as a multicentre project (see www.snp.chbl.org, Thorisson and Stein, 2002) sponsored by all of the major pharmaceutical companies, with the data freely available in the public domain.

Because of the genetic diversity of the general patient population, several SNPs will be needed to give satisfactory correlations of SNP haplotypes with drug response phenotypes. Single SNPs will give interpretable answers only if the genes responsible for the response variation are known, so that alleles of these genes can be selected for testing.

Correlating human genotypes with phenotypic characteristics (including drug responses), as well as being a statistically complex task, raises profound ethical problems that go far beyond the application to therapeutics discussed here. It should also be remembered that environmental factors (e.g. diet, age, co-administered drugs, and doubtless many other factors not yet recognized) can profoundly influence drug responses, and so genotyping cannot be expected to account for all of the observed variability. In some fields, such as cancer, genotyping is likely to emerge as a practical guide to therapeutic choice (McLeod and Yu, 2003), but in other fields, such as diabetes or psychiatric disorders, progress will be much slower, and genotyping may never become quite the infallible lodestar to therapeutic choice that some suggest. Conducting rigorous trials to determine whether or not genotyping can significantly improve therapeutic outcome in a particular disease and treatment will be far from straightforward, but will undoubtedly be required before genotyping can be approved as part of the therapeutic protocol. A recent review (Valdes et al., 2003) discusses the potential and problems of using pharmacogenomics as a clinical tool.

Summary

The complete nucleic acid sequence of the human genome is now known. A great deal of technology had to be invented to accomplish this feat (Cantor and Smith, 1999), and even more is being developed to manipulate the unprecedented volume of information flowing from the Human Genome Project, as well as the genomes of other organisms. The genome over the lifetime of an organism represents a static set of possibilities, whereas physiology is, by necessity, dynamic. Derived subsets of this library – the various 'omes' such as the transcriptome, the proteome and others – aim to bridge this gap, thereby linking physiology to the genetic blueprint.

Complex genetic diseases are studied in populations of patients in an attempt to understand the multiple factors involved in the pathology. Whole genome linkage mapping with anonymous nucleotide markers is used to localize disease-related genes to regions of chromosomes. From the mapping studies and the available genome sequence, candidate genes can be identified. The gene products or pathways they influence represent potential therapeutic targets. Reaching this point often takes a long time, and there is the risk that the identified target(s) will not be 'druggable'.

Pharmacogenetics and pharmacogenomics are applications of genomic technologies that seek to understand the variations in patient responses to drugs. In this approach anonymous or gene-associated polymorphisms are associated with patient therapeutic response or with adverse effects (toxicogenomics). Besides resulting in more effective treatments for patients, this allows smaller, and thus cheaper and faster, clinical trials of efficacy. Recognizing non-responders and possible toxicological issues in advance should improve data quality and reduce the likelihood of adverse reactions[1].

Expression profiling of mRNAs and proteins in tissues affected by disease is a popular way to directly assess the pathological state. Differentiating between cause and effect in observed changes can become an issue. mRNA expression is most readily monitored with commercial chip microarrays of cDNAs or oligonucleotides which sample thousands of genes, and could soon have all genes represented. Proper interpretation of the data is the difficult part, and is often not done well. Informatics support plays a crucial role in analysing the data and organizing it in ways that highlight pathways and connectivities from which therapeutic targets may be chosen. Proteomics, the analysis of the protein products of mRNAs, is the most direct readout, but unfortunately is more complex than nucleic acid analysis. Some protein microarray procedures, mainly antibody-based, are available. Two-dimensional gels complemented by sequencing of relevant spots can be used, but the technology is complex and expensive.

Functional genomics is the most difficult part of the process of validating a therapeutic target. Genetic manipulation of cells and animals has proved to be very effective in generating models for testing putative drug targets. Genetically knocking out the function of the protein of interest can provide information on whether a mutant phenotype is reproduced in cells or in animals. The mechanism of action of a drug impinging on a particular protein can be confirmed if eliminating or disabling the protein eliminates the drug effect in cells or whole animals. Transgenic animals can provide models of the disease, or used to introduce 'humanized' drug targets, so that drugs designed to act on human targets can be tested in animal models.

A revolution in biomedical sciences is under way, and none can doubt that it will radically change the science of drug discovery. Currently, pharmaceutical companies are in the process of trying to find ways of making use of this expanded information landscape in the quest for the next generation of drugs. Many have taken the risk of investing heavily in technology and expertise, to ensure that they are not left behind, realizing that it will take some years before the investment can pay off in terms of drugs on the market. The mounting costs and dwindling productivity of pharmaceutical R&D in recent years have undoubtedly fuelled some scepticism about the impact of the genomic revolution on the business of pharmaceuticals. Realistically, what can be expected is that drug discovery can be speeded up, new targets identified, and diseases redefined, allowing drugs to be used more selectively and effectively for individual patients. Many believe that this will signal the end of the 'blockbuster' drugs that have dominated the commercial ambitions of pharmaceutical companies in recent years, requiring a U-turn in their strategic planning.

Bioinformatics

What is bioinformatics?

Molecular biology generates data that differs from traditional biological data in being relatively simple in format and hugely voluminous. Intuitive interpretations, and descriptive written presentations of data, on which the biological literature has relied in the past, are of little use with genomic data: advanced computational methods are necessary. The field of bioinformatics has evolved to meet this need, taking advantage of advances in computer technology, in particular the Internet.

As molecular biology moves into the post-genomic era, so the data sets handled in the bioinformatics environment become more complex, involving protein structure and function, and even cellular signalling pathways, rather than just strings of DNA sequence. Bioinformatics is a highly elastic discipline which is set to become the core technology for storing and handling all kinds of biological data. As a discipline it has strong links to electronic publishing, chemical informatics and laboratory information management systems. A key principle in all of these systems is to achieve compatibility, so that data can be readily exchanged between them. Needless to say, scientists being what they are, it can be difficult to reach the necessary agreement on such matters as nomenclature and data formats, and to accommodate scientific and technological advances, but organizations such as the National Institutes of Health (NIH), the European Molecular Biology Organization (EMBO) and others have been very successful in laying down standards, and the public domain databases set up under their auspices represent a vital scientific resource. Regrettably, from a scientific point of view, many

---

[1]Needless to say, a trial conducted on a group of genetically preselected subjects can only be used to support registration of the drug for use in preselected patients, which may not be feasible in everyday clinical use. The purpose is therefore to obtain quick and conclusive proof of efficacy before proceeding to large-scale trials on a broader patient group.

of the data generated by pharmaceutical and bio-technology companies never find their way into the public domain. The recently established SNP Consortium (see above) is a welcome break from this tradition.

Informatics and drug discovery

From the perspective of a drug discovery scientist, Informatics Heaven is the situation when the identification of a stretch of DNA that might – just might – represent a novel drug target for treating, say Alzheimer's disease, can lead by database queries, to information about the gene and its function, the tissues and circumstances in which it and any splice variants are expressed, the 3D structure of the protein or proteins encoded by it, the structure of ligands known to bind to it or to closely related proteins, and – most importantly – whether anyone else has published the idea or, worse still, patented it. Although that Heaven still seems a long way off, the high priests of bioinformatics have undoubtedly set out on the road.

In the context of drug discovery, three kinds of 'high-throughput' technology now play a critical role, namely, genomics and studies related to it, as discussed in this chapter; high-throughput screening (Chapter 8); and combinatorial chemistry (Chapter 9). All of these depend heavily on computer-based informatics systems, and expertise in this important area is much in demand. Most informatics experts currently have a background in computer technology, molecular biology or, less often, chemistry. The essential task that lies ahead for the pharmaceutical industry is to build data structures that efficiently link the key high-throughput drug discovery disciplines and provide a bridge to public domain databases, and to the conventional biomedical literature where current knowledge and understanding are recorded. Bioinformatics as currently practised is just one part of this broader informatics framework, and will undoubtedly expand further to embrace aspects such as in vivo pharmacology, toxicology, clinical trials and regulatory affairs to become the glue that binds the whole multidisciplinary exercise together. Paper is already giving way to electronic documentation with built-in data links, and the language is changing from formal prose to scientific shorthand, graphics and managerial bullet points.

It is beyond the scope of this book to describe the principles and tools of bioinformatics in any detail. Below, we give a short description of some of the main data resources and their organization. Excellent publications that go into much greater depth include books by Lesk (2002), Krane and Raymer (2002) and Lengauer (2002). The various web-based resources referred to are listed in Table 7.3.

Organizing bioinformatics data: resources and databases

With the introduction of the World Wide Web in the early 1990s, Internet-based services and databanks quickly became popular in the biological sciences. Individual laboratories started sharing their collected data, and huge central repositories for the systematic collection of biological data were created. At the time of writing the database catalogue of such repositories (DBCAT), maintained by the Centre de Resources Infobiogen lists 511 entries.

Databases relating to molecular and cell biology cover the following broad areas:

● Nucleic acid sequence and genomics
● Protein sequence and structure, including specialized 'boutique' databases relating to specific protein families (e.g. GPCRs, kinases etc.)
● Gene and protein expression profiles
● Functional pathways (e.g. signal transduction, metabolism)
● Genetics.

Given this polyglot collection of archives, many of which will contain fragments of information relevant to a particular question that a researcher might wish to ask (e.g. Is this piece of rat DNA sequence that I have found likely to represent the phosphatase that I am interested in, and if so, has it already been described, and how similar is it to the human enzyme?), it is essential to have a 'gateway' similar to the kind of literature retrieval software familiar to every scientist. '**Entrez**' is a system developed by the US National Center for Biotechnology Information (NCBI), designed for this purpose, which provides access through a simple query language to the main data archives, including the published literature. Although the landscape of databases appears at first glance to be scattered, the major resources are closely 'hyperlinked', allowing integrated access via a single entry point. Other popular access packages include GeneCards, provided by the Weizmann Institute, and the Source database developed at Stanford University.

In addition to the main public domain databases, many commercial providers (e.g. BioBase, Celera Genomics, Compugen, Derwent, Inpharmatica, GeneLogic and Incyte Genomics) maintain proprietary data collections accessible to subscribers, some of which are much more extensive than those in the public domain. For any computational scientist or molecular biologist in biomedical research a good knowledge of these databases and resources is mandatory. Here we can give no more than a brief overview, and a list of useful websites. For more detailed information see Letovsky (1999), Lesk (2002) and Lacroix and Critchlow (2003). A useful online source of information is the Genome Web facility.

Table 7.3
Bioinformatics websites

General

ENTREZ (useful bioinformatics search engine)	http://www.ncbi.nlm.nih.gov/Entrez/
DBCAT (catalogue of bioinformatics databases)	http://www.infobiogen.fr/services/dbcat/
EBI services and Genome Web (general information and access to key bioinformatics websites)	http://www.ebi.ac.uk/services http://www.hgmp.mrc.ac.uk/genomeweb
GeneCards (human genes, products and involvement in diseases)	http://bioinfo.weizmann.ac.il/cards/
SOURCE (generates simple formatted report summarizing all published data on genes or proteins)	http://genome-www5.stanford.edu/cgi-bin/SMD/source/sourceSearch

Sequence repositories

Genbank, EMBL Nucleotide Sequence DB, DNA databank of Japan (all published sequences)	http://www.ncbi.nlm.nih.gov/ http://www.ebi.ac.uk/embl/ http://www.ddbj.nig.ac.jp/
RefSeq (edited version of GenBank)	http://www.ncbi.nlm.nih.gov/LocusLink/refseq.html
UniGene (nucleotide sequences, mainly ESTs, assigned to clusters, tentatively representing individual genes)	http://www.ncbi.nlm.nih.gov/UniGene/
Ensembl (fully annotated gene database)	http://www.ensembl.org/
EGO	http://www.tigr.org/tdb/tgi/ego/ego.shtml
TIGR Gene Indices	http://www.tigr.org/tdb/tgi/
OMIM	http://www.ncbi.nlm.nih.gov/entrez/query.fcgi?db=OMIM
STACK	http://www.sanbi.ac.za/Dbases.html
Swissprot (published protein sequences, fully annotated)	http://www.expasy.ch/sprot/
DbSNP, JSNP (single nucleotide polymorphism databases)	http://www.ncbi.nlm.nih.gov/SNP/ http://snp.ims.u-tokyo.ac.jp/

Protein databases

General

PIR, PIR-NREF (actual and predicted sequences)	http://pir.georgetown.edu/
SWISS-PROT/TrEMBL (actual and predicted proteins) sequences)	http://www.expasy.ch/sprot/ http://www.ebi.ac.uk/trembl/index.html
PROSITE, SMART (protein database revealing sequence and domain homologies)	http://www.expasy.org/prosite/ http://smart.embl-heidelberg.de/
PDB, SCOP, CATH (databases of 3D protein structures)	http://www.rcsb.org/pdb/ http://scop.mrc-lmb.cam.ac.uk/scop/ http://www.biochem.ucl.ac.uk/bsm/cath_new/index.html

Specific protein families

TRANSFAC (transcription factors)	http://transfac.gbf.de/TRANSFAC/index.html
BRENDA (enzyme information)	http://www.brenda.uni-koeln.de/
GPCRDB (G-protein-coupled receptors, including mutations and binding data)	http://www.gpcr.org
MEROPS (proteolytic enzymes)	http://merops.iapc.bbsrc.ac.uk/
S/MARtDB (scaffold and matrix proteins)	http://transfac.gbf.de/SMARtDB/index.html

Table 7.3
Bioinformatics websites—cont'd

Comparative genomics	
COG (classification of orthologous proteins in different genomes)	http://www.ncbi.nlm.nih.gov/COG/
EuGenes (general information on eukaryotic genes)	http://iubio.bio.indiana.edu:8089/
Genome Information Broker (general information on microbial genomes)	http://gib.genes.nig.ac.jp/
Genome News Network (Regularly updated list of fully sequenced genomes, plus other genome news)	http://www.genomenewsnetwork.org
Comprehensive Microbial Resource, CMR (annotated genomes of microorganisms)	http://www.tigr.org
Gene expression	
BodyMap (tissue-specific expression, mouse, human)	http://bodymap.ims.u-tokyo.ac.jp/
Stanford Microarray Database (compilation of microarray data in various organisms under different experimental conditions)	http://genome-www5.stanford.edu/MicroArray/SMD/
HugeIndex (human gene expression data)	http://www.hugeindex.org/
Mutations	
DbSNP (database of single nucleotide polymorphisms)	http://www.ncbi.nlm.nih.gov/SNP/
OMIM (human genetic diseases)	http://www.ncbi.nlm.nih.gov/Omim/
HGMD (gene lesions underlying human genetic diseases)	http://www.hgmd.org/
TBASE (transgenic animals, mainly mouse)	http://tbase.jax.org/
JAXMICE (details of mouse strains available from Jackson Laboratory)	http://jaxmice.jax.org
Pathways	
BIND, MINT (interactions between biomolecules)	http://www.bind.ca/ http://cbm.bio.uniroma2.it/mint/
DIP (protein–protein interactions)	http://dip.doe-mbi.ucla.edu/
PathDB (pathways)	http://www.ncgr.org/pathdb/

Nucleic acid sequence and genomics database

Nucleotide sequencing is fundamental to modern biology, and the task of collecting all public known nucleotide sequences has been taken over by the International Nucleotide Sequence Database Collaboration (INSD), involving the US National Center for Biotechnology Information (NCBI), the European Bioinformatics Institute and the Japanese National Institute of Genetics. Sequence data are collected worldwide on a daily basis from individual authors or sequencing projects. Complete releases are published frequently and made freely available.

The primary data collected by the INSD serves as input for many other derived databases (Figure 7.3) that organize, curate or transform the sequence data according to a number of principles.

Genbank, which is built and maintained by NCBI, is the most widely used sequence database. In mid-2004 it contained more than 37 million individual sequence records, annotated in a standard format, and over 100 000 species. Genbank is accessible through NCBI's retrieval system Entrez (see above), which integrates DNA, RNA and protein sequence data with genomic, mapping, taxonomy, protein structure data and literature information. Sequence similarity searches in the database can be conducted by the BLAST family of programs.

Genbank aims to be comprehensive, but because it is not highly curated, sequence data can be redundant and of uncertain quality. Data-mining projects based on Genbank sequences have to take account of these limitations.

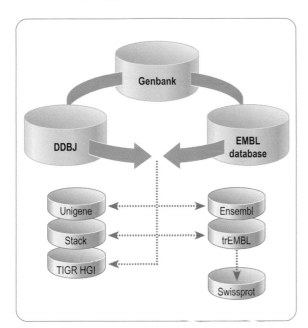

Fig. 7.3
Flow of public sequence data between major sequence repositories. Shown in blue are the components of the International Nucleotide Sequence Database Collaboration (INSDC) comprising Genbank (USA), the European Molecular Biology Laboratory (EMBL) Database (Europe) and the DNA Data Bank of Japan (DDBJ). These databases and some of those derived from them (shown in red) are described in the text.

To overcome these problems, NCBI has created a curated, non-redundant set of reference sequences, **RefSeq**, derived from Genbank.

The **EMBL Nucleotide Sequence Database** (Stoesser et al., 2002) and the **DNA Data Bank of Japan** are the European and Japanese counterparts of Genbank, containing almost identical sequence data and access to similar search and analysis algorithms.

Derived from these primary sequence repositories are many other useful databases, of which a few are shown in red in Figure 7.3.

Unigene, derived from Genbank, contains non-redundant sequences divided into 'clusters', each of which represents a single gene in a particular species. Unigene clusters consist largely of expressed sequence tags (ESTs), which are short stretches of transcribed mRNA sequence from either the 5′ or the 3′ end of the gene. Gene expression profiling experiments generally detect ESTs rather than full length mRNA sequences, and Unigene helps by assigning them to clusters that may allow the parent gene sequence to be identified. Many of the genes are uncharacterized functionally, which makes Unigene a useful resource for the discovery of novel genes.

The large number of ESTs creates a challenge for the computation of clusters, and the number of Unigene clusters considerably overestimates the actual number

of genes and splice variants. Assignments of sequence fragments to Unigene clusters are liable to change as new data are entered, so users of this database need to keep their wits about them.

The **Ensembl** databases are a combined project of the Wellcome Trust Sanger Institute and the European Bioinformatics Institute, the aim being to provide a complete bioinformatics framework, subdivided into databases representing different species.

Ensembl combines genomic DNA, expressed sequence information and computational de novo gene prediction in order to identify genes within the genome sequences, determine gene structures and predict alternative transcripts. All Ensembl genes are extensively annotated: sequence homologies with other database entries are identified, and the predicted genes are classified by protein families, gene ontologies and protein domains. Chromosome mapping data are included, as well as mapping of individual exons and splice sites, and gene entries are cross-referenced to other databases. Valuable features of Ensembl include its web-based user interface, and its extensive graphical viewing capabilities allow for easy navigation across the whole genome, chromosomal overviews, zooming into specific regions, complete evidence records for genes such as nucleotide or protein sequence matches, gene predictions, genetic markers or SNP maps (Figure 7.4).

Stack (Sequence Tag Alignment and Consensus Knowledgebase) is similar to Unigene, but uses different clustering algorithms, resulting in less redundancy.

The Institute for Genomics Research (TIGR) provides another set of organism-specific gene-oriented sequence cluster databases, the **TIGR Gene Indices**, covering (July 2002) 54 animal, plant, protist and fungal species. Another useful resource integrated with the TIGR Indices is **EGO** (Eukaryotic Gene Orthologs), a database that provides instant access to precomputed orthologous genes in eukaryotes.

SwissProt and **TrEMBL** (Figure 7.3) are described below.

The growing catalogue of SNPs representing interindividual differences, which is likely to play a major role in customizing therapies on an individual basis, is accessible as a database – **SNPDB** – maintained by NCBI.

Protein sequence and structure databases

The protein equivalents of Genbank are the SwissProt database (Bairoch and Apweiler, 2000), maintained jointly by the Swiss and European Bioinformatics Institutes, and the **Protein Information Resource** (PIR) database maintained by Georgetown University. SwissProt is a curated protein sequence database containing currently (mid-2004) over 160 000 entries, well annotated in relation to protein domains, functions, splice variants

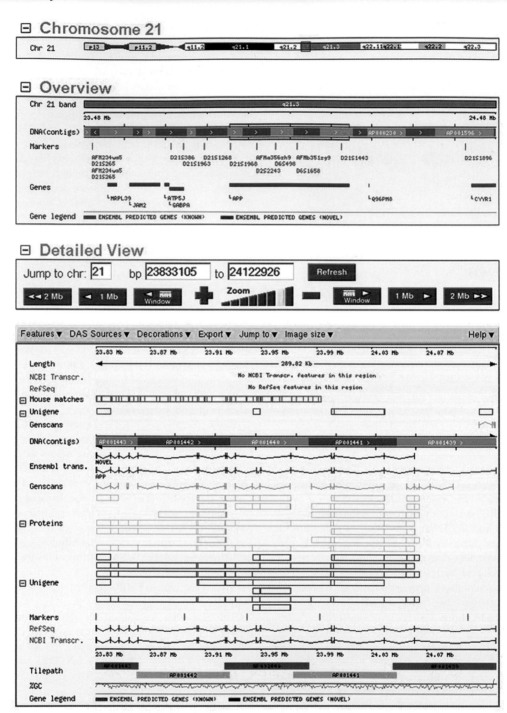

Fig. 7.4
Screenshot from the Ensembl website. Shown is a chromosomal overview and a regional view of chromosome 21 surrounding the gene APP, the Alzheimer's disease amyloid A4 protein precursor. In the detailed view the precise exon–intron structure of the gene is shown, including sequence homology matches to a variety of databases or de novo gene predictions. The viewer is highly customizable and users can easily navigate along the genomic axis.

and post-translational modifications. Associated with it is TrEMBL, which collates *predicted* translations (currently about 1.4 million) of identified DNA coding sequences. **PIR-PSD** and **PIR-NREF** are sequence and

translation databases very similar to SwissProt and TrEMBL.

Information on the possible functions and architecture of novel protein sequences is provided by

Table 7.4
Estimates of genome sizes for selected organisms (data from Ensembl website)

	Species	Genome size (megabases)	Estimated number of genes
Bacteria	*Helicobacter pylori*	1.7	1550
Protozoa	*Plasmodium* (malaria parasite)	23	5300
Invertebrates	*Caenorhabditis elegans*	97	19 099
	Drosophila melanogaster	180	13 600
Vertebrates	*Danio rerio* (zebrafish)	1600	~20 000
	Fugu rubribe (pufferfish)*	400	~30 000
	Mus musculus (mouse)	2700	~30 000
	Homo sapiens (human)	3200	~35 000

*The pufferfish (Fugu) genome is of particular interest, as it includes a similar number of genes (~30 000) to those of other vertebrates, including human, although its genome is only about 1/8 of the size of the human genome. The low proportion of non-coding DNA in this species makes gene identification much easier.

various databases and tools, for example **ProSite** and **SMART**, which reveal sequence homologies with known protein families and domains, and predict their likely topologies.

Databases specifically related to 3D-protein structures include **Protein Data Bank** (PDB), **Structural Classification of Proteins** (SCOP) and **Classification/Architecture/Topology/Homology** (CATH).

There are also many 'boutique' databases, accessible via the general gateways, that provide detailed information on specific protein families, such as antibodies, G-protein-coupled receptors, ion channels, proteases, kinases, transcription factors etc., which are likely to be of particular interest in the context of drug discovery.

Gene and protein expression databases

Gene and protein expression profiling (see Chapter 6) is increasingly being used as a tool to investigate many aspects of biology, such as growth and development, tumorigenesis, immune responses, brain function, drug effects, neurodegeneration, tissue repair, transgene effects, and much else. The data generated are massive in volume and much more heterogeneous than the kind of data discussed above, partly because the quality tends to be inconsistent and different methods do not always give comparable results, and partly because of the great variability in the number and nature of the test conditions that are investigated. Expression databases are therefore more heterogeneous and fragmented than sequence databases. **BodyMap** and **HugeIndex** catalogue expressed genes in various mouse and human tissues, whereas more specialized databases contain expression data relating to pathological disturbances.

Genome analysis

The first genome of a free-living organism, *Haemophilus influenzae*, was fully sequenced in 1995; since then about 180 additional genomes have been finished, and many more are in progress. Most have dedicated websites, which track progress in sequencing, gene identification and functional annotation. Some important ones are listed in Table 7.4. What use can be made of this comparative genomic data in the context of drug discovery?

The comparison of whole genomes can reveal important insights. The conserved order of co-located, adjacent genes may indicate that the genes play a common role in a basic process such as gene expression regulation or chromatin organization, or that they participate in a common biochemical pathway. Comparison of the DNA sequence between species may help in predicting genes where transcription data is lacking and where computational gene prediction is uncertain. Intergenic regions that are highly conserved between closely related species can point to *cis*-acting regulatory elements such as promoters. Comparison of prokaryotic and mammalian genomes can be a guide to new anti-infective drug targets, which are not present in the host. Genes of unknown function which are conserved across evolution may play key physiological roles and can be involved in disease processes in a way yet to be discovered.

Microbial genomes are available in **CMR (Comprehensive Microbial Resource)**, which contains a systematic collection of more than 170 microbial genomes. Other organism-specific genome databases are listed in Table 7.4.

Functional pathways

Linking genes and proteins into functional (as distinct from structural) groups relies greatly on existing knowledge of the enzymes, transporters, transcription factors etc. involved in particular physiological or biochemical processes, and codifying such functional data presents a more difficult informatics challenge than codifying structural data.

A first step is to collate information on molecular interactions involving proteins, nucleotides and small molecules, as these specific interactions are the basis of all biological processes. The **BIND**, **MINT** and **DIP** databases cover this area. The main areas where biochemical knowledge is sufficiently detailed for pathways to be mapped meaningfully at the molecular level, and comprehensive databases created (e.g. **PathDB**, **WIT**), are signal transduction at the cellular level, and intermediary metabolism.

Genetics

Among many resources in this category, two particularly useful ones are **OMIM**, which collates data on inherited diseases in humans, and **TBASE**, which catalogues and describes the rapidly growing number of transgenic animal (mainly mouse) strains that have been produced.

Summary and conclusions

Bioinformatics is one component of the general informatics infrastructure upon which drug discovery now depends. Initially conceived as a way of collating and sharing DNA and protein sequence data, bioinformatics quickly grew to encompass gene organization and protein structure and function. The growth of genomics and other '-omics' disciplines would have been inconceivable without web-based bioinformatics databases and analytical tools.

Sequence-based bioinformatics resources have reached a high level of development, and the procedures for capturing, collating and disseminating new data on a worldwide basis run impressively well. Distinguishing genes within genomic DNA sequences remains a problem, as evidenced by the continuing uncertainty about how many genes are actually present in humans.

Moving from the 'fixed' one-dimensional world of gene and protein sequence to the 'dynamic' multi-dimensional world of function presents a real challenge. Pattern-recognition algorithms of various kinds are an important first step along this road. Using them, we can deduce, for example, that particular genes are present in a highly conserved form in many organisms, whereas others are species specific. We can also recognize characteristic 'domains' in genes and proteins, which allows us to classify them logically. Algorithms for predicting protein structure from sequence already exist, and are being developed to create a further important link to function. Finding out what lies on the surface of a protein molecule, and is therefore accessible to drug molecules, has obvious relevance to drug design.

Profiling gene and protein transcription patterns is a powerful approach to understanding function, but reducing such information to standardized database formats is difficult, mainly because of its inherent complexity and dependence on experimental conditions.

As a final word, bioinformatics now occupies a key role in drug discovery – and indeed the whole of biology – and as computer and Internet technology develop further, its role is set to increase. So, watch this space.

References

Bairoch A, Apweiler R (2000) The SWISS-PROT protein sequence database and its supplement TrEMBL. Nucleic Acids Research 28: 45–48.

Bandara LR, Kennedy S (2002) Toxicoproteomics – a new preclinical tool. Drug Discovery Today 7: 411–418.

Baranzini SL, Elfstrom C, Chang SY et al. (2000) Transcriptional analysis of multiple sclerosis brain lesions reveals a complex pattern of cytokine expression. Journal of Immunology 165: 6576–6582.

Bedell MA, Jenkins NA, Copeland NG (1997a) Mouse models of human disease. Part I: techniques and resources for genetic analysis in mice. Genes and Development 11: 1–10.

Bedell MA, Largaespada DA, Jenkins NA et al. (1997b) Mouse models of human disease: Part II: recent progress and future directions. Genes and Development 11: 11–43.

Burbaum J, Tobel GM (2002) Proteomics in drug discovery. Current Opinion in Chemical Biology 6: 427–433.

Cantor CR, Smith CL (1999) Genomics. the science and technology behind the Human Genome Project. New York: John Wiley and Sons.

Chandra SK, Caldwell JS (2003) Fulfilling the promise: drug discovery in the post-genomic era. Drug Discovery Today 8: 168–174.

Cutler P (2003) Protein arrays: the current state of the art. Proteomics 3: 3–18.

Dopazo J, Zanders E, Dragoni I et al. (2001) Methods and approaches in the analysis of gene expression data. Journal of Immunologic Methods 250: 93–112.

Drews J (2003) Strategic trends in the drug industry. Drug Discovery Today 8: 411–420.

Dwek MV, Rawlings SL (2002) Current perspectives in cancer proteomics. Molecular Biotechnology 22: 139–152.

Frank R, Hargreaves R (2003) Clinical biomarkers in drug discovery and development. Nature Reviews Drug Discovery 2: 566–580.

Friend SH, Stoughton RB (2002) The magic of microarrays. Scientific American February: 44–53.

Greenbaum D, Luscombe NM, Jansen R et al. (2001) Interrelating different types of genomic data, from proteome to secretome: 'oming in on function. Genome Research 11: 1463–1468.

Griffiths A J F, Gelbart W M, Lewontin R C, Wessler S R, Suzuki D T, Miller J H (2000) Introduction to genetic analysis, 7th Ed. W H Freeman, New York

Harrison PJ, Owen MJ (2003) Genes for schizophrenia? Recent findings and their pathophysiological implications. Lancet 361: 417–419.

Hunt SP, Livesey FJ, eds. (2000) Functional genomics. Practical approach. Oxford: Oxford University Press.

International Human Genome Sequencing Consortium (2004) Finishing the euchromatic sequence of the human genome. Nature 431: 931–945.

Jeffrey DA, Bogyo M (2003) Chemical proteomics and its application to drug discovery. Current Opinion in Biotechnology 14: 87–95.

Kennedy S (2002) The role of proteomics in toxicology: identification of biomarkers of toxicity by protein expression analysis. Biomarkers 7: 269–290.

Kim V N (2003) RNA interference in functional genomics and medicine. Journal of Korean Medical Science 18: 309–318.

Kramer R, Cohen D (2004) Functional genomics to new drug targets. Nature reviews Drug Discovery 3: 965–972.

Krane D, Raymer M (2002) Fundamental concepts of bioinformatics. San Francisco: Benjamin Cummings.

Lacroix Z, Critchlow T (eds) (2003) Bioinformatics: managing scientific data. San Francisco: Morgan Kaufmann.

Lander ES, Linton LM, Birren B et al. (2001) Initial sequencing and analysis of the human genome. Nature 409: 860–921.

Latchman DS (2002) Gene regulation: a eukaryotic perspective. Cheltenham: Thomas Nelson.

Lee J, Nam S, Hwang SB et al. (2004) Functional genomic approaches using the nematode *Caenorhabditis elegans* as a model system. Journal of Biochemistry and Molecular Biology 37: 107–113.

Lengauer T (ed) (2002) Bioinformatics: methods and principles in medicinal chemistry. Chichester: John Wiley.

Lesk A M (2002) Introduction to bioinformatics. Oxford: Oxford University Press.

Letovsky S (ed) (1999) Bioinformatics: databases and sytems. Amsterdam: Kluwer Academic.

Liggett SB (2000) The pharmacogenetics of beta2-adrenergic receptors: relevance to asthma. Journal of Allergy and Clinical Immunology 105: 487–492.

Lindpaintner K (2002) The impact of pharmacogenetics and pharmacogenomics on drug discovery. Nature Reviews Drug Discovery 1: 463–469.

Liu BH (1998) Statistical genomics. Linkage, mapping, and QTL analysis. Boca Raton, FL: CRC Press.

Maelicke A, Lubbert H (2002) DEPD, a high resolution gene expression profiling technique capable of identifying new drug targets in the central nervous system. J Recept Signal Transduct Res. 22: 283–295.

Marshall A, Hodgson J (1998) DNA chips: an array of possibilities. Nature Biotechnology 16: 27–31.

McLeod HL, Yu J (2003) Cancer pharmacogenomics: SNPs, chips, and the individual patient. Cancer Investigation 21: 630–640.

Michaud GA, Snyder M (2002) Proteomic approaches for the global analysis of proteins. Biotechniques 33: 1308–1316.

Mitchell P (2002) A perspective on protein microarrays. Nature Biotechnology 20: 225–229.

Munder T, Hinnen A (1999) Yeast cells as tools for target-oriented screening. Applied Microbiology Biotechnology 52: 311–320.

Offermanns S, Hein L (eds) (2004) Transgenic models in pharmacology. Handbook of experimental pharmacology. Vol 159. Berlin: Springer-Verlag.

Pinkert CA (2002) Transgenic animal technology. London: Academic Press.

Powell J (2000) SAGE. The serial analysis of gene expression. Methods in Molecular Biology 99: 297–319 .

Quackenbusch J (2001) Computational analysis of microarray data. Nature Reviews Genetics 2: 418–427.

Ramsay G (1998) DNA chips: state of the art. Nature Biotechnology 16: 40–44.

Riordan J R, Rommens JM, Kerem B et al. (1989) Identification of the cystic fibrosis gene: cloning and characterization of complementary DNA. Science 245: 1066–1073.

Rocchi A, Pellegrini S, Siciliano G, Murri L (2003) Causative and susceptibility genes for Alzheimer's disease: a review. Brain Research Bulletin 61: 1–24.

Schafer AJ, Hawkins JR (1998) DNA variation and the future of human genetics. Nature Biotechnology 16: 33–39.

Scriver CR (2001) The metabolic and molecular bases of inherited disease, 8th edn. New York: McGraw-Hill.

Stoesser G, Baker W, van den Broek A et al. (2002) The EMBL nucleotide sequence database. Nucleic Acids Research 30: 21–26.

Thorisson GA, Stein LD (2002) The SNP consortium website: past present and future, Nucleic Acids Research 31: 124–127.

Tribut O, Lessard Y, Reymann JM et al. (2002) Pharmacogenomics. Medical Science Monitor 8: 152–163.

Valafar F (2002) Pattern recognition techniques in microarray data analysis. Annals of the New York Academy of Sciences 980: 41–64.

Valdes R, Linder MW, Jortani SA (2003) What is next in pharmacogenomics? Translating it into clinical practice. Pharmacogenomics 4: 499–505.

Velculescu V, Zhang L, Vogelstein B, Kirzler K (1995) Serial analysis of gene expression. Science 270: 484–487.

Venter JC, Adams MD, Myers EW et al. (2001) The sequence of the human genome. Science 291: 1304–1351.

Virlon B, Cheval L, Buhler JM, Billon E, Doucet A, Elalouf JM (1999) Serial microanalysis of renal transcriptomes. Proceedings of the National Academy of Sciences of the USA 96: 15286–15291.

Weinshilboum R (2003) Inheritance and drug response. New England Journal of Medicine 348: 529–537.

Wulfkuhle JD, Liotta LA, Petricoin EF (2003) Proteomic applications for the early detection of cancer. Nature Reviews Cancer 3: 267–275.

8 High-throughput screening

K Stoeckli
H Haag

Introduction: a historical and future perspective

Systematic drug research began about 100 years ago, when chemistry had reached a degree of maturity that allowed its principles and methods to be applied to problems outside the field, and when pharmacology had in turn become a well-defined scientific discipline. A key step was the introduction of the concept of selective affinity through the postulation of 'chemoreceptors' by Paul Ehrlich. He was the first to argue that differences in chemoreceptors between species may be exploited therapeutically. This was also the birth of chemotherapy. In 1907, Ehrlich tested 605 compounds and finally identified number 606, salvarsan (diamino-dioxy-arsenobenzene), which was brought to the market in 1910 by Hoechst for the treatment of syphilis, and hailed as a miracle drug (Figure 8.1).

This was the first time extensive pharmaceutical screening had been used to find drugs. At that time

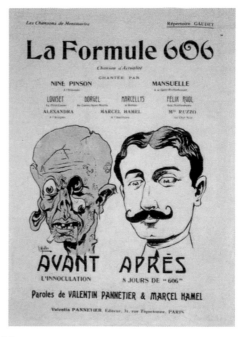

Fig. 8.1
In France, where Salvarsan was called 'Formule 606', true miracles were expected from the new therapy.

screening was based on phenotypic readouts (antimicrobial effect), a concept which has since led to unprecedented therapeutic triumphs in anti-infective and anticancer therapies, based particularly on natural products. In contrast, today's screening is largely driven by distinct molecular targets and relies on biochemical readout.

In the further course of the 20th century drug research became influenced primarily by biochemistry. The dominant concepts introduced by biochemistry were those of enzymes and receptors, which were empirically found to be drug targets. In 1948 Ahlquist made a crucial, further step by proposing the existence of two types of adrenoceptor (α and β) in most organs. The principle of receptor classification has been the basis for a large number of diverse drugs, including β-adrenoceptor agonists and antagonists, benzodiazepines, angiotensin antagonists, and ultimately monoclonal antibodies.

All today's marketed drugs are believed to target about 120 human biomolecules (see Chapter 6), ranging from various enzymes and transporters to G-protein-coupled receptors (GPCRs) and ion channels. At present the GPCRs are the predominant target family, and more than 600 genes encoding these biomolecules have been identified in the human genome (Hopkins and Groom, 2002). Although the target portfolio of a pharmaceutical company can change from time to time, the newly chosen targets are likely to belong still to one of the main therapeutic target classes. The selection of targets and target families (see Chapter 6) plays a pivotal role determining the success of today's lead molecule discovery.

Over the last 10 years significant technological progress has been achieved in genomic sciences (Chapter 7), high-throughput medicinal chemistry (Chapter 9), cell-based assays and high-throughput screening. These have led to a 'new' concept in drug discovery. Hypothetical targets are incorporated into biochemical or cell-based assays which are exposed to large numbers of compounds, each representing a given chemical structure space. Massively parallel screening, called high-throughput screening (HTS), was first introduced by pharmaceutical companies in the early 1990s and is now a routine process. HTS is the most widely applicable technology for identifying chemistry starting points for drug discovery programmes.

Nevertheless, HTS remains only one of the possible lead discovery strategies (see Chapter 9). In the best case it can provide an efficient way to obtain useful data on the biological activity of large numbers of test samples by using high-quality assays and high-quality chemical compounds. Today's lead discovery departments are typically composed of the following units: (1) compound logistics; (2) assay development; (3) automated screening; (4) tool production; and (5) profiling. In addition, some companies are interested in exploring natural products and thus have dedicated research departments, which work closely with HTS groups.

Compared with HTS in the 1990s there is now much more focus on quality-oriented output. At first, screening throughput was the main emphasis, but it is now only one of many performance indicators. In the 1990s the primary concern of a company's compound logistics group was to collect all its historic compound collections in sufficient quantities and of sufficient quality to file them by electronic systems, and store them in the most appropriate way in compound archives. This resulted in huge collections that range from several hundred thousand to a few million compounds. Today's focus has shifted to the application of defined electronic or physical filters for compound selection, before they are assembled into a library for testing. The result is a customized ensemble of either newly designed or historic compounds for use in screening, otherwise known as 'cherry picking'.

In assay development there is a clear trend towards mechanistically driven high-quality assays that capture the relevant biochemistry (e.g. stochiometry, kinetics) or cell biology. Homogeneous assay principles, along with sensitive detection technologies, have enabled the miniaturization of assay formats. Even subcellular resolution can be achieved with today's imaging technology. This in turn has led to high-content screening (HCS) methods which allow the study of intracellular pharmacology through spatiotemporal resolution, and the quantification of signalling and regulatory pathways.

In automated screening there is a clear trend away from large linear-track 'production line' robotics towards integrated networks of workstation-based instrumentation. Typically, the screening unit of a large pharmaceutical company will generate tens of millions of single point determinations per year, with fully automated data acquisition and processing. Following primary screening, there has been an increasing need for secondary/complementary screening to confirm the primary results and to refine them further. Typical data formats include half-maximal concentrations at which a compound causes a defined modulatory effect in functional assays, or binding/inhibitory constants. Recently, post-HTS selectivity profiling has been introduced, active compounds being profiled on panels of related target families. Data harmonization and standardization play a crucial role when it comes to data analysis and data mining. In the past, lead-finding activities were mainly directed towards seeking maximal potency and selectivity irrespective of molecular properties and compound suitability. On the other hand, it is well recognized that a proportion of compounds identified and confirmed as active from HTS, often do not turn out to be suitable for the initiation of further medicinal chemistry exploration. Many do not fulfil certain quality criteria, and so quality assessment at all key points in the discovery process is crucial. Late-stage attrition of drug candidates, particularly in development and beyond, is extremely expensive and such failures must be kept to a minimum. This is typically done by an extensive assessment of chemical integrity, synthetic accessibility, functional properties, structure–activity relationship (SAR) and biophysicochemical properties, and related absorption, distribution, metabolism and excretion (ADME) characteristics, as discussed further in Chapter 10.

In summary, significant technological progress has been made over the last 10 years in HTS. Major concepts such as automation, miniaturization and parallelization have been introduced in almost all areas and steps of the lead discovery process. This has led to a great increase in screening capacities, to significant savings in compound or reagent consumption, and ultimately to improved cost-effectiveness. More recently, stringent quality assessment in library management and assay development, along with data harmonization in automated screening, has led to much higher-quality screening outcomes. The future HTS will be even more information driven than it has been to date (Figure 8.2). Various statistical, informatics and filtering methods have recently been introduced to foster the integration of experimental and in silico screening, and so maximize the output in lead discovery. As a result, future lead-finding activities will benefit greatly from a more unified and knowledge-based approach to biological screening, in addition to the many technical advances towards even higher-throughput screening.

Lead discovery and high-throughput screening

A lead compound is generally defined as a new chemical entity that could potentially be developed into a new drug by optimizing its beneficial effects and minimizing its side effects (see Chapter 9 for a more detailed discussion of the criteria). High-throughput screening (HTS) is currently the main approach for the identification of lead compounds. In a random approach large numbers of compounds are tested for their biological activity against a disease-relevant target. However, there are other techniques in place for lead discovery that are complementary to HTS.

Besides the conventional literature search (identification of compounds already described for the desired activity), structure-based virtual screening is an evolving technique (Lyne, 2002). Molecular recognition events are simulated by computational techniques based on knowledge of the molecular target and, by applying this information, pharmacophore models can be developed. These allow the identification of potential leads in silico, without experimental screening. Similarly, X-ray analysis of the target can be applied to guide the de novo synthesis and design of bioactive molecules.

Typically, in HTS, large compound libraries are screened ('primary' screen) and numerous bioactive compounds ('primary hits' or 'positives') are identified. These compounds are taken through successive, further screening ('secondary' screens) to confirm their potency. Once a handful of leads has been identified they are advanced into the 'lead optimization' process, during which the drug-like properties (e.g. specificity, pharmacokinetics or bioavailability) are further improved by medicinal chemistry (Figure 8.3).

HTS is multidisciplinary and has to integrate many different functions, which are all critical to the success of drug discovery programmes: assay development, reagent preparation (protein expression and purification), high-throughput library screening, compound management and informatics (Figure 8.4).

Assay development and validation

The target validation process (see Chapter 6) establishes the relevance of a target in a certain disease pathway. In the next step an assay has to be developed, allowing the

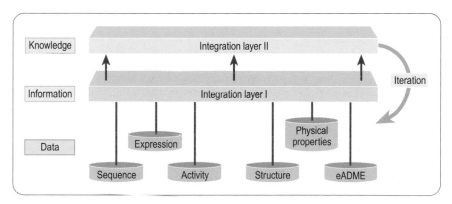

Fig. 8.2
Future lead discovery will be information driven.

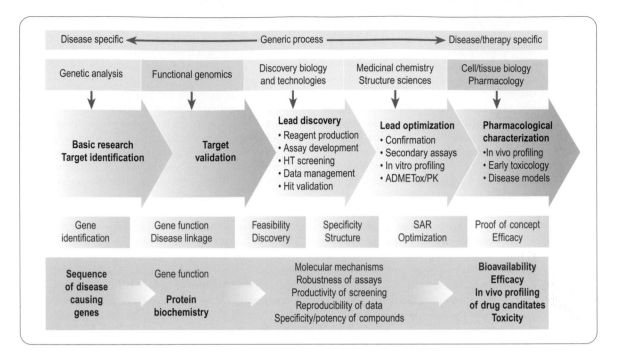

Fig. 8.3
The drug discovery process.

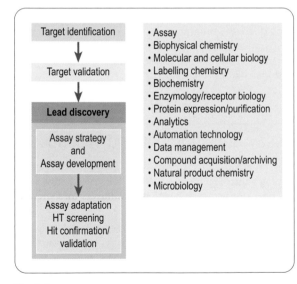

Fig. 8.4
Lead discovery and skills.

quantification of the interaction of molecules with the chosen target. This interaction can be inhibition, stimulation, or simply binding. There are numerous different assay technologies available, and the choice for a specific assay type will always be determined by factors such as type of target, sensitivity, robustness, ease of automation and cost. Assays can be carried out in different formats based on 96-, 384- or 1536-well microtitre plates.

The format to be applied depends on various parameters, e.g. readout, desired throughput, or existing hardware in liquid handling and signal detection. In all cases the homogeneous type of assay is preferred, as it is quicker, easier to handle and cost-effective, allowing 'mix and measure' operation without any need for further separation steps.

Next to scientific criteria, cost is a key factor in assay development. The choice of format has a significant effect on the total cost per data point: the use of 384 low-volume microtitre plates instead of a 96-well plate format results in a significant reduction of the reaction volume. This reduction correlates directly with costs per well. The size of a typical screening library is between 500 000 and 1 million compounds. Costs per well can easily vary between US$0.05 and more than U$0.5 per data point, depending on the type and format of the assay. Therefore, screening an assay with a 500 k library will cost either US$25 000 or US$250 000, depending on the selected assay design – a significant difference!

Once a decision on the principal format and readout technology is taken, the assay has to be validated for its sensitivity and robustness. Biochemical parameters, reagents and screening hardware (e.g. detectors, microtitre plates) must be optimized. To give a practical example, in a typical screen designed for inhibitors of protease activity, test compounds are mixed together with the enzyme and finally substrate is added. The substrate consists of a cleavable peptide linked to a fluorescent label, and the reaction is quantified by measuring the change in fluoresecence intensity that accompanies the enzymic cleavage. In the process of validation, the best available labelled substrate (natural or synthetic) must be selected, the reaction conditions optimized (for example reaction time, buffers and temperature), enzyme kinetic measurements performed to identify the linear range, and the response of the assay to known inhibitors (if available) tested. Certain types of compound or solvent (which in most cases will be dimethylsulfoxide, DMSO) may interfere with the assay readout and this has to be checked. As some assay formats require a long incubation time the stability of assay reagents is an important parameter to be determined during assay validation.

At this point other aspects of screening logistics have to be considered. If the enzyme is not available commercially it has to be produced in-house by process development, and batch-to-batch reproducibility and timely delivery have to be ensured. With cell-based screens it must be guaranteed that the cell production facility is able to deliver sufficient quantities of consistently functioning, physiologically intact cells during the whole screening campaign.

The principal goal of developing HTS assays is the fast and reliable identification of active compounds ('positives' or 'hits') from chemical libraries. Most HTS programmes test compounds at only one concentration. In order to identify hits with confidence, only small variations in signal measurements can be tolerated. The statistical parameters used to determine the suitability of assays for HTS are the calculation of standard deviations, the coefficient of variation (CV), signal-to-noise (S/N) ratio or signal-to-background (S/B) ratio. The inherent problem with using these last two is that neither takes into account the dynamic range of the signal (i.e. the difference between the background (low control) and the maximum (high control) signal), or the variability in the sample and reference control measurements. A more reliable assessment of assay quality is achieved by the z'-factor equation (Zhang et al., 1999):

$$z' = 1 - \frac{3 \,(\text{SD of high control}) + 3 \,(\text{SD of low control})}{[\text{mean of high control} - \text{mean of low control}]}$$

where SD = standard deviation. The maximum possible value of z is 1: a value greater than 0.5 represents a good assay whereas a value less than 0.5 is generally unsatisfactory for HTS.

This equation takes into account that the quality of an assay is reflected in the variability of the high and low controls, and the separation band between them (Figure 8.5). z'-Factors are obtained by measuring plates containing 50% low controls (in our protease example: assay plus reference inhibitor, minimum signal to be measured) and 50% high controls (assay without inhibitor; maximum signal to be measured). In addition inter- and intra-plate coefficients of variation (CV) are determined to check for systematic sources of variation. All measurements are normally made in triplicate. Once an assay has passed these quality criteria it can be transferred to the robotic screening laboratory.

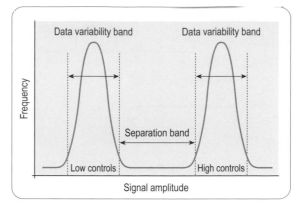

Fig. 8.5
Illustration of data variability and the signal window, given by the separation band between high and low controls.

Biochemical and cell-based assays

There are two major types of assay used in HTS, **biochemical** and **cell-based**.

Biochemical assays (Figure 8.6) involve the use of cell-free in vitro systems to model the biochemistry of a subset of cellular processes. The assay systems vary from simple interactions, such as enzyme/substrate reactions, receptor binding or protein–protein interactions, to more complex models such as in vitro transcription systems. In contrast to cell-based assays, biochemical assays give direct information on the nature of the molecular interaction (e.g. kinetic data). However, biochemical assays lack the cellular context, and are insensitive to properties such as membrane permeability, which determine the effects of compounds on intact cells.

Unlike biochemical assays, cell-based assays (Figure 8.7) mimic more closely the in vivo situation and can be adapted for targets that are not suited for screening in biochemical assays, such as those involving signal transduction pathways, membrane transport, cell division cytotoxicity or antibacterial actions. Parameters measured in cell-based assays range from growth, transcriptional activity, changes in cell metabolism or morphology to changes in the level of an intracellular messengers such as cAMP (Moore and Rees, 2001). Importantly, cell-based assays are able to distinguish between receptor antagonists and agonists, which cannot be done by measuring binding affinity in a biochemical assay.

Many cell-based assays have quite complex protocols, for example removing cell culture media, washing cells, adding compounds to be tested, prolonged incubation at 37°C, and finally reading the cellular response. Therefore, screening with cell-based assays requires a sophisticated infrastructure in the screening laboratory (including cell cultivation facilities, and robotic systems equipped to maintain physiological conditions during the assay procedure) and the throughput is generally lower.

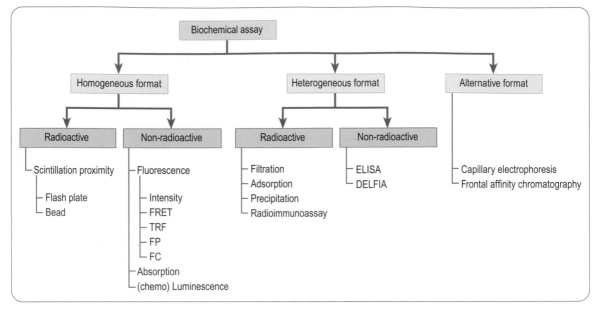

Fig. 8.6
Types of biochemical assay.

Cell-based assays frequently lead to higher hit rates, because of non-specific and 'off-target' effects of test compounds that affect the readout. Primary hits therefore need to be assessed by means of secondary assays in order to determine the mechanism of the effect (Moore and Rees, 2001).

Although cell-based assays are generally more troublesome than cell-free assays to set up and run in high-throughput mode, there are many situations in which they are needed. For example, assays involving membrane transporters and ion channels generally require intact cells, or at least membranes prepared from intact cells. In other cases, the production of biochemical

targets such as enzymes in sufficient quantities for screening may be difficult or costly compared to cell-based assays directed at the same targets. The main pros and cons of cell-based assays are summarized in Table 8.1.

Assay readout and detection

Radioactive assays

Assays based on radiolabelled compounds are sensitive and robust and are widely used for ligand-binding assays. The assay is based on measuring the ability of the test compound to inhibit the binding of a radiolabelled ligand to the target, and requires that the assay can distinguish between bound and free forms of the radioligand. This can be done by physical separation of bound from unbound ligand (*heterogeneous* format) by filtration, adsorption or centrifugation. The need for several washing steps makes it unsuitable for fully automated HTS, and generates large volumes of radioactive waste, raising safety and cost concerns over storage and disposal. Such assays are mainly restricted to 96-well format.

In recent years *homogeneous* formats for radioactive assays have been developed and are replacing heterogeneous assays. Reducing the overall reaction volume and eliminating separation steps reduces the problem of waste disposal and increases throughput.

The majority of homogenous radioactive assay types are based on the scintillation proximity principle. This relies on the excitation of a scintillant incorporated in a matrix, in the form of either *microbeads* ('SPA') or *microplates* ('FlashPlate'; Picardo and Hughes, 1997), to

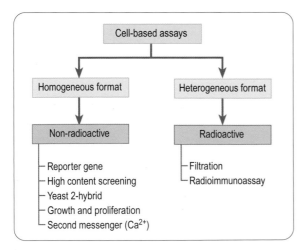

Fig. 8.7
Types of cell-based assay.

Table 8.1
Advantages and disadvantages of cell-based assays

Advantages	Disadvantages
Cytotoxic compounds are detected and eliminated at the outset	Require high-capacity cell culture facilities and more complex robotics to control long incubations
In receptor studies, agonists can be distinguished from antagonists	Often require specially engineered cell lines
Binding and different functional readouts can be used in parallel – high information content	Cells liable to become detached from support
They can be used for screening when the molecular target is unknown (e.g. to detect compounds that affect cell division, growth, differentiation or metabolism)	High rate of false positives due to non-specific effects of test compounds on cell function
	More difficult to miniaturize
	Assay conditions (e.g. use of solvents, pH) limited by cell viability

the surface of which the target molecule is also attached (Figure 8.8). Binding of the radioligand to the target brings it into close proximity to the scintillant, resulting in light emission, which can be quantified. Unbound radioactivity is too distant from the scintillant and no excitation takes place. Isotopes such as ^{3}H or ^{125}I are typically used, as they produce low-energy particles that are absorbed over short distances (Cook, 1996). Test compounds that bind to the target compete with the radioligand, and thus reduce the signal.

With bead technology (Figure 8.8A), polymer beads of ~5 μm diameter are coated with antibodies, streptavidin, receptors or enzymes (Beveridge et al., 2000; Bosworth and Towers, 1989). Ninety-six- or 384-well plates can be used. Limitations are the sensitivity to colour quench by test compounds, and the variable efficiency of scintillation counting, due to sedimentation of the beads.

LEADseeker (Amersham Bioscience) is a variation of the scintillation proximity principle that uses a quantitative imaging system to scan the whole plate, resulting in a higher throughput and increased sensitivity. A CCD camera is used instead of a scintillation counter, for detection of the light emitted, together with modified beads containing europium yttrium oxide or europium polystyrene as scintillants. LEADseeker assays have been developed successfully in 1536-well format (Sorg et al., 2002).

In microplate assays (Figure 8.8B) the target protein (e.g. an antibody or receptor) is coated on to the floor of a plate well to which the radioligand and test compounds are added. The bound radioligand causes a microplate surface scintillation effect (Brown et al., 1997). Flash Plate has been used in the investigation of protein–protein (e.g. radioimmunoassay) and receptor–ligand (i.e. radioreceptor assay) interactions (Birzin and Rohrer, 2002), and in enzymatic (e.g. kinase) assays (Braunwaler et al., 1996). Applicable formats are 96- or 384-well, which allow middle-range throughput, but costs per well are high.

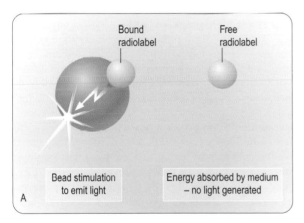

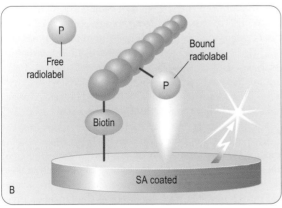

Fig. 8.8
Principle of scintillation proximity assays. (a) Bead format. (b) Plate format.

Fluorescence technologies

In recent years more and more radioactive assays have been replaced by fluorescence assays (Sittampalam et al., 1997; Hemmilä and Webb, 1997).

The simplest fluorescence techniques involve excitation of a sample with light at one wavelength and measurement of the emission at a different wavelength. The difference between the absorbed wavelength and the emitted wavelength is called the *Stokes shift*, the magnitude of which depends on how much energy is lost in the fluorescence process (Lakowizc, 1999). A large Stokes shift is advantageous as it reduces optical crosstalk between photons from the excitation light and emitted photons.

Fluorescence techniques currently applied for HTS can be grouped into five major categories:

- Fluorescence intensity
- Fluorescence resonance energy transfer
- Time-resolved fluorescence
- Fluorescence polarization
- Fluorescence correlation.

Fluorescence intensity

In fluorescence intensity assays the change of total light output is monitored and used to quantify the biochemical reaction. This type of readout is frequently used in enzymatic assays (e.g. proteases, lipases). There are two variants: *fluorogenic assays* and *fluorescence quench assays*. In the former type the reactants are not fluorescent but the reaction products are, and their formation can be monitored by an increase in fluorescence intensity.

In fluorescence quench assays a fluorescent group is covalently linked to a substrate. In this state, its fluorescence is quenched. Upon cleavage the fluorescent group is released, producing an increase in fluorescence intensity (Haugland, 2002).

Fluorescence intensity measurements are easy to run and cheap. However, they are sensitive to fluorescent interference resulting from the colour of test compounds, organic fluorophores in assay buffers, and even fluorescence of the microplate itself (Wedin, 1999).

Fluorescence resonance energy transfer (FRET)

In this type of assay (Figure 8.9) a *donor* fluorophore is excited, most of the energy being transferred to an *acceptor* fluorophore, resulting in photon emission by the acceptor. The amount of energy transfer from donor to acceptor depends on the fluorescent lifetime of the donor, the distance between donor and acceptor (10–100 Å), and the dipole orientation between donor and acceptor. The transfer efficiency can be calculated using the equation of Förster (Clegg, 1995).

Usually the emission wavelengths of donor and acceptor are different, and FRET can be determined either by the quenching of the donor fluorescence by the acceptor or by the fluorescence of the acceptor itself.

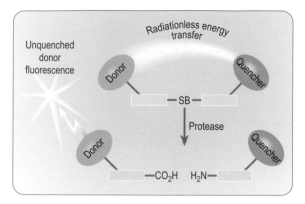

Fig. 8.9
Protease assay based on FRET. The donor fluorescence is quenched by the neighbouring acceptor molecule. Cleavage of the substrate separates them, allowing fluorescent emission by the donor molecule.

Typical applications are for protease assays based on quenching of the uncleaved substrate. With simple FRET techniques interference from background fluorescence is often a problem, which is largely overcome by the use of time-resolved fluorescence techniques, described below.

Time resolved fluorescence (TRF)

TRF techniques (Hemmilä and Webb, 1997) use lanthanide chelates (samarium, europium, terbium and dysprosium) that give an intense and long-lived fluorescence emission (>1000 µs). Fluorescence emission is elicited by a pulse of excitation and measured after the end of the pulse, by which time short-lived fluorescence has subsided. This makes it possible to eliminate short-lived autofluorescence and reagent background, and thereby enhance the signal-to-noise ratio. Lanthanides emit fluorescence with a large Stokes shift when they coordinate to specific ligands. Typically, the complexes are excited by UV light, and emit light of wavelength longer than 500 nm.

Europium (Eu^{3+}) chelates have been used in immunoassays by means of a technology called DELFIA (dissociation-enhanced lanthanide fluoroimmuno assay). DELFIA is a heterogeneous time-resolved fluorometric assay based on *dissociative fluorescence enhancement*. Cell- and membrane-based assays are particularly well suited to the DELFIA system because of its broad detection range and extremely high sensitivity (Valenzano et al., 2000).

High sensitivity – to a limit of about 10^{-17} moles/well – is achieved by applying the dissociative enhancement principle. After separation of the bound from the free label, a reagent is added to the bound label which causes the weakly fluorescent lanthanide chelate to dissociate and form a new highly fluorescent chelate inside a protective micelle. Though robust and very sensitive, DELFIA assays are not ideal for HTS, as the process involves several binding, incubation and washing steps.

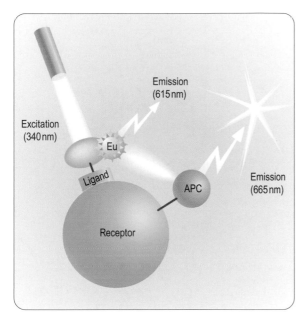

Fig. 8.10
HTRF assay type: the binding of a europium-labelled ligand
(= donor) to the allophycocyanine (APC = acceptor)-labelled receptor
brings the donor–acceptor pair into close proximity and energy
transfer takes place, resulting in fluorescence emission at 665 nm.

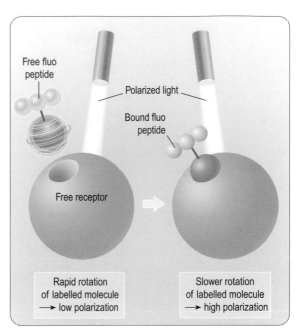

Fig. 8.11
Principle of fluorescence polarization assays.

The need for homogeneous ('mix and measure')
assays led to the development of LANCE (Perkin Elmer
Life Sciences) and HTRF (Homogeneous Time-Resolved
Fluorescence; Cisbio). LANCE, like DELFIA, is based on
chelates of lanthanide ions, but in a homogeneous
format. The chelates used in LANCE can be measured
directly without the need for a dissociation step.
However, in an aqueous environment the complexed
ion can spontaneously dissociate and increase background fluorescence (Alpha et al., 1987).

In HTRF (Figure 8.10) these limitations are overcome
by the use of a *cryptate* molecule, which has a cage-like
structure, to protect the central ion (e.g. Eu$^+$) from dissociation. HTRF uses two separate labels, the donor (Eu)K
and the acceptor APC/XL665 (a modified allophycocyanine from red algae).

In both LANCE and HTRF, measurement of the ratio
of donor and acceptor fluorophore emission can be
applied to compensate for non-specific quenching of
assay reagents. HTRF assays can be adapted for use in
plates up to 1536-well format. The variants and applications of these methods are discussed by Hemmilä and
Webb (1997) and Hemmilä and Hurskainen (2002).

Fluorescence polarization (FP)
When a stationary molecule is excited with plane-
polarized light it will fluoresce in the same plane. If it is
tumbling rapidly, in free solution, so that it changes its
orientation between excitation and emission, the emission signal will be depolarized. Binding to a larger molecule reduces the mobility of the fluorophore so that the
emission signal remains polarized, and so the ratio
of polarized to depolarized emission can be used to
determine the extent of binding of a labelled ligand
(Figure 8.11; Nasir and Jolley, 1999). The rotational relax-
ation speed depends on the size of the molecule, the
ambient temperature and the viscosity of the solvent,
which usually remain constant during an assay.

The method requires a significant difference in size
between labelled ligand and target, which is a major
restriction to its application. FP-based assays can be
used in 96-well up to 1536-well formats.

Fluorescence correlation methods
The most widely applied readout technology, *fluorescence correlation spectroscopy*, allows molecular interactions to be studied at the single-molecule level in real
time (Figure 8.12), allowing analysis of biomolecules
at extremely low concentrations. In contrast to other
fluorescence techniques, the parameter of interest is not
the emission intensity itself, but rather intensity fluctuations. By confining measurements to a very small detection volume, achieved by the use of confocal optics, and
low reagent concentrations, the number of molecules
monitored is kept small, and the statistical fluctuations
of the number contributing to the fluorescence signal at
any instant become measurable. Analysis of the frequency components of such fluctuations can be used
to obtain information about the kinetics of binding

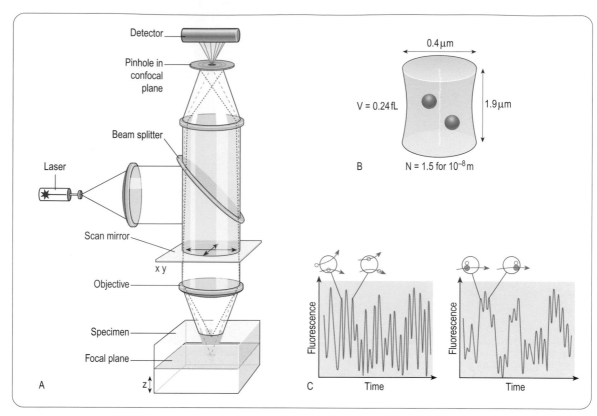

Fig. 8.12
Principle of fluorescence correlation method for single molecules. (A) Optical system. (B) Detection volume. (C) Physical origins of fluorescence correlation spectroscopy data. Free fluorescent ligands move in and out of the detecting volume (open circle) and are detected as a series of short, randomized fluorescence bursts (left panel). Macromolecule-bound ligands are less mobile, producing a more slowly fluctuating (i.e. more highly autocorrelated) time-dependent fluorescence pattern (right panel).

reactions. For example, binding of a fluorescently labelled ligand to its target will increase its effective molecular weight and thus reduce its diffusion coefficient, and increase the average time for which the molecule remains within the detection volume. Intensity fluctuations associated with bound label will therefore occur at lower frequencies than those of unbound label, allowing the ratio of bound to unboundlabel to be determined. Recording photon bursts in a time-resolved manner following a brief pulse of excitation by a laser light source can also be used.

Single molecule detection

Standard fluorescence measurement techniques capture the overall fluorescence of entire ensembles of molecules. These types of signal, no matter whether intensity or anisotropy is measured, represent the total of specific signals and are subject to interference of many kinds (inner filter effects, quenching, autofluorescence, light scattering, photobleaching) that can contribute to fluorescence noise. With help of the confocal microscopy technique and laser technologies, it has become possible to measure molecular interactions at single molecule level. Single molecule detection (SMD) technologies

provide a number of advantages: significant reduction of signal-to-noise ratio, high sensitivity and time-resolution. Furthermore they enable the simultaneous readout of various fluorescence parameters at the molecular level. SMD readouts include fluorescence intensity, translational diffusion (fluorescence correlation spectroscopy, FCS), rotational motion (fluorescence polarization), fluorescence resonance energy transfer, and time-resolved fluorescence. SMD technologies are ideal for miniaturization and have become amenable to automation (Moore et al., 1999). Further advantages include very low reagent consumption and broad applicability to a variety of biochemical and cell-based assays.

Single molecular events are analysed by means of confocal optics with a detection volume of approximately 1 fL (Figure 8.12A), allowing miniaturization of HTS assays to 1 μL or below. The probability is that, at any given time, the detection volume will have a finite number of molecular events (movement, intensity, change in anisotropy), which can be measured and computed. The signal-to-noise ratio typically achieved by these methods is high, while interference from scattered laser light and background fluorescence are largely eliminated (Eigen and Rigler, 1994).

The most widely applied readout technology, *fluorescence correlation spectroscopy*, allows molecular interactions to be studied at the single-molecule level in real-time (see below). In essence it is a high-resolution spatial and temporal analysis of biomolecules at extremely low concentrations. In contrast to other fluorescence techniques, the parameter of interest is not the emission intensity itself, but rather intensity fluctuations (see above).

An ideal reaction system consists of one small labelled ligand and a comparatively large, non-fluorescent counterpart. Diffusion coefficients will change on binding events between the ligand and its receptor, as the mass ratio will change. More recently proprietary 2D fluorescence intensity distribution analysis (2D-FIDA) of anisotropy (Kask et al., 2000) and liquid handling technology has been described (Wright et al., 2002). This technology platform was used in a kinase assay to measure fluorescence polarization (FP) on the single microlitre scale. The steady-state kinetic parameters derived from this assay format correlated well with those generated using a radiometric assay. 2D-FIDA anisotropy provides superior performance statistics (typical $z' = \sim 0.5$) relative to conventional FP (typical $z' = 0.3$) and enables very cost-effective drug screening.

Fluorescence cross-correlation spectroscopy (FCCS) differs from FCS in that two detection channels and laser systems are used, allowing the monitoring of two spectrally different fluorescent groups at one time. FCCS, using different labelled molecules, can be used to elucidate inhibitory mechanisms and to measure association/dissociation or enzyme kinetics. By applying FCCS, Kettling et al. (1998) demonstrated the characterization of enzyme kinetics at extremely low enzyme concentrations (>1.6 pm). Different types of single molecule detection are summarized in Table 8.2.

Cell-based assays

Readouts for cell-based assays

The readouts that can be used for cell-based assays are many and varied. In some cases, such as radioligand binding or enzyme activity, the readouts are essentially the same as those described above. Here we describe three cell-based readout technologies that have found general application in many types of assay, namely *fluorometric methods*, *reporter gene assays*, and *yeast complementation assays*. Some informative case histories of cell-based assays based on different readout prin-

Table 8.2
Different fluorescence techniques used for single molecule detection

Technique/Name	Abbreviation	Parameter/Species resolved	Hardware requirement	Amenability to current HTS
Fluorescence correlation spectroscopy	FCS	Translation diffusion	1 detector CW laser	Limited
Fluorescence cross-correlation spectroscopy	FCCS	Colour	2 detectors CW laser	No
Fluorescence intensity distribution analysis 2-Dimensional FIDA	FIDA	Brightness / Anisotrophy and brightness	1 detector CW laser / 2 detectors CW laser	Yes
Fluorescence intensity multiple distribution analysis	FIMDA	Brightness and diffusion time	1 detector CW laser	No
Confocal fluorescence lifetime analysis	cFLA	Fluorescence lifetime	1 detector Pulsed laser	Yes
Fluorescence intensity and lifetime distribution analysis	FILDA	Fluorescence lifetime and brightness	1 detector Pulsed laser	Yes
Confocal time-resolved anisotropy	cTRA	Fluorescence lifetime and anisotrophy	2 detectors Pulsed laser	Yes
Combination cTRA + 2D-FIDA	FIDTRA	Fluorescence lifetime, anisotrophy and brightness	2 detectors Pulsed laser	In development

ciples have been presented by Johnston and Johnston (2002).

Fluorometric assays are widely used to monitor changes in the intracellular concentration of ions or other constituents such as cAMP. A range of fluorescent dyes has been developed which have the property of forming reversible complexes with ions such as Ca^{2+} or Na^+. Their fluorescent emission changes when the complex is formed, allowing changes in the free intracellular ion concentration, for example in response to activation or block of membrane receptors or ion channels, to be monitored. Other membrane-bound dyes are available whose fluorescence signal varies according to the cytoplasmic or mitochondrial membrane potential. Membrane-impermeable dyes which bind to intracellular structures can be used to monitor cell death, as only dying cells with leaky membranes are stained. The jellyfish photoprotein *aequorin* (see below), which emits a strong fluorescent signal when complexed with Ca^{2+}, is also used to monitor changes in $[Ca^{2+}]_i$. Cell lines can be engineered to express this protein, or it can be introduced by electroporation. Such methods find many applications in cell biology, particularly when coupled with confocal microscopy to achieve a high level of spatial resolution. For HTS applications, the Fluorescence Imaging Plate Reader (FLIPR, Molecular Devices Inc., described by Schroeder and Negate, 1996), allows the simultaneous application of reagents and test compounds to multi-well plates, and the capture of the fluorescence signal from each well elicited by a brief laser pulse by means of an imaging system. Repeated measurements can be made at intervals of less than 1 s, to determine the time course of the response, and confocal imaging can be used if necessary. Cellular responses, such as changes in $[Ca^{2+}]_i$ or membrane potential, are often short-lasting, so that monitoring the time profile rather than taking a single snapshot measurement is essential.

Reporter gene assays

Gene expression in transfected eukaryotic cells can be quantified by linking a promoter sequence to a reporter gene, whose level of expression is readily monitored, and reflects the degree of activation or inhibition of the promoter (Alam and Cook, 1990). Compounds activating or inhibiting the promoter itself, or interfering with a signal pathway connected to that promoter, can thus be detected. By using two different reporter constructs (e.g. firefly and *Renilla* luciferase; see below), different targets can be screened simultaneously. The principle of a reporter gene assay for GPCR activity, based on luciferase, is shown in Figure 8.13.

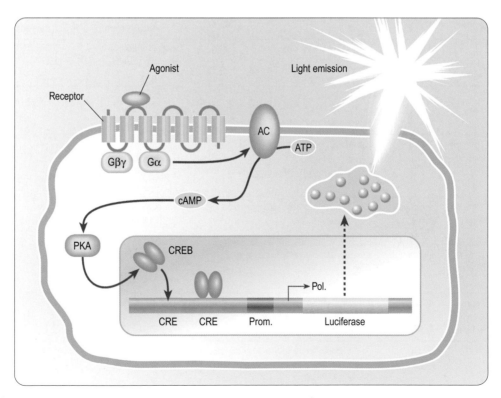

Fig. 8.13
Reporter gene (luciferase) assay for the screening of a ligand receptor (G-protein-coupled receptor) interaction in a mammalian cell. Upon binding of a small molecule to the receptor, the luciferase expression will change, mediated through a signal transduction cascade.

Commonly used reporter genes are CAT (chloramphenicol acetyltransferase), GAL (β-galactosidase), LAC (β-lactamase) (Zlokarnik et al., 1998), LUC (luciferase, Kolb and Neumann, 1996) and GFP (green fluorescence protein, Kain, 1999). CAT, GAL and LAC products can be assayed radiometrically or colorimetrically. A recently developed LAC substrate is composed of two fluorophores attached to cephalosporin, which brings them close together to allow fluorescence resonance energy transfer (FRET). β-Lactamase activity cleaves off the acceptor fluorophore, resulting in loss of the FRET emission.

Luciferase (LUC), isolated from the light organs of the North American firefly, produces light (yellow-green, 560 nm) during the oxidation of its chemical substrate, luciferin. In cell-based reporter assays luciferase is released into the assay medium after cellular lysis. Upon addition of the substrate, luciferin, the oxidation is quantified by a luminometer.

A different luciferase from the sea pansy *Renilla reniformis* catalyses the oxidation of coelenterazine and produces light as a byproduct. The activities of firefly and *Renilla* luciferase can be measured sequentially, allowing screening on two different targets in one sample.

The jellyfish *Aequorea victoria* emits light by transferring energy from the Ca^{2+}-activated photoprotein aequorin to GFP. Wildtype GFP and a number of red shifted variants have been cloned and expressed in heterologous systems. GFP provides an excellent method for monitoring gene expression and protein location. However, the production of signal by this protein is non-catalytic, and so the number of molecules required to overcome the autofluorescence background is relatively high (Niswender et al., 1995).

Yeast complementation assay

Yeast is a well-characterized organism for investigating mammalian systems, and particularly convenient for genetic engineering. The yeast two-hybrid assay is a powerful method for measuring the protein–protein and protein–DNA interactions that underlie many cellular control mechanisms. Widely used in cell biological studies, the yeast two-hybrid system (Figure 8.14) can also be used to screen small molecules for their interference with protein–protein and protein–DNA interactions, and has recently been adapted for other types of drug–target interactions (Fields and Song, 1989; Young et al., 1998; Serebriiskii et al., 2001). Conventional in vitro measurements, such as immunoprecipitation or chromatographic co-precipitation (Regnier, 1987; Phizicky and Fields, 1995), require the interacting proteins in pure form and at high concentrations, and therefore are often of limited use.

The yeast two-hybrid system uses two separated peptide domains of transcription factors: a DNA-specific binding part (DNB) and a transcription activation domain (AD). The DNB moiety is coupled to one protein (the 'bait'), and the AD moiety to another (the 'prey'). If the prey protein binds to the bait protein, the AD moiety is brought into close association with the reporter gene, which is thereby activated, producing a product (e.g. GAL or LAC, as described above, or an enzyme which allows the yeast to grow in the presence of cycloheximide). The addition of a test compound that blocks the specific protein–protein interaction prevents activation of the reporter gene. Serebriiskii et al. (2001) describe a project in which lead compounds able to block the activation of a specific N-type voltage-gated Ca^{2+} channel have been identified with a yeast two-hybrid assay. The bait and prey proteins contained domains of two different channel subunits which need to associate to form a functional channel.

High content screening

High content screening (HCS) is a further development of cell-based screening in which multiple fluorescence readouts are measured simultaneously in intact cells by means of imaging techniques. Repetitive scanning provides temporally and spatially resolved visualization of cellular events. HCS is suitable for monitoring such events as nuclear translocation, apoptosis, GPCR activation, receptor internalization, changes in $[Ca^{2+}]_i$, nitric oxide production, apoptosis, gene expression, neurite outgrowth and cell viability (Giuliano et al., 1997).

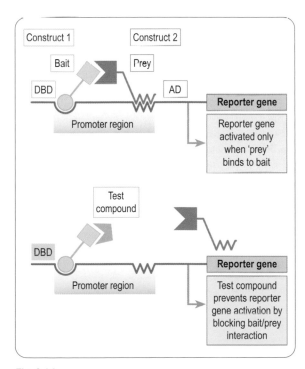

Fig. 8.14
Principle of yeast two-hybrid assay.

The aim is to quantify and correlate drug effects on cellular events or targets by simultaneously measuring multiple signals from the same cell population, yielding data with a higher content of biological information than is provided by single-target screens (Liptrot, 2001).

The instrumentation involves a fluorescence-based laser scanning reader (96–1536-well format) able to detect fluorescent structures against a less fluorescent background. These detectors (Kapur, 2002) acquire multicolour fluorescence image datasets of cells at a preselected spatial resolution. High content screening relies heavily on powerful image pattern recognition software.

The concept of gathering all the necessary information about a compound at one go has obvious attractions, but the very sophisticated instrumentation and software produce problems of reliability. Furthermore, the principle of 'measure everything and sort it out afterwards' has its drawbacks: interpretation of such complex data sets can be very difficult. The experimenter may not know in advance which cellular effects, among the many that can be measured, are most relevant for identifying lead compounds in a particular project. For routine purposes, conventional screening methods are therefore likely to remain the most useful approach.

Biophysical methods in high-throughput screening

Conventional bioassay-based screening remains a mainstream approach for lead discovery. However, during recent years alternative biophysical methods have been developed for drug discovery whose main purpose is the detection of low-affinity low molecular weight compounds.

Affinity-based screening techniques (Siegel, 2002; Wabnitz and Loo, 2002) can help in ranking small molecules on the basis of their binding affinity towards a target macromolecule. They can also be applied to eliminate hit compounds exhibiting unfavourable binding affinities to other macromolecules.

Mixtures of compounds are combined with a target, followed by a physical separation of unbound molecules and protein–compound complexes. This is accomplished by the use of size exclusion or restricted access separation media. The macromolecule–compound complexes are trapped and, after dissociation of the complex, the chemical structure of the released molecules is determined by online HPLC-coupled mass spectrometry. Alternatively, the target protein is immobilized on the separation column itself (Chan and Hueso-Rodriguez, 2002).

Other biophysical methods, such as X-ray crystallography (Carr and Jhoti, 2002) or nuclear magnetic resonance (NMR) (Hajduk and Burns, 2002), are applied in a different approach to high-throughput screening, namely *fragment-based screening*. Hits from HTS usually already have drug-like properties, e.g. a molecular weight of ~ 300 Da). During the following lead optimization synthesis programme an increase in molecular weight is very likely, leading to poorer drug-like properties with respect to solubility, absorption or clearance. Therefore, it may be more effective to screen small sets of molecular fragments (~10 000) of lower molecular weight (100–250 Da) which can then be chemically linked to generate high affinity drug-like compounds. Typically, such fragments have much weaker binding affinities than drug-like compounds and are outside the sensitivity range of a conventional HTS assay. NMR- or X-ray crystallography-based assays are better suited for the identification of weak binders, as well as providing information on the exact binding site on the protein.

As discussed in Chapter 9, the chemical linkage of weak binding fragments can generate a high-affinity lead without violating the restrictions in molecular weight. The efficiency of this strategy has been demonstrated by several groups (Nienaber et al., 2000; Lesuisse et al., 2002).

Assay formats – miniaturization

Multiwell plates began to be used for screening in the early 1980s, before which time tube-based assays were routinely used in a low-throughput mode. Their introduction, starting with 96-well plates and progressing to 384-well and 1536-well formats, culminating in recent 'lab-on-a-chip' technology, allowed the automation and miniaturization of biochemical experiments, to the point where screening operations are no longer a bottleneck in drug discovery.

The establishment of the standard 96-well plate format initiated a tremendous development in liquid dispensing technology, stacking devices and plate readers.

Steady improvements in instrumentation, liquid handling and detection technology have now made the 384-well plate the standard of choice in most pharmaceutical screening laboratories. Further miniaturization to the 1536-well format, with reaction volumes typically 2–10 μL, is possible (Table 8.3) and is used for some

Table 8.3
Reaction volumes in microtitre plates

Plate format	Typical assay volume
96	100–200 μL
384	25–50 μL
384 low volume	5–20 μL
1536	2–10 μL

assays. With the development of detection technologies such as CCD imaging, the readout of 1536-well plates can be performed quickly enough for screening purposes. There are attendant disadvantages, however. Liquid handling in the low or submicrolitre range is still a challenge, and is further complicated by the need for a humidified environment to reduce evaporation. Miniaturization to 1536-well format often results in higher variability of data and loss in quality. The necessary large investments in hardware may outweigh savings in reagents and other costs. The introduction of the 384-well low-volume plate provides an attractive compromise (Garyantes, 2002), realizing significant savings in costs, reagents and compounds without requiring large investments in liquid handling and reader technology.

Robotics in HTS

After successful validation the screening assay is installed in a robotic workstation that can operate in high-throughput mode (typically up to 100 000 compounds per day at a single concentration). The robotic system consists of devices for storage, incubation and transportation of plates in different format; instruments for liquid transfer; and a series of plate readers for the various detection technologies.

A typical robotic system is illustrated in Figure 8.15. Rotating arms (2) and transport systems (13) move plates between different devices. Hotels (6) and incubators (4, 10) are used for storage and incubation of microplates. Incubators can be cooled or heated; for mammalian cell cultivation they can also be supplied with CO_2. Plates are automatically transferred in and out. A piercer perforates

the sealed lids of compound plates; compounds and other liquid assay reagents are transferred by pipetters (1) or dispensers (3). Stackers are sequential storage units for microtitre plates, connected to automated pipetting instruments. Various detection devices (with different detection systems) are located at the output of the system. Finally, plates are automatically discarded into waste (12).

Before primary screening can start sample plates have to be prepared, which is usually done offline by separate automated liquid transfer systems (96- or 384-tip pipetters). Compound storage plates, containing the library to be screened prepared as DMSO solutions, are delivered from the compound library warehouse and samples are further diluted with aqueous buffer to reach the desired compound and DMSO concentration for the assay. Samples are usually transferred to the assay plates by the robot during the assay run.

Programming and testing of the different process steps for individual screens is the most time-consuming part of the operation. In particular, the correct timing of different steps during the assay is critical, as different devices (pipetters, incubators, readers etc.) have different cycle times and have to be coordinated in a way that is optimized for maximum throughput. In modern robotic systems efficient scheduling software optimizes the process without any manual intervention.

During the screening itself, all processes have to be monitored online to ensure the quality of the data obtained. The performance of the assay is continuously measured by calculating z' values for each plate (see earlier section). For this purpose, each screening plate includes high and low controls for quality analysis, in addition to the compounds for screening.

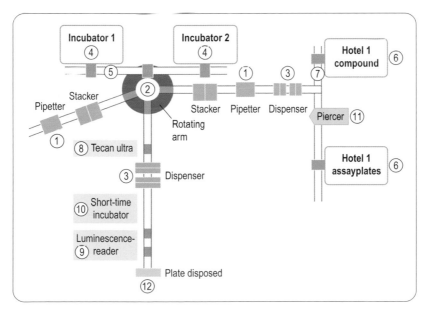

Fig. 8.15
Plan of robotic system for HTS.

For the selection of positives the 'hit limit' or threshold is usually set at least three standard deviations away from the mean of the library signal.

Data analysis and management

Owing to the large volume of data generated in HTS, efficient data management is essential. Software pack-

ages for HTS (e.g. ActivityBase, Spotfire) are available to carry out the principal tasks:

- Storage of raw data
- Quality control
- Transformation of data into information
- Documentation
- Reporting.

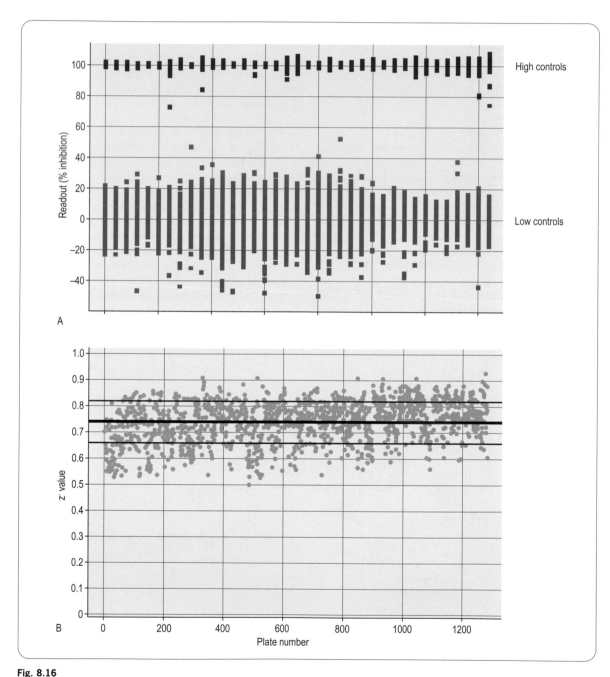

Fig. 8.16
Data validation checks in a typical screening assay.
(A) Distribution of high and low controls (% inhibition) in a set of screening plates. Each column represents one plate and each point represents one well ($n = 16\ 312$). (B) z' values during a screening campaign. Each data point reflects one test plate.

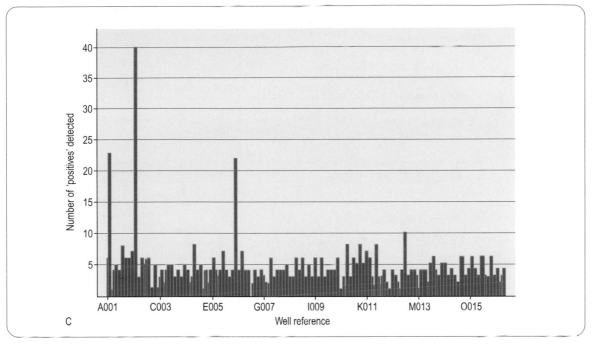

Fig. 8.16–cont'd
(C) Well-based pipetting artefacts. The y-axis shows the number of 'positive' compounds as a function of the well position, in an assay involving many plates. With randomly distributed compounds there should be an equal chance of finding positives at each well address. The high values in wells A3, B3 and F3 therefore represent artefacts due to mechanical failure.

In HTS each biochemical experiment in a single well is analysed by an automated device, typically a plate reader or other kind of detector. The output of these instruments comes in different formats depending on the type of reader. Sometimes multiple readings are necessary, and the instrument itself may perform some initial calculations. These heterogeneous types of raw data are automatically transferred into the data management software.

In a next step raw data are translated into contextual information by calculating results. Data on percentage inhibition or percentage of control are normalized with values obtained from the high and low controls present in each plate. In secondary screening IC_{50}/EC_{50} and K_i values are also calculated. The values obtained depend on the method used (e.g. the fitting algorithm used for dose–response curves) and have to be standardized for all screens within a company. Once the system captures the data it is then necessary to apply validation rules and techniques, such as trimmed means, to eliminate outliers and to apply predetermined acceptance criteria to the data, for example, the signal-to-noise ratio, the z'-value, or a test for gaussian distribution of the data. All plates that fail against one or more quality criteria are flagged and discarded.

A final step in the process requires the experimenter to monitor visually the data that have been flagged, as a final check on quality. This is to ensure the system has performed correctly. Visualization of data helps to reveal artefactual patterns in data sets and to identify false positives resulting from phenomena such as edge effects in the plate (gradients in temperature or in oxygen supply), pipetting errors, or instabilities of assay reagents. Examples of validation data obtained in a typical screening assay are shown in Figure 8.16.

In addition to registering the test data, all relevant information about the assay has to be logged, for example the supplier of reagents, storage conditions, a detailed assay protocol, plate layout, and algorithms for the calculation of results. Each assay run is registered and its performance documented.

HTS will initially deliver hits in targeted assays. Retrieval of these data has to be simple, and the data must be exchangeable between different project teams to generate knowledge from the mass of data.

Screening libraries and compound logistics

Compound logistics

In the drug discovery value chain the effective management of compound libraries is a key element and is usually handled by a dedicated compound logistics group, whose interactions with other parts of the drug discovery

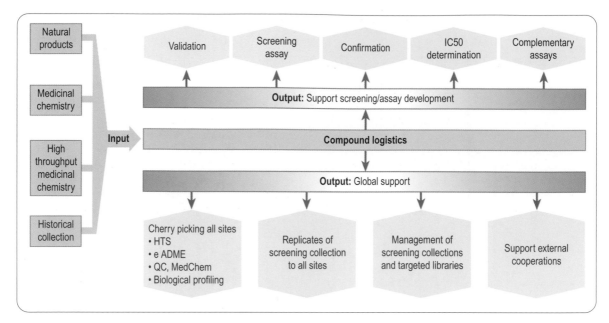

Fig. 8.17
The compound management facility had to manage various sources of compound libraries, ranging from the historical collection of synthetic compounds to natural product extract libraries. They have manifold interactions with various clients across the lead discovery chain.

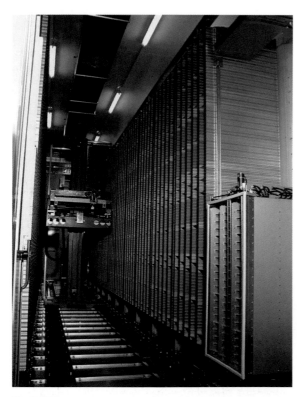

Fig. 8.18
Storage of a compound screening collection in 384-well plates at –4°C. A robot is able to move around and collect the plates or individual samples specified in the compound management software.

enterprise are summarized in Figure 8.17. The compound management facility (Figure 8.18) is the central port for transshipment of compounds in lead discovery, not only for primary screening, but also during the hit-to-lead phase. It is the unit responsible for registration of samples, their preparation, storage and retrieval. This facility has to ensure global compound accessibility, both individually and in different formats; maintain compound integrity (quality control and proper storage); guarantee error-free compound handling; guarantee efficient compound use; and guarantee a rapid response to compound requests.

Many pharmaceutical companies have greatly increased both the size of their compound collection and their screening capacity. Screening libraries frequently exceed 500 000 compounds and originate from many different sources with variable quality. This has necessitated both hardware and software automation of compound management in order to cope with the increasing demands of HTS and lead discovery.

Most advanced systems use fully automated robotics for handling compounds. Compounds used for screening are stored as liquids in microtitre plates in a controlled environment (temperature –4C° to –20°C; low humidity).

Splitting the collection into a number of copies in different formats secures a balance between fast response times to the various compound requests and optimal storage conditions. Different sets of compound libraries are needed, depending on the target and project specifications.

In many companies the 384-well plate format has become a standard in screening, and robotic storage systems also use this format.

Because library sets are not static, as new compounds are continuously being added, samples in the repository need to be individually addressable to allow a flexible and quick rearrangement of existing libraries to more specific, focused collections. Advanced compound logistic systems store compound libraries in a single tube system so that individual tubes can be accessed without the need to take out a whole plate from the storage facility.

This functionality is a prerequisite for efficient 'cherry picking'. After primary screening, positive compounds have to be confirmed in secondary assays and dose–response curves determined. The individual active compounds have to be located and reformatted in microtitre plates. With a large number of targets and projects running at any one time, a highly automated compound handling systems is needed to do this efficiently.

Profiling

High-throughput screening, the subject of this chapter, has as its first objective the identification of a few 'validated hits' (defined in Chapter 9) within large compound

libraries. The decision as to whether a particular hit is worth pursuing as a chemical lead in a drug discovery project depends on several factors, important ones being its chemical characteristics and its pharmacodynamic and pharmacokinetic properties. These aspects, broadly covered by the term 'compound profiling', are discussed in detail in the next three chapters.

The technology involved in miniaturization, automation and assay readouts needed for HTS is continuing to develop rapidly, and as it does so, the laboratory set-ups installed in HTS facilities are steadily broadening their capabilities beyond their primary function of identifying hits. As this happens, it becomes possible for HTS techniques to be applied to more diverse compound profiling assays relating not only to the target selectivity of compound libraries, but also to their pharmacokinetic characteristics. Increasingly, therefore, early compound profiling tasks on 'hit' compounds are being carried out in HTS laboratories where the necessary technological expertise is concentrated. Such assays are also very helpful in the 'lead identification' stage of a project, where focused synthetic compound libraries based on the initial hits need to be assessed. As this work generally involves testing small compound libraries, usually fewer than 1000 compounds at a time, in

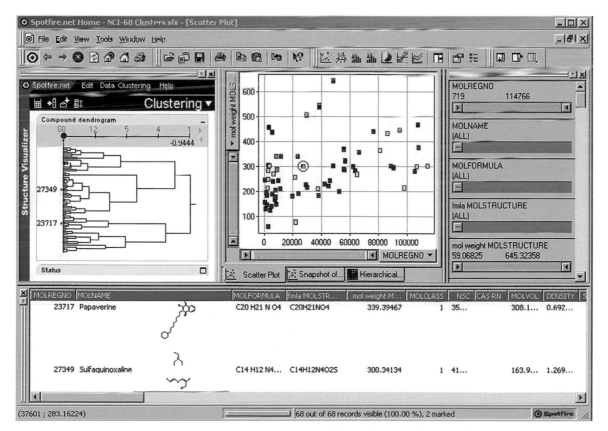

Fig. 8.19
Spotfire software for analysis of compound profiling data.

several different assays, small dedicated robotic workstations are needed, rather than the fast but inflexible factory-style robotic assemblies used for large-scale HTS.

In vitro pharmacokinetic assays (see Chapter 10), which are not generally project specific and can be automated to run in medium-throughput fashion, are very suitable for running in this environment. This extension of the work of HTS laboratories beyond the primary task of finding hits is a clear and continuing trend, for which the term 'high-throughput profiling' (HTP) has been coined. It brings the work of HTS laboratories into a close and healthy relationship with drug discovery teams. The highly disciplined approach to assay formats and data logging that is essential for HTS[1] brings the advantage that profiling data collected over a wide range of projects and drug targets is logged in standard database formats, and is therefore a valuable company-wide tool for analysing structure–activity relationships. Software packages such as 'Spotfire' (Figure 8.19) have been developed to handle data such as these.

In summary, it is clear that pharmacological profiling will be an increasing activity of HTS units in the future, and will help to add further value in the drug discovery chain.

References

Alam J, Cook JL (1990) Reporter genes: application to the study of mammalian gene transcription. Analytical Biochemistry 188: 245–254.

Alpha B, Lehn JM, Mathis G (1987) Energy-transfer luminescence of europium(III) and terbium(III) with macrobicyclic polypyridine ligands. Angewandte Chemie 99: 259–261 .

Beveridge M, Park YW, Hermes J et al. (2000) Detection of p56(lck) kinase activity using scintillation proximity assay in 384-well format and imaging proximity assay in 384- and 1536-well format. Journal of Biomolecular Screening 5: 205–212 .

Birzin ET, Rohrer SP (2002) High-throughput receptor-binding methods for somatostatin receptor 2. Analytical Biochemistry 307: 159–166.

Bosworth N, Towers P (1989) Scintillation proximity assay. Nature 341: 167–168.

Braunwaler AF et al. [aq] (1996) A solid-phase assay for the determination of protein tyrosine kinase activity of c-src using scintillating microtitration plates. Analytical Biochemistry 234: 23–26.

Brown BA, Cain M, Broadbent J et al. (1997) FlashPlate technology. In: Devlin PJ, ed. High-throughput screening. New York: Marcel Dekker, 317–328.

Carr R, Jhoti H (2002) Structure-based screening of low-affinity compounds. Drug Discovery Today 7: 522–527.

Chan JA, Hueso-Rodriguez JA (2002) Compound library management. Methods in Molecular Biology 190: 117–127.

Clegg RM (1995) Fluorescence resonance energy transfer. Current Opinion in Biotechnology 6: 103–110.

Cook ND (1996) Scintillation proximity assay: a versatile high-throughput screening technology. Drug Discovery Today 1: 287–294.

Eigen M, Rigler R (1994) Sorting single molecules: application to diagnostics and evolutionary biotechnology. Proceedings of the National Academy of Sciences of the USA 91: 5740–5747.

Fields S, Song O (1989) A novel genetic system to detect protein–protein interactions. Nature 340: 245–246.

Garyantes TK (2002) 1536-well assay plates: when do they make sense? Drug Discovery Today 7: 489–490.

Giuliano KA, de Basio RL, Dunlay RT et al. (1997) High-content screening: a new approach to easing key bottlenecks in the drug recovery process. Journal of Biomolecular Screening 2: 249–259.

Hajduk PJ, Burns DJ (2002) Integration of NMR and high-throughput screening. Combinatorial Chemistry High Throughput Screening 5: 613–621.

Haugland RP (2002) Handbook of fluorescent probes and chemical research, 9th edn. Molecular Probes. Web edition: www.probes.com/handbook.

Hemmilä IA, Hurskainen P (2002) Novel detection strategies for drug discovery. Drug Discovery Today 7: S150–S156.

Hemmilä I, Webb S (1997) Time-resolved fluorometry: an overview of the labels and core technologies for drug screening applications. Drug Discovery Today 2: 373–381.

Hopkins AL, Groom CR (2002) The druggable genome. Nature Reviews Drug Discovery 1: 727–730.

Johnston PA, Johnston PA (2002) Cellular platforms for HTS: three case studies. Drug Discovery Today 7: 353–363.

Kain RK (1999) Green fluorescent protein (GFP): applications in cell-based assays for drug discovery. Drug Discovery Today 4: 304–312.

Kapur R (2002) Fluorescence imaging and engineered biosensors: functional and activity-based sensing using high content screening. Annals of the New York Academy of Sciences 961: 196–197.

Kask P, Palo K, Fay N et al. (2000)Two-dimensional fluorescence intensity distribution analysis: theory and applications. Biophysics Journal 78: 1703–1713.

Kettling U, Koltermann A, Schwille P, Eigen M (1998) Real-time enzyme kinetics monitored by dual-color fluorescence cross-correlation spectroscopy. Proceeding of the National Academy of Sciences of the USA 95: 1416–1420.

Kolb AJ, Neumann K (1996) Luciferase measurements in high throughput screening. Journal of Biomolecular Screening 1: 85–88.

Lakowicz JR (1999) Principles of fluorescence spectroscopy. New York: Plenum Press.

Lesuisse D, Lange G, Deprez P et al. (2002) SAR and X-ray. A new approach combining fragment-based screening and rational drug design: application to the discovery of nanomolar inhibitors of Src SH2. Journal of Medicinal Chemistry 45: 2379–2387.

Liptrot C (2001) High content screening – from cells to data to knowledge. Drug Discovery Today 6: 832–834.

Lyne PD (2002) Structure-based virtual screening: an overview. Drug Discovery Today 7: 1047–1055.

Moore K, Rees S (2001) Cell-based versus isolated target screening: how lucky do you feel? Journal of Biomolecular Screening 6: 69–74.

Moore KJ, Turconi S, Ashman S et al. (1999) Single molecule detection technologies in miniaturized high throughput screening: fluorescence correlation spectroscopy. Journal of Biomolecular Screening 4: 335–354.

Nasir MS, Jolley ME (1999) Fluorescence polarization: an analytical tool for immunoassay and drug discovery. Combinatorial Chemistry High Throughput Screening 2: 177–190.

Nienaber VL, Richardson PL, Klighofer V et al. (2000) Discovering novel ligands for macromolecules using X-ray crystallographic screening. Nature Biotechnology 18: 1105–1108.

[1]But not second nature to many laboratory scientists.

Niswender KD, Blackman SM, Rohde L, Magnuson MA, Piston DW (1995) Quantitative imaging of green fluorescent protein in cultured cells: comparison of microscopic techniques, use in fusion proteins and detection limits. Journal of Microscopy 180: 109–116.

Phizicky EM, Fields S (1995) Protein–protein interactions: methods for detection and analysis. Microbiology Review 59: 94–123.

Picardo M, Hughes KT (1997) Scintillation proximity assays. High-Throughput Screening. In: Devlin PJ, ed. New York: Marcel Dekker, 307–316.

Regnier FE (1996) Chromatography of complex protein mixtures. Journal of Chromatography 418: 115–143.

Schroeder KS, Negate BD (1996) FLIPR, a new instrument for accurate high-throughput optical screening. Journal of Biomolecular Screening 1: 75–80.

Serebriiskii IG, Khazak V, Golemis EA (2001) Redefinition of the yeast two-hybrid system in dialogue with changing priorities in biological research. Biotechniques 30: 634–655.

Siegel MM (2002) Early discovery drug screening using mass spectrometry. Current Topics in Medicinal Chemistry 2: 13–33.

Sittampalam GS, Kahl SD, Janzen WP (1997) High-throughput screening: advances in assay technologies. Current Opinion in Chemistry and Biology 1: 384–391.

Sorg G, Schubert HD, Buttner FH, Heilker R (2002) Automated high throughput screening for serine kinase inhibitors using a LEADseeker scintillation proximity assay in the 1536-well format. Journal of Biomolecular Screening 7: 11–19.

Valenzano KJ, Miller W, Kravitz JN et al. (2000) Development of a fluorescent ligand-binding assay using the AcroWell filter plate. Journal of Biomolecular Screening 5: 455–461.

Wabnitz PA, Loo JA (2002) Drug screening of pharmaceutical discovery compounds by micro-size exclusion chromatography/mass spectrometry. Rapid Communications in Mass Spectrometry 16: 85–91.

Wedin R (1999) Bright ideas for high-throughput screening. Modern Drug Discovery 2: 61–71.

Wright P, Boyd HF, Bethell RC et al. (2002) Development of a 1-µl scale assay for mitogen-activated kinase 7 using 2-D fluorescence intensity distribution analysis anisotropy. Journal of Biomolecular Screening 7: 419–428.

Young K, Lin S, Sun L et al. (1998) Identification of a calcium channel modulator using a high throughput yeast two-hybrid screen. Nature Biotechnology 16: 946–950.

Zhang JH, Chung TD, Oldenburg KR (1999) A simple statistical parameter for use in evaluation and validation of high-throughput screening assays. Journal of Biomolecular Screening 4: 67–73.

Zlokarnik G, Negulescu PA, Knapp TE et al. (1998) Quantitation of transcription and clonal selection of single living cells with beta-lactamase as reporter. Science 279: 84–88.

9 The role of chemistry in the drug discovery process

C S J Walpole

The challenge

Few would dispute that the role of chemistry in the drug discovery process is pivotal. As one commentator observed, 'chemistry is one of the disciplines at the centre of the bottleneck in drug research' (Wess et al., 2001). Yet despite this central role, the impact of chemistry in drug discovery has not been marked, in recent years, by transformative breakthroughs in innovation and efficiency to the same extent as has that of bioscience (Drews, 1998), but has only enjoyed relatively steady, linear progress. This shortfall has been described as 'the pharmaceutical industry's dirty secret: new drugs are small organic molecules and small organic molecules are made by chemists' (Goodfellow, 2002). Despite this obvious need for innovation, interest in chemistry around the world, and the proportion of students studying the subject, is declining, in contrast to the exponential growth and progress seen in the biological disciplines in the last decade. New technologies, automation and better success at computational prediction of desirable properties are, however, making an impact on productivity, albeit not the quantum leaps forward which were heralded by some. The challenge of the current decade will be for chemists to transform the role of their discipline in drug discovery from that of a 'cottage industry' (Goodfellow, 2002) to a modern, technologically advanced yet creative one.

In this chapter we discuss some of the basic principles and approaches used by medicinal chemists, without going into much technical detail. For greater depth, recent textbooks by Patrick (2001), Krogsgaard-Larsen et al. (2002), and the latest edition of *Burger's Medicinal Chemistry* (Abraham, 2003) should be consulted.

The idea

Before a drug discovery project can be put into operation it is obviously necessary to define its scientific approach and goals. At one end of the innovation spectrum one can imagine that a new protein target, for example a receptor, is discovered and its function linked to potential therapeutic utility in a particular indication. It would be important to gain evidence for its expression in normal and pathological tissue, develop assays of its function, both in human cell lines and also relevant animal species (i.e. those intended to be used for in vivo testing of selected candidate compounds), and to identify chemical ligands from which lead series of compounds could be developed. At the other end of the spectrum, clinically validated drug targets might already be well established and active compounds known to exist, either in the public domain or in the hands of competitors. Indeed, drugs already on the market or in development may be taken as the starting point for a drug discovery idea. In the case of such a 'me too' or 'fast follower' project a very strong business case would be required and a high level of confidence that an improved compound, 'best-in-class' at the time of registration, could be discovered and developed quickly enough to be commercially successful. Clearly, here, patent novelty, marked superiority over the leading competitor product(s) and the existence of development capacity and the will to ensure a faster than average development would be key to success.

At either end of this innovation spectrum, however, the identification of robust, patentable chemical lead series is an essential first step. Ultimately, the goal of discovery groups in the pharmaceutical industry is to generate high-quality candidate drugs that are less likely to fail in development than compounds identified in previous decades. Such drugs can only realistically be derived by optimization of high-quality lead compounds, if lead optimization can be achieved at a reasonable cost in time and resources. 'High quality' in this context refers not only to performance in an assay, or physical property profile, but also to 'information content', such as an understanding of structure–activity relationships (SARs), which drive design efforts, or the availability of protein–small-molecule docking information that suggests fruitful design strategies. Clearly, in the increasingly competitive environment of the modern pharmaceutical industry, with the requirement for much lower attrition of candidate drugs and the expectation of constantly decreasing project lifetimes, there is a need to select projects (and therefore targets and chemical leads)

which are 'druggable'. This means that there would be a strong likelihood of success in the discovery of small drug-like molecules, which possess the desired features of a candidate drug, within a relatively short period of time. Some features that are recognized to improve 'druggability' (Wess et al., 2001) include:

- Small molecular weight (MW) lead compounds with 'drug-like' physicochemical attributes available;
- Cell surface target (no requirement for cell penetration);
- Binding affinity of the lead is dominated by a few key strong interactions, e.g. hydrophobic, ionic bonds, rather than multiple weak, highly directional interactions such as H-bonds (as is the case, for example, with adhesion molecules);
- Binding locus is not spread over a wide surface area (as is the case with cytokine receptors);
- Robust assays are available which give a primary readout on the molecular recognition event (e.g. binding or second-messenger assay);
- Chemical series is, ideally, amenable to parallel chemistry and automation;
- Availability of structural data (e.g. X-ray structure of target or NMR solution conformation), or target is a member of a well known class for which many drug-like ligands already exist, e.g. G-protein-coupled receptors (GPCRs).

The process

As outlined in Chapter 4, a typical drug discovery project consists of four main phases, summarized in Figure 9.1. Each phase has defined endpoints which are delivered at the end of one phase and provide a starting point for the next. These phases are known by different names by the different pharmaceutical companies, but the activities that take place during the phases are fairly uniform. Figure 9.1 illustrates the process up to the

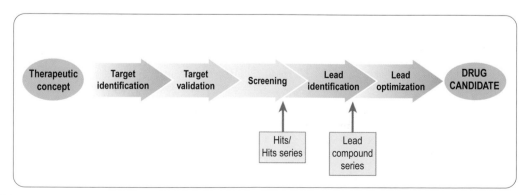

Fig. 9.1
Basic steps in drug discovery.

> ➤ **Box 9.1 Definitions used in the text**
>
> **Primary hit:** A compound giving a positive result in a screening assay.
>
> **Confirmed hit:** A compound that is confirmed as positive when the assay is repeated, and shows a degree of specificity (i.e. the positive result is not due to non-specific effects such as cytotoxicity or interference with the readout system). Frequently (see Chapter 8) such checks will be incorporated as controls in the primary screening protocol.
>
> **Validated hit:** A confirmed hit that shows selective activity and a clear concentration–effect relationship in secondary screening assays that reflect activity on the selected target. For example, if the primary screen is a receptor-binding assay, secondary screens might be cell-based assays or organ bath assays showing receptor activation. In addition, selectivity for the particular target will need to be checked, for example by testing for activity against a range of related targets (e.g. monoamine receptors, ion channels, proteases, kinases). Depending on the circumstances, a potency threshold (IC_{50} or EC_{50} <1 µM, say) may be applied. The chemical structure must be proven, unequivocally, by resynthesis.
>
> **Hit series:** A set of chemically related validated hits, providing a pointer to structure–activity relationships.
>
> **Lead compound/lead series:** A compound or series of compounds that fulfil the criteria for validated hits, and also further criteria, namely:
>
> - Complies with Lipinski Rule of 5, or other physicochemical criteria appropriate to the intended route of administration; amenable to parallel synthesis
> - No structural features known to be associated with toxicity
> - Patentable structures
> - Clear evidence of structure–activity relationships
> - Acceptable physicochemical and DMPK properties.
>
> The compounds may be members of the original screening library (i.e. a hit series), or new synthetic compounds designed on the basis of the screening results.
>
> **Drug candidate:** The end result of lead optimization, namely a compound judged suitable for preclinical and clinical development, based on the criteria defined at the outset of the project. These criteria will depend on the nature of the compound and its intended clinical use, but typically will include:
>
> - Potency and selectivity for target
> - Appropriate pharmacokinetics (see Chapter 10)
> - Relevant pharmacological activity in vitro and in vivo (see Chapter 11)
> - Acceptable safety pharmacology profile (see Chapter 16)
> - Chemical stability and compatibility with likely pharmaceutical formulations
> - Chemical scale-up feasible
> - Patentable (see Chapter 19).
>
> **Development compound:** A drug candidate that has been accepted for further development, on the basis of operational and commercial considerations, which will include assessment of the unfilled medical need, the expected size of the market and the level of competition, the 'fit' with company's franchise and business plan, the availability of resources and expertise needed to complete the project, and the timescale and probability of successful registration.

point where a drug candidate, suitable for clinical development, is delivered. Definitions of what attributes characterize hit compounds, lead compounds and drug candidates are given in Box 9.1.

The role of medicinal chemistry in lead identification

Many drug discovery chemistry groups now recognize the 'hit-to-lead' phase as a distinct part of the discovery cycle (Boguslavsky, 2001), involving different skills, working practices and objectives from the later lead optimization stage. Previously, the two phases, hit-to-lead and lead optimization were carried out as a single operation, based on 'one-at-a-time' chemical synthesis. The task of the medicinal chemistry group was to

deliver drug candidates into preclinical development through a number of activities, including analogue synthesis, delivery of material for in vivo pharmacological and drug metabolism and pharmacokinetics (DMPK) testing, route discovery for scale-up, and preformulation (see Chapter 17). In general, these groups were adept at producing relatively large quantities (i.e. grams) of relatively few compounds (on average, about 50 per chemist per year) to high purity standards. This traditional 'one-at-a-time' synthesis is, however, ill-suited to the early lead identification phase of most projects, where a large body of structure–activity relationship (SAR) data needs to be amassed before decisions can usefully be taken on where best to focus the chemical effort. However, even in 'one-at-a-time' mode, analogue synthesis was carried out repetitively by reacting a central intermediate with many reagents of a common chemical class (acid chlorides, for example) in such a way as to introduce diverse functionality into one part of the molecule. It was later recognized that the efficiency of these operations could be greatly increased by performing these reactions in parallel.

Enabling technology: parallel synthesis

During the 1990s industry groups started to experiment with technologies that would enable common chemical transformations which were usually carried out in series, one-at-a-time, to be carried out in parallel (notably former Parke-Davis's Diversomer ideas, as described by DeWitt et al. (1993). Today, there are many solutions to the problem and robotic systems are commercially available for both solution and solid-phase parallel synthesis on a variety of scales, from lead finding to lead optimization, where larger quantities of drug substance are needed.

At the same time as these fundamental changes in approach to compound synthesis were evolving it was also recognized that strict adherence to full 'publication quality' characterization of compounds for screening was unnecessary: compound quality should be 'fit for purpose'. Purification to homogeneity was realized to be unduly time-consuming and not generally necessary for the purpose of identifying active compounds. The consequence of these changes in mindset brought about a fundamental shift in the way such early SAR generation is now typically performed (the so-called 'paradigm-shift' in drug discovery; see Krebs, 1999).

Optimizing DMPK parameters

The routine provision of DMPK data in the early stages of drug discovery (see Chapter 10) has revolutionized medicinal chemistry for the better. The value of optimizing DMPK parameters at the same time as pharmacological properties is self-evident today, but until recently DMPK received much less attention than the optimization of potency and selectivity. Nowadays, the routine provision of in vitro metabolic data (such as clearance by liver microsomes or hepatocytes from human and other species) for many compounds in parallel, allows large datasets of SAR information relating to metabolic stability and clearance to be quickly generated. This information, viewed in parallel with binding or functional data and physicochemical measurements (see below), can be used to select only those compounds that fulfil the criteria most desirable for progression. In this way, much time spent exploring 'unproductive' avenues is saved, allowing resources to be concentrated on chemical series in which all the desired characteristics of a lead compound are likely to converge.

Quantitative structure–activity relationship (QSAR) models based on such large data sets of metabolic stability or clearance data, as well as in silico filtering based on CYP P450 active site structures or pharmacophores,

is now enabling 'virtual screening' of libraries prior to synthesis (van de Waterbeemd, 2002; Ekins et al., 2000). This has greatly reduced the need to make every member of a congeneric series, with considerable savings on manpower and reagents. The use of Lipinski's rules (see Box 9.3) to guide the design of orally available drug candidates has enjoyed near universal acceptance in the pharmaceutical industry, as they are so simple and are clearly based on sound scientific principles (Lipper, 1999). Measurements of drug permeability though a monolayer of cultured intestinal carcinoma cells (Caco-2) are useful as a medium-throughput screen for gastrointestinal absorption. Intrinsic clearance from hepatocytes or liver microsomes, together with Caco-2 penetration data, can be used to predict oral bioavailability with reasonable accuracy (Mandagere et al., 2002). These methods and approaches are discussed in more detail in Chapter 10.

Optimizing physicochemical parameters

To ensure that suitable physicochemical properties are achieved and maintained during the course of a lead identification (and lead optimization) project, data on lipophilicity and aqueous solubility need to be routinely available. Medium-throughput methods which allow fast evaluation of multiple compounds (comparable to DMPK optimization, above) are ideally required, such that data obtained on congeneric series synthesized in parallel can be considered alongside other attributes before compounds are selected for resynthesis. pKa measurements, at least on key compounds which exemplify 'subseries', are also very valuable in interpreting SAR and planning desired changes in properties.

Optimizing pharmacological potency and selectivity

Because by this stage considerable SAR information on the series of interest is available, further rounds of the design/test/redesign cycle are typically performed, guided by structural information on target–ligand complexes, where available, or by computational methods such as pharmacophore analysis (see below). The chemist aims to fine-tune the potency and selectivity of compounds within the structural scope defined by that subset of the series in which suitable physicochemical and DMPK attributes have been found to reside. Attractive substructures within the series are progressively defined and retained while other parts of the molecule, where the structural requirements on activity are less well known, are systematically varied. If successful, this iterative approach converges on a series of compounds in which most – if not all – of the desired characteristics coincide – a 'lead series'. With such a lead series identified, the likelihood of future successful modification in the lead optimization phase is relatively high.

Generating compounds as research tools

Target validation is a major challenge for drug discovery in the current decade, and 'chemical tools' can provide critical validation data on which decisions relating to the project's viability may be based. Selection of a novel biomolecule as a potential drug target can be greatly strengthened by showing that blocking or activating it with a selective pharmacological agent produces the required pharmacodynamic effect. Identifying selective ligands, even if they lack pharmacokinetic and other properties required in a development compound, is therefore a useful strategy for target validation. Novel compounds (small synthetic molecules or peptides) can be used as probes to provide validation of novel targets in disease models. For this purpose, Lipinski's 'rule of 5' can safely be flouted as long as sufficiently potent and selective compounds with good enough DMPK properties (given by parenteral or intrathecal routes of administration) can be found to allow reliable interpretation of their in vivo pharmacological effects. By analogy with 'hit-to-lead' chemistry, this activity could be called 'hit-to-tool' and may follow a different path from a programme that aims to generate leads. One example of such a compound is HOE-140 (Hock et al., 1991), a potent and selective peptidic antagonist of the kinin B_2 receptor which is sufficiently metabolically stable to allow proof-of-principle experiments to be carried out in animal models of inflammatory hyperalgesia, and even proof-of-concept studies in man, even though its peptidic nature precluded its further development.

> ### Box 9.2 Strategies for lead identification
>
> - Physical screening of large compound libraries. This is the needle-in-a-haystack approach, relying purely on chance to find promising leads among libraries of synthetic or natural compounds.
> - Physical screening of smaller 'lead generation' libraries, produced by combinatorial chemistry, consisting of variants of structural classes known to include compounds active on certain types of target. Chance is still involved, but the haystack is much smaller and more likely to contain needles.
> - 'Designed' molecules. The design may be based on structures (generally endogenous molecules or competitor drugs) known to be active on the target in question (ligand-based design), or on the known structure of the target. The analogy here is with archery rather than haystack hunting. Chance, in principle, is eliminated, but it is still very easy to miss and so the odds are improved further if this approach is coupled with the generation of 'targeted libraries' around the desired compound.
> - Computational methods play an increasingly important role. They are used in many ways, for example:
>   - To compute estimates of physicochemical properties, based on chemical structure
>   - To create and rank 'virtual libraries' of compounds that are unavailable or not yet synthesized
>   - To perform 'virtual screening' on structurally defined targets
>   - To generate pharmacophore models, based on established structure-activity relationships.

Finding leads: chemical starting points

The task of identifying leads is the first essential step for medicinal chemists in drug discovery. It requires two essential components: test systems in the form of screening assays (described in Chapter 8), and compounds to test.

In theory, the number of possible organic compounds of reasonable molecular weight, say <500 Da, is for practical purposes boundless. Estimates range from about 10^{30} to 10^{70}, but the number matters little, save that it is way beyond our capacity, let alone exceeding the amount of carbon on the planet, to make and test more than a minute fraction of them. The largest compound collections amassed by pharmaceutical companies (see below) contain a few million compounds.

In principle, two strategies can be used for identifying leads, namely *screening* and *design*. At one extreme (Box 9.2) lies the strategy of physically screening as many compounds as possible, typically hundreds of thousands, in the hope of finding some that look promising. At the other lies the strategy of designing

compounds fine-tuned for the chosen target, and synthesizing and testing just a few. Between these extremes lies the strategy of generating and screening 'focused' libraries of hundreds or thousands of compounds, chosen broadly with a particular target in mind. In applying design principles, computational methods play an important and increasing role, as discussed below, having the advantage that 'virtual' compound libraries can be readily accessed and evaluated before bench chemistry needs to be committed. In the following sections we discuss the various approaches to lead identification in more detail.

High-throughput screening (HTS)

The principles and technology of HTS are described in Chapter 8. Here we focus on compound sources.

Corporate small-molecule collections (synthetic chemical libraries)

A very common way to obtain a chemical starting point for a drug discovery project is by screening the chosen target, in some assay which is compatible with high-throughput automation, against a collection of com-

Drug discovery

pounds, typically the pharmaceutical company's corporate compound collection. The size and quality of such collections varies throughout the industry, but would typically consist of 0.5–2 million discrete small-molecule compounds of known structure. Such collections are the result of decades of compound synthesis and acquisition. They seldom represent uniformly high-quality collections for lead finding, arising as they do from the unplanned accumulation of compounds synthesized for various projects over many years. These are often heavily biased towards certain chemical classes or particular targets as a result of the companies' historical interests, and may be entirely unsuitable for the purpose of finding hits for unrelated targets. Old compounds, unsuitably stored, may have decomposed, and the collection evolves as compounds are consumed or discarded and new ones added.

The importance of quality in compound collections, with respect to physical purity and identity, conformity to 'drug-like' or 'lead-like' physicochemical criteria as well as biological relevance, has been increasingly recognized over the past 10 years. Until recently, most companies treated their compound collections rather casually and many did not recognize their enormous commercial value. In the last 10 years, most companies have undertaken comprehensive pruning of their collections such that only compounds meeting the required quality standards are retained, at the same time as actively enriching their collections by increasing its diversity, drug-like qualities and physical quality. Compounds are often purchased from commercial suppliers for this purpose; this is still judged worthwhile, even though other companies will in general also have access to the same compounds. Unique collections, such as those bought en masse from university departments, have proved valuable to some companies. Likewise, contract synthesis of compounds which, as a class, fill a gap in the compound collection, and may be obtained on an exclusive basis, is often undertaken.

Another route by which many companies have succeeded in increasing the quality and diversity of their compound collections is through company mergers. The collections of two medium-sized players can combine to result in a very rich resource for the new merged company. This was documented for the case of Warner-Lambert and Pfizer (Koberstein, 2000). The size of the collection, however, is not necessarily an advantage. It is now generally accepted that there is no advantage in amassing collections larger than 2 million compounds, and fewer compounds – approximately 1 million – if sufficiently diverse, can give acceptable hits rates on most targets. Pfizer, who have relied very heavily on HTS as a source of leads, and have publicly presented their philosophy and record of success, have stated that, in their experience, screening 1 million compounds would suffice, in most cases, to provide a 'good lead' for standard targets such as GPCRs and enzymes (Spencer,

1998). Somewhat at variance with this stated dogma, however, Pfizer later announced that their goal was to make available '3 million "beautiful compounds" for screening'. GlaxoSmithKline are reported to have access to a collection of around 2 million compounds (Langley, 2001). Typical primary hit rates from HTS are strongly dependent on the target class. For targets such as GPCRs and enzymes, hit rates of the order of 1 in 1000 are typical; however, some target classes, e.g. cytokine receptors, achieve a much lower hit rate, estimated at about 1 in 100 000 (Spencer, 1998). As computational power and screening technology advance, intelligent selection of subsets of collections for screening has become feasible and is certain to become more common than screening the whole collection on a new target. Selections based on diversity, record of success against a particular target class, in silico screening against a 3D pharmacophore model or some other attributes may be performed prior to screening. As a result, HTS hit rates are substantially increasing.

Typical compound collections have a normal distribution of molecular weight (MW) and calculated lipophilicity (cLogP)[1] which tends to be on the high side of optimal from the point of view of a chemical lead (Lipinski, 2000). For this reason current trends favour the collection of 'lead-like' compounds for screening (Langley, 2001). This is because whereas the majority of compounds fall within the desired range of physicochemical space described by Lipinski's 'Rule of 5' (Box 9.3) as optimal for a typical orally available drug (Lipinski et al., 1997), MW and LogP tend to increase during lead optimization. Lipinski's simple set of empirical 'rules' predicts with surprising reliability the drug-like properties required for an orally available drug.

More recently, the importance of molecular weight as a determinant of oral bioavailability has been questioned and another important parameter, molecular flexibility, introduced. In a large set of drug-like compounds the number of rotatable bonds appears to be a reliable predicting factor for oral bioavailability, even in compounds with MW significantly greater than 500 (Veber et al., 2002).

> ➤ **Box 9.3 Lipinski's 'Rule of 5' – general attributes for an oral drug**
>
> - Molecular weight < 500 Da
> - cLogP <5
> - Number of H-bond donors <5
> - Sum of number of Ns and Os <10

---

[1]P is the octanol:water partition coefficient. cLogP is the calculated value of logP, computed from the chemical structure. LogP >5 implies a partition coefficient exceeding 10^5, i.e. a highly lipophilic compound.

9

The tendency of molecular properties to move away from the ideal during lead optimization is driven by the need to access binding sites additional to those exploited by the original lead, in order to achieve higher affinity, thereby necessarily increasing molecular weight. Gaining affinity by exploiting hydrophobic binding sites (non-directional and capable of giving rise to sizeable increases in binding affinity; see Andrews, 1986) is a tried and tested strategy. For these reasons, HTS hits tend to be larger and more lipophilic than would be ideal (Lipinski, 2000). Realistically, though, there is a limit to the structural simplicity that is possible in hit compounds, as by definition they must possess the chemical information necessary for specific molecular recognition of the target, that is, at least a two-site interaction, in order to achieve micromolar affinity (Farmer, 1980; Farmer and Ariens, 1982), the practical limit at which hits can be discriminated in typical assays. Complementary approaches to HTS typified by affinity screening methods such as SAR by NMR or MS have overcome this barrier, owing to the increased sensitivity of these techniques. In such examples, ligands with millimolar affinities can be detected and then linked by various spacers (Figure 9.2) giving, in successful cases, compounds with micromolar or even nanomo-

lar affinities. Certain targets, such as SH2 domains, are known to achieve low hit rates from HTS programmes, presumably because the chemical information necessary for recognition is distributed diffusely over a wide surface area and generally consists of mulptiple low-energy directional interactions (e.g. H-bonds), which may be difficult to mimic in small molecules. Nevertheless, it is possible to discover low molecular weight ligands for such targets, albeit much more rarely. One successful example where a small molecule was found for such a target using HTS is provided by the work on selectin inhibitors described by a group at Ontogen (Slee et al., 2001). Although the original HTS hit had an IC_{50} of 17 µM in a P-selectin assay, it proved possible to generate from this hit potent ligands with oral availability in anti-inflammatory models. Impressive though this case history is, it represents the exception rather than the rule. Because HTS and combinatorial libraries synthesized for the purpose of lead generation may not always deliver useful hits for all targets, another valuable source of compounds which are screened by most large pharmaceutical companies is natural products.

Natural product collections

In order to establish natural products collections, plant material, bacteria, fungi and marine organisms, usually originating from one or more of 12 biologically 'megadiverse' countries (Australia, Mexico, Colombia, Ecuador, Peru, Brazil, Zaire, Madagascar, China, India, Malaysia, Indonesia), are collected. These countries have more than 70% of world biodiversity (McNeely et al., 1990). Natural product drug discovery programmes have traditionally targeted those organisms that can be easily collected or cultured, and include plants, dominant marine organisms and culturable microbes. Samples are typically stored as dried material and extracted prior to a screening campaign. Some companies favour testing crude extracts, whereas others purify and characterize major components prior to screening. Alternatively, the crude extracts may be fractionated chromatographically to generate samples containing several compounds. The fractions are assayed, and those showing activity are further analysed to identify the active compound in the mixture.

Occasionally, breakthrough medicines of exceptional novelty and great scientific significance are discovered by screening natural products (see Chapter 4). Examples include many antibacterial drugs, following on from the accidental discovery of penicillin, and more recently the immunosuppressant ciclosporin A (Wenger, 1984), obtained from culture of soil microbes, and the statin class of cholesterol-lowering drugs, first discovered in fungal extracts. Historically, natural products have been a significant contributor to drug discovery pipelines. In 1996, eight of the top 20 selling pharmaceuticals were natural product derived. There has been a particularly high success rate of natural products in oncology, with

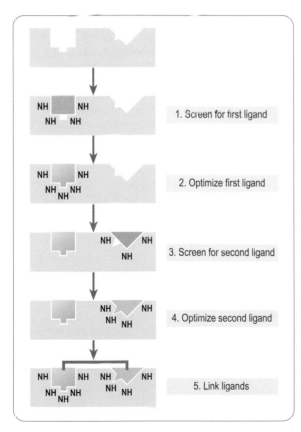

Fig. 9.2
Affinity screening by NMR spectroscopy (SAR by NMR).

1. Screen for first ligand
2. Optimize first ligand
3. Screen for second ligand
4. Optimize second ligand
5. Link ligands

61% of new compounds introduced between 1983 and 1994 being natural product derived, taxol/taxotere (see Chapter 4) being a recent major success (Cragg et al., 1997).

Although natural products account for several best-sellers, such success stories are actually relatively rare. Nevertheless, natural product libraries are still often screened in parallel with synthetic compound collections as a means of diversifying the 'chemical space' covered. Diversity analysis by Bayer of its 350 000-compound synthetic library plus other databases indicated that 40% of natural products were not represented in the synthetic compound library (Henkel et al., 1999). Of course, natural products often differ from small-molecule collections in undesirable ways, in that they typically have high MW, are structurally complex with several chiral centres, and are often highly lipophilic. In order to increase the odds of discovering more drug-like molecules, fractionation based on lipophilicity is sometimes carried out prior to screening of extracts.

Most, if not all, of the major pharmaceutical companies have some degree of involvement in natural product screening. The R&D pipelines of GlaxoSmithKline, Merck and Bristol Myers Squibb in particular, all of which run bioprospecting projects in tropical countries, contain a large proportion of compounds originating from natural products. AstraZeneca has an extensive natural products collection and an isolation group based in Australia. Pfizer, for a long time non-participants in the natural products arena, has recently begun to adopt this strategy through a collaboration with the New York Botanical Garden.

Historically, success in the field of discovery of lead compounds and drugs derived from natural products has come from the screening of extracts. The move to screening of single purified compounds is a recent initiative by some companies, with the intention of shortening the time between screening and structure elucidation. Strategies to prepare libraries of pure compounds invariably involve exhaustive C-18 HPLC fractionation (as practised by Xenova UK, for example). The prefractionation strategy is time-consuming and, moreover, biases the process to major constituents. There is a chance that active compounds are discarded and never screened, and so the value of biodiversity can be lost.

Lead generation libraries

Lead generation libraries differ from typical corporate compound collections in that they are libraries of compounds generated by combinatorial chemistry techniques, and are specifically designed and synthesized for the purpose of lead finding.

Combinatorial chemistry has revolutionized the synthesis of chemical libraries since its inception in the early 1990s (for exhaustive historical reviews see Thompson and Ellman, 1996; Balkenhohl et al., 1996).

The historical roots of combinatorial chemistry lie in the automated solid-phase synthesis of peptides, but the modern capability to synthesize multiple small organic molecules in parallel reached a turning point with the pioneering work of DeWitt and coworkers at Parke-Davis, who first described the design and use of an apparatus for the parallel synthesis of small organic molecules – the so-called 'Diversomer' approach (DeWitt et al., 1993).

Combinatorial chemistry has undergone many conceptual redefinitions and has been subject to several changes in fashion in its short history. The initial explosion of effort in the mid-1990s favoured solid-phase synthesis, evolved from its peptide ancestry. These approaches are typified by the 'split and mix' approach (Thompson and Ellman, 1996) to solid-phase library synthesis, in which solid-phase resins are derivatized with multiple different chemical units in separate pools, then recombined and mixed and subsequently treated with another set of 'diversity reagents', and the procedure is repeated until the library has been synthesized. It is an inherent feature of such techniques that the final product cleaved from the resin is a mixture, and complex 'deconvolution' strategies needed to be devised so that useful information could be gleaned from screening such libraries (Balkenhohl et al., 1996). This method was ideal for creating very large chemical libraries for 'prospective' screening, but the complexity and time demands imposed by the necessary deconvolutions before a confirmed active compound could be identified were found to be prohibitive for many lead generation purposes. More recently, the combinatorial synthesis of individual compounds (one compound per well) has found favour because of these practical concerns, and because of a shift towards the synthesis of smaller, less diverse libraries biased towards 'medicinally relevant' chemical space.

During the late 1990s emphasis shifted away from large, chemically diverse libraries to smaller libraries, especially those focused on chemical substructures known to have biological relevance. In the early days of combinatorial chemistry it was assumed that if libraries were diverse enough, hits would be found for the majority of targets; however, in more recent years the critical question has been raised as to how biologically relevant is the diversity created in chemistry (Hill, 2001). Despite the former dominant philosophy that diversity would resolve all lead-finding problems, theoretical considerations have indicated that sufficient atoms do not exist in the universe to fill all available 'biological space' (Fenniri, 1996; Lipinski, 2000). Molecular design, preferably based on structural information from the target or, at least existing ligands, is therefore the only answer to improving the current paucity of suitable chemical leads. The bottleneck in lead generation, then, has not been resolved simply by high-throughput screening and combinatorial chemistry (Wess et al., 2001). A new era in which knowledge-based molecular design is used in conjunction with high-throughput chemistry and screening is absolutely required – in short, we have to be more intelligent but just as fast in our discovery efforts.

Terms such as 'library design', 'drug-like' properties, 'diversity', 'in silico screening', 'virtual library' and 'pharmacophore generation' abound in discussions of library approaches. The following scheme describes the approach used by AstraZeneca to generate libraries directed towards G-protein-coupled receptors (GPCRs) and uses these terms in context, such that their significance can be appreciated.

Library design

By studying compounds which are known from the literature to be GPCR-acting it is possible to identify common molecular fragments ('privileged fragments'; Lewell et al., 1998) that occur more frequently in GPCR ligands than in those for other biological targets. Libraries containing scaffolds which incorporate these fragments can then be designed. Accessible high-yielding chemistry and the availability of sufficient variable positions into which diversity elements can be incorporated are attributes that guide the selection of scaffold to be used. Libraries are then planned and synthesized around these scaffolds, as detailed below.

'In silico' screening

A 'virtual library' of several tens of thousands of compounds is generated computationally, from which a feasible number of compounds (usually fewer than 5000) are selected for practical synthesis. The selection process on the virtual ('in silico') library is achieved by computational filtration to remove compounds with inappropriate molecular weight, lipophilicity (Log P), solubility and number of rotatable bonds. Compounds that do not have these drug-like properties (i.e. do not conform to the 'Rule of 5') or have predicted aqueous solubility <50 µg/mL or have more than eight rotatable bonds are filtered out. Finally, a 'diversity analysis' is performed to eliminate redundant compounds from the library. 'Diversity', as the term is used here, refers to an analysis of structural descriptors by which 'similarity' or 'likeness' between two molecules or molecular fragments can be recognized and ranked by computational algorithms. The most common measurement of 'diversity' is called the Tanimoto distance or index (Butina, 1999).

Synthesis

A typical library size is 1000–2000 compounds and, depending on the synthetic sequence, either solid- or solution-phase syntheses can be used. The compounds are prepared as individual compounds on a scale of about 5 mg per well in 96-well microtitre plates. The chemical steps used for library construction are those that are sufficiently well validated for the scaffold reagents used that sufficient purity for screening (>60%)

can be achieved without exhaustive purification. Purity analysis and verification of structure are carried out, and the structures and analytical data are registered in a suitable database. Each compound is given a unique identifier, such as compound number, plate barcode and well number, and the library is then ready for screening.

Screening

Libraries so produced are then screened against selected GPCR assays (typically receptor-binding assays), either singly or pooled so as to make more efficient use of screens. In the case of pooled screening libraries deconvolution is straightforward, as the constituent compounds in a given 'hit' well can simply be tested individually to identify the true 'confirmed hit'. Once identified, the component of the active well is then resynthesized in order to confirm identity and activity (a 'validated hit'). Resynthesis is only performed on confirmed hits, and so is not unduly time-consuming if the cut-offs for percentage inhibition are adjusted such that hit rates are in a range that can be effectively followed up.

Information gathering and analysis

Typical hit rates from such GPCR-oriented libraries are in the 1–5% range, much higher than those typically observed with 'random' high-throughput screening. The hits that come from screening are then used to prepare pharmacophore and QSAR models that can be used to refine the library design further. 'Focused' libraries (which typically aim to vary in parallel one or two diversity elements in a 'hit series') may be generated at this stage to gain sufficient SARs to establish the likely breadth of tolerated functionality. Once sufficient SARs are evident and reproducible biological activity has been observed with resynthesized compounds of known structure, the active compounds are called a 'hit series' for the receptor under study.

A very similar approach to the generation of ion-channel libraries using knowledge-based design has been described by Wess et al. (2001). This approach also afforded hit rates (~4%) much higher than those expected from random screening.

Affinity screening methods

These methods, based on physical techniques such as nuclear magnetic resonance (NMR) spectroscopy or mass spectrometry (MS), are complementary to the HTS methods described in Chapter 8 and are particularly useful for identifying low-affinity binding to soluble targets. In the context of library design, the aim is to identify low-affinity 'warheads' (i.e. low molecular weight entities which have weak binding interactions with soluble drug targets) that can be linked to generate composite molecules with high affinity (see Figure 9.2). The potency sought in the initial screen may be too low for the compounds to represent 'hits' as conventionally defined. These assays require abundant supplies of soluble target proteins, and so the methods are of limited use for conventional screening purposes. These approaches, dubbed SAR by NMR and SAR by MS, have been successfully used in recent years (Ringe, 1996; Shuker et al., 1996; Wabnitz and Loo, 2001), particularly for soluble enzyme targets such as proteases or kinases. SAR by NMR, for example, has been used to evaluate ligand binding to a protein target by observing changes in the protein's NMR spectrum when incubated with a binding ligand, or changes in a ligand's spectrum when incubated with a target protein. NMR studies can identify the location of the binding site and, in some cases, provide atomic coordinates of the protein–ligand complex.

Using this approach, Fesik and coworkers (Shuker et al., 1996) discovered inhibitors for the immuno-modulation target FKBP with affinities as low as 19 nM. NMR screening gave two fragment leads with affinities of 2 μM and 100 μM, respectively, which were then combined in a single molecule and optimized to high-affinity leads.

With the introduction of electrospray ionization, mass spectrometry (MS) has proved to be a useful means of detecting non-covalent protein–ligand complexes. When a protein–ligand complex is formed the observed molecular weight of the protein increases by the mass of the ligand, and so the complex can be discriminated from unliganded protein. MS can be combined with size exclusion gel chromatography as a simple means of screening small-molecule mixtures for protein binding (Wabnitz and Loo, 2001). Compared with NMR screening, SAR by MS has the advantage of increased speed, sensitivity, and the ability to provide stoichiometric information.

A severe restriction, however, to the general utility of these techniques is that only a minority of attractive therapeutic targets are available as purified, soluble proteins which can be studied in their biologically active conformation, and which are available in sufficient quantity to enable study. The applicability of these useful approaches to a wider range of targets, such as GPCRs, ion channels and other membrane receptors, awaits substantial advances in spectroscopic techniques and protein engineering.

Computational approaches in lead discovery

Computational chemistry has developed rapidly since its beginnings in the 1970s, and now plays an important part in most drug discovery projects. Here we describe some of the techniques and approaches that have proved effective.

Virtual screening

In virtual screening (as distinct from screening for physicochemical and other properties, as described earlier) compounds are 'docked' into a 3D model of a structurally defined biological target and the binding energy of the resulting complex is estimated, allowing compounds to be rank-ordered. This technique has proved most successful where the target structure has been determined at high resolution (e.g. by X-ray crystallography). Computational models of membrane proteins such as GPCRs do not as yet have sufficient precision to allow this technique to be useful.

Virtual screening does not, of course, need physical test samples, or even previously synthesized compounds. In one application of virtual screening, structure-based-focusing (Kick et al., 1997; Kirchoff et al., 2001), a virtual library (e.g. all possible compounds that could be made by established methods from available starting materials) can be screened computationally against an experimentally determined 3D structure in which binding site interactions are understood. In others, compounds that exist physically in a collection (e.g. a compound collection used for HTS) can be computationally screened prior to the selection of a subset, which would then be physically screened against the target. Virtual screening and HTS offer strongly complementary approaches to hit identification, as screening resources can be focused on those compounds most likely to provide hits. Although at present the science of virtual screening is in its infancy, computational efforts aimed at providing more reliable 'scoring functions', from which predictive rank orders can be derived, are progressing rapidly (Stahl and Rarey, 2001).

Drug design

The de novo design of molecules to create drugs has a long and illustrious history, starting with Ehrlich's discovery of the first antimicrobial drugs early in the 20th century. Indeed, design was the mainstay of drug discovery for many years, and many of the familiar therapeutic classes, such as diuretics, ACE inhibitors, antihistamines, antiepileptics, oral hypoglycaemics, proton pump inhibitors etc, emerged from drug-design programmes that did not involve screening for leads[2].

Drug design can in principle be *ligand based* or *target based*. Until recently only the former approach was possible, as there was little knowledge about target structure, and it remains the most appropriate strategy in most cases. Until about 1960, very few drug targets had been defined at the biochemical or pharmacological level. We did not know about phosphodiesterases, monoamine transporters, cyclooxygenase, calcium channels or dopamine receptors as drug targets, though drugs acting on all of them were in use. With the exception of

---

[2]The term '*rational* drug design' is often used, apparently to emphasize the intellectual high ground on which the strategy is supposed to rest, and to distance it from the supposedly more mindless approach of screening. However, as there is no such thing as *irrational* drug design, the qualifier is redundant.

a few pioneers (see Chapter 1), such as Hitchings and Elion working on metabolic pathways, and Black working on receptors, drug design at this time was based largely on producing imaginative chemical variations of existing therapeutic agents, such as phenothiazine antipsychotics, diuretics and non-steroidal anti-inflammatory drugs, a strategy which in many cases proved highly successful. The current situation is that most of the targets for existing therapeutic drugs have been identified at the biochemical level, as well as many potential new targets not yet covered therapeutically. For these new targets, various ligands – endogenous molecules and synthetic drugs – may be available as starting points for ligand-based drug design, even though high-resolution structures of the target molecules are not available. Even now, only a few targets, such as HIV protease, have been characterized structurally in sufficient detail to be used as a basis for de novo drug design.

Ligand-based approaches

One obvious strategy for deriving a chemical starting point applicable to projects that aim to mimic or block the effects of a natural mediator, a monoamine neurotransmitter or bioactive peptide for example, is to use the mediator itself as the lead compound.

Such natural ligands are seldom good starting points for optimization, however, and usually the task of modifying the endogenous ligand to generate a high-quality drug candidate involves herculean effort. It has nevertheless produced some striking successes, including the design of the first registered β-adrenoceptor antagonist, *pronethalol*, by modifying the structure of *isoproterenol*, a synthetic agonist closely related to norepinephrine. Similarly, the first 5HT₃-receptor antagonist, *ondansetron*, was chemically inspired by the 5HT molecule. Still, the success of such projects is typically slower and less predictable than approaches based on lead generation libraries or HTS optimization programmes. To add to the challenges faced by medicinal chemists, natural mediators have attributes whose optimization requires almost diametrically opposed strategies from those employed with HTS hits. They are usually too highly polar, too highly ionized, too conformationally flexible, and often have unacceptably high molecular weight and chemical complexity. Figure 9.3 shows some famous examples of drugs developed by modifying endogenous mediators, and we consider below some of the chemical strategies that have been used to pull off this difficult trick.

Make physicochemical attributes of the ligand more 'drug-like'

- Reduce the highly ionized or zwitterionic nature of the mediator. *Example*: (see Figure 9.3, entry 1) (Prout et al., 1977; Ganellin, 1981). Production of histamine H₂ receptor antagonists (antiulcer drugs *cimetidine* and *ranitidine*) from histamine.

Replacement of the primary ammonium group in histamine by non-basic dipolar H-bond donors led to selectivity over H₁ receptors, as well as making the molecules more 'drug-like'.

Removal of unnecessary functionality

- Reduce MW, reduce the number of polar OH groups, eliminate chiral centres where possible. *Example*: (see Figure 9.3, entry 2) (Barrio et al., 1980). Removal of non-essential polar groups in nucleoside antiviral drugs such as the antiherpes drug *aciclovir*. In addition to improving the drug-like features of the molecule, this transformation also brought about two other effects which are critical for the drug's mode of action, namely selectivity for the viral DNA polymerase with respect to the host enzyme, and chain-terminating activity during the DNA polymerase reaction, because the drug lacks the critical 3'-hydroxyl group and so cannot substitute for the natural nucleoside.

Remove metabolically labile groups

- Simple removal of labile functionality or replacement with more stable 'bioisosteric' groups. In biological mediators metabolically labile groups may be evolutionarily conserved, as the very brief lifetime of the mediator is essential to avoid inappropriate second-messenger signalling. In a drug aimed, for example, at blocking the effects of such a mediator, much greater stability is usually required. *Example*: (see Figure 9.3, entry 3) (Humphrey et al., 1988; Street et al., 1995). *Sumatriptan*, an antimigraine drug, which is a selective agonist at 5-HT₁D receptors, derived from *5-hydroxytryptamine*.

Introduce conformational constraints

- Torsional constraints in simple monoamines brought about by cyclization. *Examples:* 7-OH DPAT (potential neuroleptic drug) derived from dopamine (see Figure 9.3, entry 4) (Chidester et al., 1993; Ma et al., 1987), also (not shown) ergolines such as *pergolide* from 5HT.

Append pharmacophoric groups to a more 'druggable' template

- Peptidomimetics (Olson et al., 1997). *Example:* (see Figure 9.3, entry 5) (Blackburn et al., 1997). Fibrinogen antagonists (potential antithrombotic drugs) from RGD peptide.
- 'Peptoid' approach to non-peptide ligands from peptides. *Example:* (see Figure 9.3, entry 6)

131

Mediator		Drug or drug-like ligand	
1	Histamine	Cimetidine	
		Ranitidine	
2	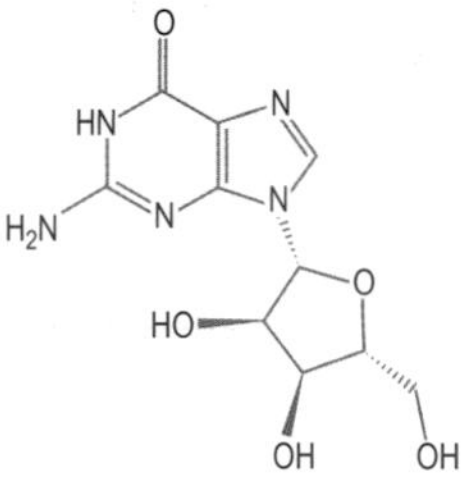 Guanosine	Aciclovir 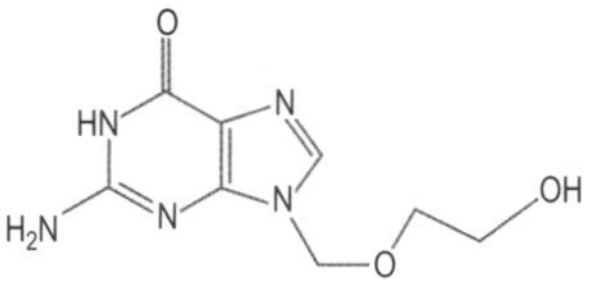	
3	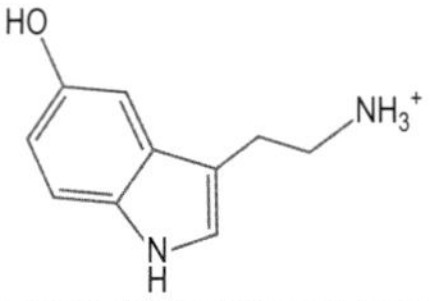 Serotonin (5-HT)	Sumatriptan 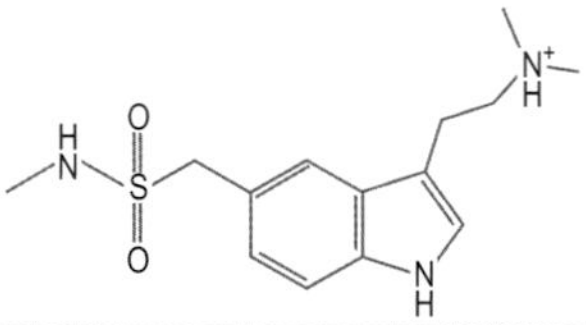	
4	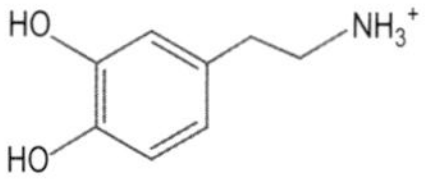 Dopamine	7-Hydroxy DPAT 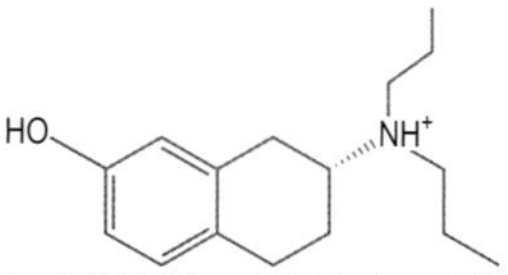	
5	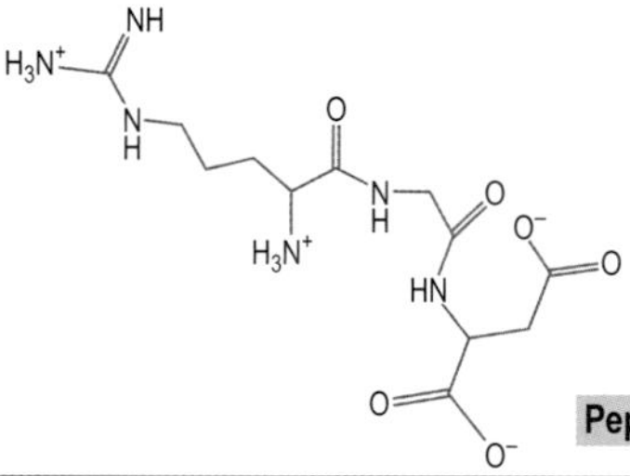 Peptide: Arg-Gly-Asp	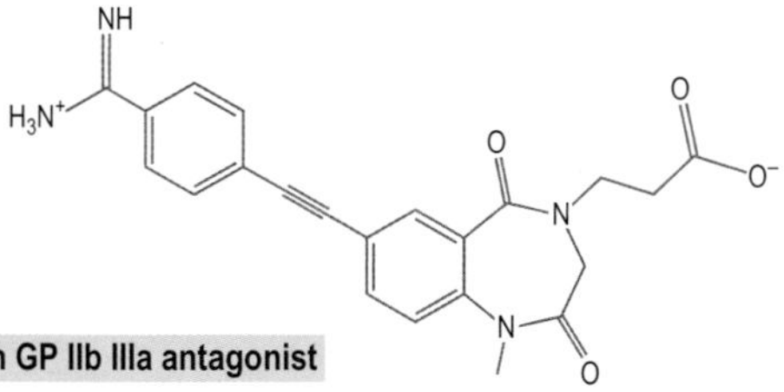 Genentech GP IIb IIIa antagonist	
6	Peptide (CCK-4): Trp-Met-Asp-Phe-NH₂	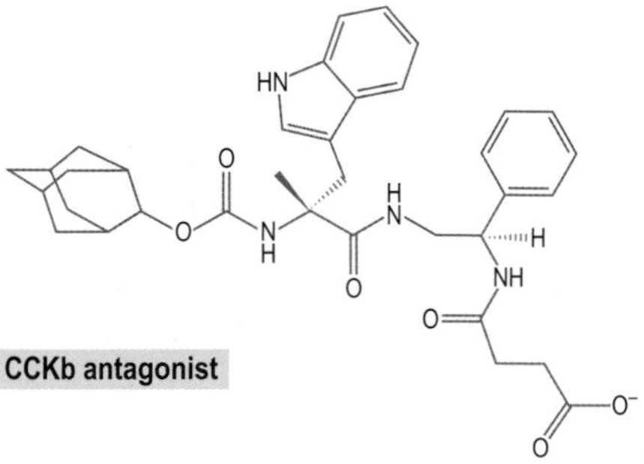 Parke-Davis CCKb antagonist	

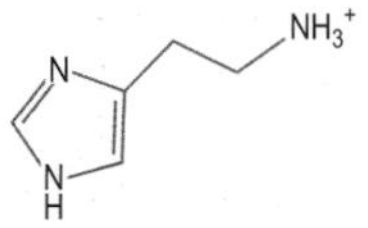

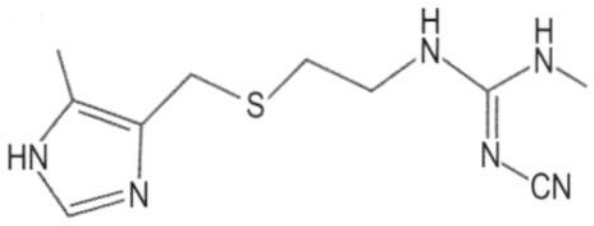

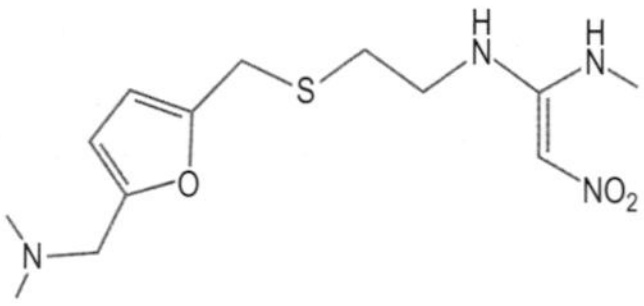

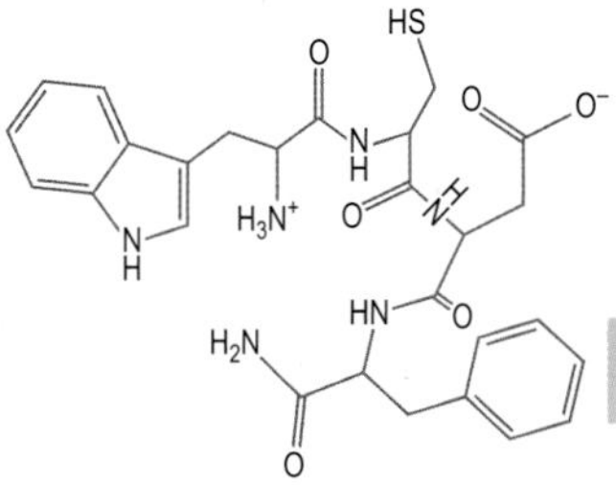

Fig. 9.3
Examples of drug structures based on endogenous mediators.

(Horwell et al., 1991; Boyle et al., 1994; Horwell, 1996) Use of α-alkylated amino acids in ligands for cholecystokinin CCK$_b$ receptors and tachykinin NK-1 receptors (potential analgesic/psychiatric drugs).

Other examples of rational design are those in which the chemical starting point is already optimized – a competitor drug candidate or an existing drug. These approaches are variously known as 'fast follower', 'best in class' or 'me too' approaches. Because the lead compound is already a viable drug candidate, the requirement for design creativity is apparently minimal. Nevertheless, discovery of a successful 'me-too' drug usually requires considerable creativity in other areas, such as finding and exploiting patent loopholes, or improving on weaknesses in process chemistry and in pharmaceutical formulation,

to generate a competitive advantage. These approaches remain very important and have spawned many commercially successful drugs (Prout et al., 1977; Patchett et al., 1980; Heel et al., 1980; Ganellin, 1981; Greenlee et al., 1985; Schmidt and Smith, 2002). The structures of the leading product and follower are often extremely similar, as can be seen from Figure 9.4. Despite this, if sufficient advantage can be gained, usually with respect to safety or pharmacokinetics, this can result in drugs of blockbuster potential if the timing of the market introduction is right. Sometimes, successful follower drugs are structurally unrelated to the leading product. For example, fluvastatin, a recently introduced cholesterol-lowering drug, has the advantage over earlier statins shown in Figure 9.3 (to which it is chemically unrelated) of being more reliably absorbed orally.

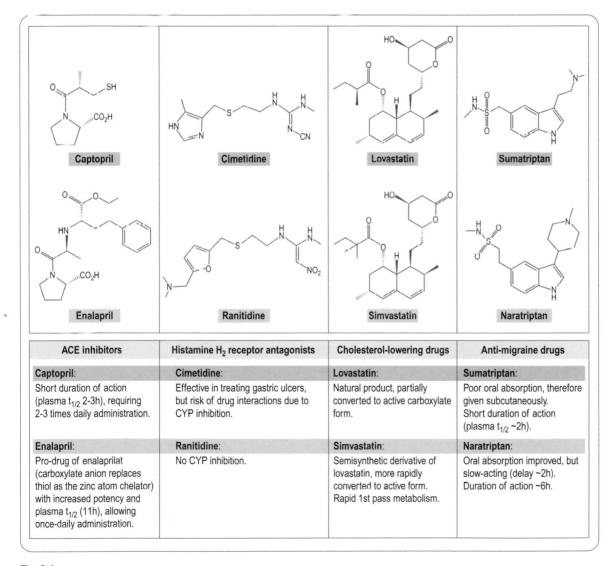

ACE inhibitors	Histamine H$_2$ receptor antagonists	Cholesterol-lowering drugs	Anti-migraine drugs
Captopril:	Cimetidine:	Lovastatin:	Sumatriptan:
Short duration of action (plasma t$_{1/2}$ 2-3h), requiring 2-3 times daily administration.	Effective in treating gastric ulcers, but risk of drug interactions due to CYP inhibition.	Natural product, partially converted to active carboxylate form.	Poor oral absorption, therefore given subcutaneously. Short duration of action (plasma t$_{1/2}$ ~2h).
Enalapril:	Ranitidine:	Simvastatin:	Naratriptan:
Pro-drug of enalaprilat (carboxylate anion replaces thiol as the zinc atom chelator) with increased potency and plasma t$_{1/2}$ (11h), allowing once-daily administration.	No CYP inhibition.	Semisynthetic derivative of lovastatin, more rapidly converted to active form. Rapid 1st pass metabolism.	Oral absorption improved, but slow-acting (delay ~2h). Duration of action ~6h.

Fig. 9.4
Examples of successful 'me-too' drugs.

Pharmacophore models

The principle of attempting to identify the common structural features of molecules that bind to specific targets is a familiar one to medicinal chemists. The aim is to generate a pharmacophore model defining the necessary features (e.g. disposition of lipophilic, hydrogen-bonding and ionic groups) of molecules active on the target in question, and a corresponding complementary model of the binding site. Traditionally, this was done by inspection of 2D molecular structures. In recent years computer methods have taken over, and now play an essential part in most drug discovery projects.

The first requirement is a set of known compounds, preferably structurally diverse, with varying degrees of affinity for the selected target. Families of minimum energy conformations are computed, so that relative spatial positions of the groups likely to be involved in binding interactions can be defined. The molecules are then overlaid in silico, to provide the best possible correspondence in the spatial arrangement of these groups. The process is made more complicated by the flexibility of the test molecules, which means that several conformations are possible, and it cannot be assumed that the calculated minimum energy conformation corresponds to the state of the molecule when docked with the target. In programs such as CATALYST, iterative calculations are used to establish which of the possible binding groups are actually determinants of binding, and also to identify space-occupying groups which can impede binding by steric hindrance even though the binding groups are appropriately located. On the basis of the pharmacophore model so generated, the activity of further actual or hypothetical compounds can be predicted, and the pharmacophore model can be used as a basis for selecting compounds for screening or synthesis. The precision and usefulness of this kind of approach depend greatly on the size and diversity of the set of compounds used to generate the pharmacophore model, and the methods are demanding in terms of computing power. The pharmacophore approach has been widely used in drug design, for example in developing ligands for a range of GPCRs, such that designing a β-adrenoceptor antagonist, for example, is now fairly straightforward – though not of much interest commercially. A more recent application of the pharmacophore principle led to the development of selective tyrosine

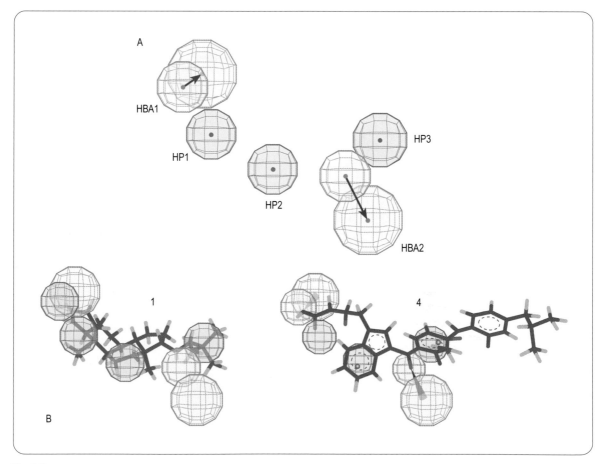

Fig. 9.5
Pharmacophore model of the enzyme 5α-reductase.

kinase inhibitors, such as *imatinib* (see Chapter 4). An example of a pharmacophore model of the enzyme 5α-reductase involved in testosterone biosynthesis is shown in Figure 9.5.

De novo design techniques, as exemplified by the use of the program 'Ludi' (Böhm, 1992), involve creating 'virtual ligands' that can provide chemical starting points directly or, more likely, can serve to evoke previously unconsidered structural possibilities. These 'idea generation' approaches are distinct from virtual screening approaches and complement them by attempting to build new molecules directly into the active site, rather than simply testing a given virtual library. Like virtual screening, this method is most successful when an experimentally derived 3D structure, such as an X-ray crystal structure, is used, but it can also be applied to refined 3D pharmacophore models in cases where receptor crystal structures are not available.

Quantitative structure–activity relationship (QSAR) models

Pharmacophore models generally aim to distinguish ligands that can bind to the target from those that cannot, but they generally give no estimates of the strength of binding, i.e. potency. QSAR models seek to correlate potency with the physicochemical and steric attributes of a family of active compounds, and are therefore useful mainly in the lead optimization phase of a project. The basis of QSAR consists of obtaining quantitative estimates of a range of different physicochemical and structural attributes of a family of test molecules of varying potencies, and using statistical techniques to determine which of these molecular descriptors is correlated to biological activity. The physicochemical descriptors include measures of hydrophobicity (e.g. cLogP), polarity and ionization properties and steric properties (e.g. van der Waals radii, molecular volume). Analysis of the test set of compounds by such techniques as *multiple regression analysis* or *principal components analysis* assigns coefficients to the various descriptors in a regression equation, indicating which are the main determinants of potency, and allowing the potency of new compounds to be estimated. The success of this kind of approach depends greatly on the number and diversity of the compounds included, and it cannot be expected to predict the activity of compounds that are structurally unrelated to the test set. It is therefore most useful in guiding the chemical synthesis programme once a lead series has been identified.

The QSAR approach described above takes no account of the 3D structure of the molecule, a shortcoming addressed by more recent developments in the form of 3D-QSAR models, implemented in software packages such as CoMFA (Comparative Molecular Field Analysis). These models start by overlaying the predicted 3D structures of known active compounds, each of which is placed in a 3D grid and probed with charged or uncharged atoms located at each point in the grid, allowing interaction forces to be calculated, and plotted as a 3D contour map. The descriptors defining this contour are then, as in conventional QSAR modelling, assigned coefficients representing their influence as determinants of biological activity.

These advanced computational QSAR methods are far from being simple push-button solutions to the problem of designing new drug molecules, and their effective use depends greatly on the judgement and expertise of computational chemists, and on the amount and quality of the experimental data on which the modelling rests. Comprehensive reviews of the QSAR field are available (see Gundertofte and Jorgensen, 2000; Akamatsu, 2002).

Structure-based design

Structure-based design (SBD) has been defined as 'a general term for using protein structural information from X-ray crystallography or NMR spectroscopy to assist in the design of novel therapeutic agents' (Murcko et al., 1999). Historically, this approach has most commonly been applied to enzyme targets (Kubinyi, 1998), the best-known successful examples being the design of inhibitors of the various families of proteases. These include the serine and cysteine proteases (Yamashita et al., 1997; DesJarlais et al., 1998), aspartyl proteases and related enzymes (e.g. HIV protease; Greer et al., 1994) and matrix metalloproteases (Summers and Davidson, 1998). More recently, the X-ray crystal structures of other biologically important enzymes, such as nitric oxide synthase (NOS) (Crane et al., 1997), histone acetyltransferase (Dutnall et al., 1998), kinases such as JNK3 (Xie et al., 1998) and non-enzymic targets such as the transcription factor NFκB (Cramer et al., 1997), have become accessible, and an explosion of structural data on therapeutically interesting targets is promised as structural genomics initiatives advance.

In the most successful SBD case histories design is based directly on the structure of the protein of interest, but approaches based on homology modelling from closely related enzymes has also proved successful (Greer, 1990). A typical SBD approach commonly contains the following steps (Yamashita et al., 1997; DesJarlais et al., 1998):

- The X-ray crystal structure of the target in its biologically active form is first determined.
- A ligand (typically a non-selective inhibitor which is active across the whole enzyme class) is co-crystallized with the target protein, and the complex analysed to reveal the binding domain.
- Essential binding interactions between ligand and protein, and other binding pockets which are not optimally exploited, are identified.
- The biological relevance of the identified interactions is often confirmed by the use of site-directed mutagenesis of the target protein.

- An iterative cycle of ligand redesign and co-crystallization is then undertaken, based on optimizing the interactions between the ligand and the critical amino acid residues that make up the binding site.

In the past, ligands that have arisen from SBD programmes, especially those designed for the serine, cysteine and aspartyl proteases, where the binding pockets are linear clefts which have evolved to recognize linear peptides, have tended to be peptidic or 'peptoidic' in nature (Farmer, 1980) and are consequently rather un-drug-like. Starting from such unpromising ligands as leads it has typically been a major challenge to develop orally available drug candidates, even with the benefit of structural information to guide the process. This is amply demonstrated by the severe challenges faced by a number of large programmes in the 1990s aimed at discovering orally available inhibitors of renin, which largely failed to deliver compounds compatible with oral dosing. More recently (see above), SBD has been successful in generating various non-peptidic protease and kinase inhibitors, and its importance will grow further as more target structures become available.

Lead optimization

Lead optimization is that part of the drug discovery process in which a defined lead compound (or series) is optimized to generate a drug candidate for preclinical development. The criteria that need to be fulfilled for promotion of a compound to drug candidate status (see Box 9.1, p. 125) vary from project to project, but invariably include properties related to pharmacokinetics and safety, as well as potency and selectivity. In addition, chemical aspects need to be addressed, for example stability, chirality and ease of synthesis. Despite perhaps giving the impression of being the most trivial of the phases of the drug discovery process, the optimization of a lead compound into a drug candidate, suitable for clinical development, is actually the hardest and least 'road-mapped' aspect (Brennan, 2000; Hill, 2001; Wess et al., 2001), because multiple requirements have to be satisfied simultaneously.

Typically, during the lead optimization phase the affinity and selectivity of the lead need to be improved, as well as DMPK parameters such as plasma half-life, oral bioavailability and CNS penetration; in practice, achieving satisfactory DMPK properties without losing potency is often difficult. This optimization must be achieved while controlling physicochemical properties (especially aqueous solubility), which will exert a strong influence over a particular compound's suitability for formulation. These properties must be closely monitored and the structural features of the compound changed in order to bring about the required balance, as dictated by the targeted profile that has been decided upon for nomination of a drug candidate for preclinical development (i.e. critical attributes of the eventual product).

In the early stages of lead optimization the structures of a chosen chemical class are typically varied rather widely in an attempt to define the boundaries imposed by SARs for the series, within which the project team will work, and also to enable broad patent coverage on series of interest. In this phase it is often more efficient to use parallel synthesis techniques (as in the lead identification stage) to prepare analogues in which key structural features are varied systematically, than to synthesize compounds one at a time, as in the past. As in the lead identification phase, pharmacological, physicochemical and metabolic data (such as intrinsic clearance (CL_{int}, see Chapter 10) by human and rat liver microsomes or hepatocytes) are often collected on all the compounds in a congeneric series before the decision is made as to which individual compounds to resynthesize. Resynthesis of selected compounds is typically performed on a scale of hundreds of milligrams.

Chirality

As a general rule, chemical series or individual compounds which are achiral, or which have fewer chiral centres, are preferred over those in which a chiral centre is found to be critical for biological activity or other required attributes. This is especially true where bond-forming reactions that generate chiral centres are an essential part of the synthesis, because of the likely higher cost and complexity of controlling this stereochemistry on a production scale in the future drug. Even if the chiral part of the structure can be incorporated from a commercially available source, it is usually more costly than achiral alternatives, and so considerable efforts are usually made to establish SAR in relation to the chiral moiety in order to establish whether it is an absolute requirement or whether an achiral alternative could be substituted. The development of racemic compounds usually presents considerable obstacles, and nowadays is rarely undertaken.

Pharmacological and pharmacokinetic considerations

In the later stages of lead optimization, where most compounds synthesized are expected to be subjected to in vivo tests for DMPK and pharmacological activity, it is more practicable to synthesize compounds singly, or a few at a time, on a scale of hundreds of milligrams. In this phase, fine-tuning of the physicochemical and pharmacokinetic parameters may be necessary if, for example, access to or exclusion from the CNS is required. As optimization progresses, selected compounds are also tested for other critical attributes to ensure that functionality is not added which is likely to be problematic. Such tests might include broad receptor screening, Caco-2 cell permeability, cytochrome P450 (CYP) isoform inhibition, genotoxicity, and in vitro screens indicative of a safety concern (blockade of the cardiac ion-channel hERG , for example (see Chapter 16; Netzer et al., 2001).

Pharmaceutical considerations

As well as the above pharmacokinetic and pharmacodynamic concerns, other attributes also need to be considered in selecting potential drug candidates. These include characteristics that contribute to ease of formulation, particularly intrinsic solubility, dissolution rate and stability. These factors are critical to the eventual pharmaceutical product but are extremely difficult to design in. Here, exploitation of 'know-how' amassed over years of experience is critical and there is often no substitute for considerable trial and error experimentation, for example in finding the best pharmaceutically acceptable salts of basic or acidic compounds. Crystallinity, lack of hygroscopicity and a sufficiently high melting point (so as to avoid local melting during drug processing, with consequent unpredictable solubility and stability characteristics) are especially important variables to consider. Pharmaceutical products which are otherwise extremely promising may fail at this stage for the seemingly trivial reason that they cannot be crystallized in a reproducible manner.

Clearly, satisfying these many challenging requirements for a potential medical product in a single molecule is far from straightforward, but it is also evident from the discussion above that the likelihood of success is much higher if these many attributes are monitored routinely in the course of lead optimization project so that the chemical strategy can be amended, iteratively, in a timely manner. This ability to change focus dynamically is essential to avoid the project being irretrievably led in the wrong chemical direction by focusing excessively on only one dimension of the problem, for example by optimizing potency to the exclusion of all else. Recording and analysing the many features being modified during the course of lead optimization, and predicting the need for and likely effect of a chemical modification, requires the use of sophisticated databases and informatics capabilities to avoid the team's losing its way as a result of information overload. In addition to this technological support, strong project management is vital to keep the project focused on overcoming the many obstacles en route to the identification of a drug candidate, and to evaluate and communicate to the team the often rapidly changing priorities.

Concluding remarks

In conclusion, it can be seen that, despite the marked impact of 'parallel technologies' for compound synthe-

sis and testing, automation and more predictive computational methods, medicinal chemistry remains an endeavour for which a clear 'process roadmap' cannot usually be written. Compared with a decade ago, we are now much more aware of the importance of 'frontloading' essential attributes of the eventual product at an increasingly early stage. Despite these advances, the dimensionality of the problem of finding a truly high-quality drug candidate seems inexorably to increase with time. A continually escalating challenge awaits future generations of medicinal chemists.

Acknowledgement

The author is indebted to Dr Mirek Tomaszewski and Dr Ron Quinn, both of AstraZeneca, for help with sections of the manuscript.

References

Abraham D J (ed) (2003) Burger's medicinal chemistry and drug discovery, 9th edn. Hoboken NJ, John Wiley.

Akamatsu M (2002) Current status and perspectives of 3D-QSAR. Current Topics in Medicinal Chemistry 2: 1381–1394.

Andrews P (1986) Functional groups, drug–receptor interactions and drug design. Trends in Pharmacological Science 7: 148–151.

Balkenhohl F, von dem Bussche-Hünnefeld C, Lansky A, Zechel C (1996) Combinatorial synthesis of small organic molecules. Angewandte Chemie [Intl edn Engl] 35:2288–2337.

Barrio JR, Bryant JD, Keyser GE (1980) A direct method for the preparation of 2-hydroxyethoxymethyl derivatives of guanine, adenine, and cytosine. Journal of Medicinal Chemistry 23: 572–574.

Blackburn BK, Lee A, Baier M et al. (1997) From peptide to non-peptide. 3. Atropoisomeric GPIIbIIIa antagonists containing the 3,4-dihydro-1h-1,4-benzodiazepine-2,5-dione nucleus Journal of Medicinal Chemistry 40: 717–729.

Boguslavsky J (2001) Minimising risks in 'hits to leads'. Drug Discovery and Development 4: 26–30.

Böhm H-J (1992) The computer program Ludi: a new method for the de novo design of enzyme inhibitors. Journal of Computer-Aided Molecular Design 6: 61–78.

Boyle S, Guard S, Higginbottom M et al. (1994) Rational design of high affinity tachykinin NK1 receptor antagonists. Bioorganic and Medicinal Chemistry 2: 357–370.

Brennan MB (2000) Drug discovery. Filtering out failures early in the game. Chemical Engineering News 78: 63–74.

Butina D (1999) Unsupervised data base clustering based on Daylight's fingerprint and Tanimoto similarity: a fast and automated way to cluster small and large data sets. Journal of Chemical Information and Computer Sciences 39: 747–750.

Chidester CG, Lin C-H, Lahti A, Haadsma-Svensson SR, Smith MW (1993) Comparison of 5-HT1A and dopamine D2 pharmacophores. X-ray structures and affinities of conformationally constrained ligands. Journal of Medicinal Chemistry 36: 1301–1315.

Cragg GM, Newman D, Snader KM (1997) Natural products in drug discovery and development. Journal of Natural Products 60: 52–60.

Cramer P, Larson CJ, Verdine GL, Muller CW (1997) Structure of the human NF-kappaB p52 homodimer-DNA complex at 2.1 A resolution. EMBO Journal 16: 7078–7090.

Crane BR, Arvai AS, Gachhui R et al. (1997) The structure of nitric oxide synthase oxygenase domain and inhibitor complexes. Science 278: 425–431.

DesJarlais RL, Yamashita DS, Oh H-J et al. (1998) Use of X-ray co-crystal structures and molecular modeling to design potent and selective non-peptide inhibitors of cathepsin K. Journal of the American Chemical Society 120: 9114–9115.

DeWitt SH, Keily JS, Stankovic CJ, Schroeder MC, Reynolds Cody DM, Pavia MR (1993) 'Diversomers': an approach to nonpeptide, nonoligomeric chemical diversity. Proceedings of the National Academy of Sciences of the USA 90: 6909–6912.

Drews J (1998) Innovation deficit revisited: reflections on the productivity of pharmaceutical R&D. Drug Discovery Today 3: 491–494.

Dutnall RN, Tafrov ST, Sternglanz R, Ramakrishnan V (1998) Structure of the histone acetyltransferase Hat1: a paradigm for the GCN5-related N-acetyltransferase superfamily. Cell 94: 427–435.

Ekins S, Waller CL, Swaan PW, Cruciani G, Wrighton SA, Wikel JH (2000) Progress in predicting human ADME parameters in silico. Journal of Pharmacological and Toxicological Methods 44: 251–272.

Farmer PS (1980) Bridging the gap between bioactive peptides and nonpeptides: some perspectives in design. In: Ariens EJ (ed) Medicinal chemistry 11. London: Academic Press; 119–143.

Farmer PS, Ariens EJ (1982) Speculations on the design of nonpeptidic peptidomimetics. Trends in Pharmacological Sciences 3: 362–365.

Fenniri H (1996) Recent advances at the interface of medicinal and combinatorial chemistry. Views on methodologies for the generation and screening of diversity and application to molecular recognition and catalysis. Current Medicinal Chemistry 3: 343–378.

Ganellin CR (1981) Medicinal chemistry and dynamic structure–activity analysis in the discovery of drugs acting at histamine H_2 receptors. Journal of Medicinal Chemistry 24: 913–920.

Goodfellow P (2002) The pharmaceutical industry harbours a dirty secret. 'Comment' in Chemistry in Britain, March, p3.

Greenlee WJ, Allibone PL, Perlow DS, Patchett AA, Ulm EH, Vassil TC (1985) Angiotensin-converting enzyme inhibitors: synthesis and biological activity of acyltripeptide analogs of enalapril. Journal of Medicinal Chemistry 28: 434–442.

Greer J (1990) Comparative modeling methods; application to the family of mammalian serine proteases. Proteins 7: 317–334.

Greer J, Erickson JW, Baldwin JJ, Varney MD (1994) Application of the three-dimensional structures of protein target molecules in structure-based design. Journal of Medicinal Chemistry 37: 1035–1054.

Gundertofte K, Jorgensen FS (2000) Molecular modeling and prediction of bioactivity. Dordrecht: Kluwer Academic.

Heel RC, Brogden RN, Speight TM, Avery GS (1980) Captopril: a preliminary review of its pharmacological properties and therapeutic efficacy. Drugs 20: 409.

Henkel T, Brunne RM, Müller H, Reichel F (1999) Statistical investigation into the structural complementarity of natural products and synthetic compounds. Angewandte Chemie [Intl edn Engl] 38: 643–647.

Hill SA (2001) Biologically relevant chemistry. Drug Discovery World (Spring): 19–25.

Hock FJ, Wirth K, Albus U et al. (1991) HOE 140, a new potent and long acting bradykinin antagonist; in vitro studies. British Journal of Pharmacology 102: 769–773.

Horwell DC (1996) Use of the chemical structure of peptides as the starting point to design nonpeptide agonists and antagonists at peptide receptors: examples with cholecystokinin and tachykinins. Bioorganic and Medicinal Chemistry 4: 1573–1576.

Horwell DC, Hughes J, Hunter JC et al. (1991) Rationally designed 'dipeptoid' analogs of CCK. α-Methyltryptophan derivatives as highly selective and orally active gastrin and CCK-B antagonists with potent anxiolytic properties. Journal of Medicinal Chemistry 34: 404–414.

Humphrey PPA, Fenuik W, Perren MJ et al. (1988) GR43175, a selective agonist for the 5-HT1-like receptor in dog isolated saphenous vein. British Journal of Pharmacology 94: 1123–1132.

Kick EK, Roe DC, Skillman AG et al. (1997) Structure-based design and combinatorial chemistry yield low nanomolar inhibitors of cathepsin D. Chemistry and Biology 4: 297–307.

Kirchhoff PD, Brown R, Kahn S, Waldman M, Venkatachalam CM (2001) Application of structure-based focusing to the estrogen receptor. Journal of Computational Chemistry 22: 993–1003.

Koberstein W (2000) Standing on scale. Pharmaceutical Executive 20: 40.

Krebs R (1999) Novel technology to improve pharmaceutical productivity. Current Opinion in Drug Discovery and Development 2: 239–243.

Krogsgaard-Larsen P, Liljefors T, Madsen U (2002) Textbook of drug design and discovery, 3rd edn. London: Taylor and Francis.

Kubinyi H (1998) Structure based design of enzyme inhibitors and receptor ligands. Current Opinion in Drug Discovery and Development 1: 4–15.

Langley D (2001) In: Van der Goot H (Ed) Trends in Drug Research, Nodwijkerhout-Camarino 13th Symposium. Amsterdam: Elsevier.

Lewell XQ, Judd D, Watson S, Hann M (1998) RECAP – Retrosynthetic Combinatorial Analysis Procedure: a powerful new technique for identifying privileged molecular fragments with useful applications in combinatorial chemistry. Journal of Chemical Information and Computer Sciences 38: 511–522.

Lipinski CA (2000) Drug-like properties and the causes of poor solubility and poor permeability Journal of Pharmacological and Toxicological Methods 44: 235–249.

Lipinski CA, Lombardo F, Dominy BW, Feeney PJ (1997) Experimental and computational approaches to estimate solubility and permeability in drug discovery and development settings. Advances in Drug Delivery Review 23: 3–25.

Lipper RA (1999) How can we optimize selection of drug development candidates from many compounds at the discovery stage? Modern Drug Discovery 2: 55–60.

Ma LYY, Camerman N, Swartzendruber JK, Jones ND, Camernan A (1987) Stereochemistry of dopaminergic ergoline derivatives: structures of pergolide and pergolide mesylate. Canadian Journal of Chemistry 65: 256–260.

Mandagere AK, Thompson TN, Hwang K-K (2002) Graphical model for estimating oral bioavailability of drugs in humans and other species from their Caco-2 permeability and in vitro liver enzyme metabolic stability rates. Journal of Medicinal Chemistry 45: 304–311.

McNeely JA, Miller KR, Reid WV, Mittermeir RA, Werner TB (1990) Conserving the world's biodiversity. IUCN, Gland, Switzerland.

Murcko MA. Caron PR. Charifson PS. 1999 Structure-based drug design. Annual Reports in Medicinal Chemistry l 34, 297–306.

Netzer R, Ebneth A, Bischoff U, Pongs O (2001) Screening lead compounds for QT interval prolongation. Drug Discovery Today 6: 78–84.

Olson GL, Bolin DR, Bonner MP et al. (1997) Perspective. Journal of Medicinal Chemistry 36: 3039–3049.

Patchett AA, Harris E, Tristram EW et al. (1980) A new class of angiotensin-converting enzyme inhibitors. Nature 288: 280–283.

Patrick GL (2001) An introduction to medicinal chemistry, 2nd edn. Oxford: Oxford University Press.

Prout K, Critchley SR, Ganellin CR, Mitchell RC (1977) Crystal and molecular structure of the histamine H2-receptor antagonists, N-methyl-N'-{2-[(5-methylimidazol-4-yl)methylthio]ethyl}thiourea (metiamide) and N-{2-[(imidazol-4-yl)methylthio]ethyl}-N'-

methylthiourea (thiaburimamide). Journal of the Chemical Society Perkin Transactions 2: 68–75.

Ringe J (1996) An experimental approach to mapping the binding surfaces of crystalline proteins. Physical Chemistry 100: 2605–2611.

Schmidt EF, Smith DA (2002) Discovery, innovation and the cyclical nature of the pharmaceutical business. Drug Discovery Today 10: 663–568.

Shuker SB, Hajduk PJ, Meadows RP, Fesik SW (1996) Discovering high-affinity ligands for proteins: SAR by NMR. Science 274: 1531–1534.

Slee DH, Romano SJ, Yu J et al. (2001) Development of potent non-carbohydrate imidazole-based small molecule selectin inhibitors with antiinflammatory activity. Journal of Medicinal Chemistry 44: 2094–2107.

Spencer RW (1998) High-throughput screening of historic collections: observations on file size, biological targets, and file diversity. Biotechnology and Bioengineering Combinatorial Chemistry 61: 61–67.

Stahl M, Rarey M (2001) Detailed analysis of scoring functions for virtual screening. Journal of Medicinal Chemistry 44: 1035–1042.

Street LJ, Baker R, Davey WB et al. (1995) Synthesis and serotonergic activity of *N,N*-dimethyl-2-[5-(1,2,4-triazol-1-ylmethyl)-1H-indol-3-yl]ethylamine and analogs: potent agonists for 5-HT1D receptors. Journal of Medicinal Chemistry 38: 1799–810.

Summers JB, Davidsen SK (1998) Matrix metalloproteinase inhibitors and cancer. Annual Report in Medicinal Chemistry 33: 131–140.

Thompson LA, Ellman A (1996) Synthesis and applications of small molecule libraries. Chemical Reviews 96: 555–600.

Traxler PM, Furet P, Matt H, Buchdunger E, Meyer T, Lydon N (1996) 4-(phenylamino)pyrrolopyrimidines: potent and selective, ATP site directed inhibitors of the EGF-receptor protein tyrosine kinase. Journal of Medicinal Chemistry 39: 2285–2292.

van de Waterbeemd H (2002) High-throughput and in silico techniques in drug metabolism and pharmacokinetics. Current Opinion in Drug Discovery and Development 5: 33–43.

Veber DF, Johnson SR, Cheng H-Y, Smith BR, Ward KW, Kopple KD (2002) Molecular properties that influence the oral bioavailability of drug candidates. Journal of Medicinal Chemistry 45: 2615–2623.

Wabnitz PA, Loo JA (2001) Drug screening of pharmaceutical discovery compounds by micro-size exclusion chromatography/mass spectrometry. Rapid Communications in Mass Spectrometry 6: 85–91.

Wenger RM (1984) Synthesis of cyclosporine. Total syntheses of cyclosporin A and cyclosporin H, two fungal metabolites isolated from the species *Tolypocladium inflatum*. Gams Helv Chim Acta 67: 502–525.

Wess G, Urmann M, Sickenberger B (2001) Medicinal chemistry: challenges and opportunities. Angewandte Chemie [Intl edn Engl] 40: 3341–3350.

Xie X, Gu Y, Fox T et al. (1998) Crystal structure of JNK3: a kinase implicated in neuronal apoptosis. Structurel 6: 983–991.

Yamashita DS, Smith WW, Zhao B et al. (1997) Structure and design of potent and selective cathepsin K inhibitors. Journal of the American Chemical Society 119: 11351–11352.

10 Pharmacokinetic issues in drug discovery

J Ducharme
A J Dudley
R A Thompson

Introduction

To succeed as a product, a new drug needs to be efficacious, safe and convenient to use. All three requirements – the last very largely – depend on pharmacokinetics, so it is essential that the pharmacokinetic properties of a drug candidate are appropriate to its intended use.

In 1988, Prentiss et al. identified inappropriate pharmacokinetics in man as the major reason for discontinuing the clinical development of new chemical entities (NCEs), and Kennedy (1997) reported that 39% of failures in clinical development resulted from problems with pharmacokinetics (Table 10.1). Until the early 1990s, NCEs were optimized for primary pharmacology (in vitro and in vivo) and a very limited number of molecules were progressed further to drug metabolism and pharmacokinetics (DMPK) and toxicology evaluations. The latter were conducted according to predetermined protocols, mostly in vivo, in rodents and non-rodents, and reported as a series of observations, with little emphasis on explanations or possible solutions. The whole process was not amenable to successive iterations designed to improve the drug's profile, and as a result imperfect molecules were progressed to humans in the hope that some of the attributes would be improved.

Table 10.1 Reasons for failure in clinical development. (Data for 198 development compounds analysed by the Centre for Medicines Research; see Kennedy (1997))	
Reason for failure	**Percentage**
Pharmacokinetics	39
Lack of efficacy	30
Toxicology	11
Adverse effects in man	10
Commercial considerations	5
Others	5

Note: Of the 198 compounds that failed in development, 77 were anti-infective drugs; if these are excluded, lack of clinical efficacy was the main cause of failure (49%), and pharmacokinetic failures were less common (7%).

Drug discovery

With the realization that appropriate DMPK properties are critical to the success of candidate drugs in the clinic, DMPK hurdles were progressively introduced earlier and earlier in the drug discovery process, the main stages of which are described in Chapter 4 (see Figure 4.2). Nowadays, all pharmaceutical companies carry out DMPK testing during lead optimization, and many are moving towards DMPK-driven chemistry strategies during the lead identification phase (see Chapter 9). The goal of frontloading DMPK activities is not only to build in quality ('druggability') at an early stage, but also to increase the efficiency of drug discovery by compressing timelines and shortening development cycles (Kaplita et al., 2002). As NCEs that fail at the end of phase III have incurred 90% of their development costs (Price-WaterhouseCoopers, 1997), there is growing pressure to discontinue inadequate candidate drugs during preclinical rather than clinical testing ('fail, but fail early').

A series of technical and scientific advancements have transformed DMPK and the early stages of drug development, driven partly by cost reduction and the need to minimize animal experimentation: The main trends are:

- Progress in genomics and molecular biology, allowing the characterization of human drug-metabolizing enzymes and the development of 'humanized' in vitro tests;
- The development of combinatorial chemistry and high-throughput screening (HTS), leading to a steep increase in the number of new compounds to be tested;

- A new generation of analytical technologies that combine faster method development, higher throughput and increased sensitivity allowed the routine use of faster DMPK screens.

As discussed in Chapter 8, therapeutic efficacy is nowadays sought mainly by achieving satisfactory potency and selectivity for a single identified protein target. Pharmacokinetic properties, in contrast, depend on a wide range of different molecular interactions. There are many active and passive mechanisms, not just one target. This complexity, summarized in Figure 10.1, is the main obstacle faced by the campaign to address pharmacokinetic issues earlier in the discovery process. In some cases, such as predicting drug interactions mediated through cytochrome P450 (CYP), there is an identified molecular target, amenable to high-throughput screening, but in most cases such a molecular starting point is lacking, and so recourse is made to relatively slow functional screens (e.g. permeability assays), or to empirical correlations with the physicochemical properties of the molecule, either measured (which is often slow) or computed. As Figure 10.1 shows, correlating such measured or computed properties with pharmacokinetics as encountered in the clinic is made difficult by the number of interacting mechanisms that can influence the overall pharmacokinetic profile of a compound. In this chapter we describe approaches that are being developed to predict the pharmacokinetic properties of unknown compounds, and to use this information much earlier in the discovery process than has hitherto been customary.

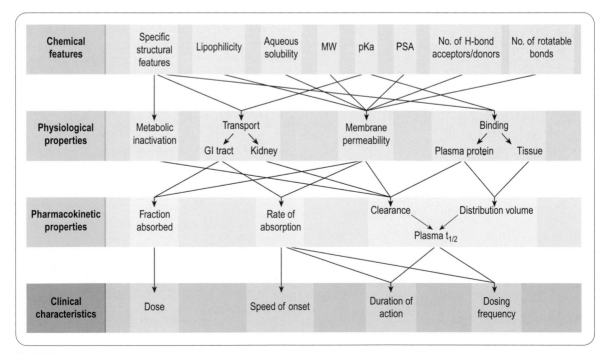

Fig. 10.1
Drug properties contributing to pharmacokinetic characteristics.

Scientific and technical drivers for early DMPK studies

Genomics

Because laboratory animals do not handle drugs the way humans do, it was important to develop predictive models of drug metabolism in man. One of the most significant advances in helping to bridge the gap between animals and man was the establishment of 'humanized' in vitro tests.

The availability of human genetic information led to the development of recombinant protein tools, which can provide an unlimited supply of human proteins. In vitro data on human metabolism allowed the judicious selection of toxicology species and the scaling of in vitro to in vivo pharmacokinetic parameters (clearance).

Combinatorial chemistry and high-throughput screening

Starting in the early 1990s, HTS rapidly grew as a major source of lead compounds for drug discovery projects. This approach was highly successful in providing novel structures with high affinity for a selected target. However, there is a current trend away from screening very large compound libraries in favour of smaller, more focused screening libraries (see Chapter 8; Lipinski, 2000). At the same time, there is a realization that suitable DMPK properties are as important as target affinity in the search for drugs with real therapeutic potential (Lipinski, 2000).

In most pharmaceutical companies, screening for DMPK properties currently takes place after the higher-capacity biological screening. However, recent progress in robotics has increased the throughput of DMPK screens, and nowadays hundreds to thousands of samples can be processed in a week. The real challenge now is to optimize our screening systems so that we can obtain the most relevant biological information possible. In 1997, Rodrigues had pointed out the need for a more rational approach to drug screening ('intelligent drug screening', or 'applying the right model to the right problem or to the right number of compounds').

New analytical technologies

Until the early 1990s, DMPK testing was carried out on one compound at a time, and was generally slow and labour-intensive in terms of both method development and sample processing (Plumb et al., 2001). Chromato-graphic separations and sample preparation (often based on lengthy liquid–liquid or solid-phase extractions) coupled to UV, fluorescence or electrochemical detection had to be carefully optimized to ensure sufficient resolution between the analytes and metabolites of interest, and to control for biological interferences. Column run times of 15–30 minutes were normal, even longer if mobile phase gradients were used.

Two technologies in particular – the coupling of liquid chromatography (LC) to mass spectrometry (LC/MS) and the introduction of atmospheric pressure electrospray ionization (ESI) – have enabled DMPK issues to be addressed much earlier in the drug discovery process than was possible hitherto. The first change was seen in the area of metabolite identification, followed by rapid advances since the late 1990s in the speed of quantitative analysis. The traditional application of quantitative LC analyses, where the column provides the selectivity and the detector the sensitivity, has given way to the use of mass spectrometry to provide both selectivity and sensitivity. The generic working procedures used today in most pharmaceutical companies allow for fast routine analysis of large numbers of new compounds.

Fast gradient reversed-phase chromatography on short columns coupled to MS with single ion monitoring or selected reaction monitoring to give greater selectivity, is now in general use. Although ESI allowed the creation of these generic methods, it is also the major obstacle to LC/MS becoming a true generic technique. ESI is a complex process (Cech and Enke, 2001) where the signal obtained depends not only on the analyte, but also on the sample matrix. Compound variables such as surface activity, proton affinity, pKa and solvation energy, as well as the presence of co-eluting compounds, all affect the degree of ionization of the analyte and hence the signal. The methods commonly used today minimize these problems by optimizing sample work-up, chromatographic conditions and ESI parameters.

The major sample work-up process in routine use is protein precipitation. This has the advantage of simplicity (the addition of cold solvent to the sample, followed by centrifugation), works for most compounds, gives a fairly good sample extraction efficiency, and can be easily automated in 96-well format. The alternative technique of solid-phase extraction (SPE) can also be automated, but requires optimization for individual compounds and thus has less general use in early drug discovery.

Chromatography is a basic component in almost all procedures. LC is no longer used to provide selectivity by physical separation of the analytes, this role now being performed by MS. The primary function of LC is to concentrate the analyte into a chromatographic peak to give increased sensitivity, and to separate it from polar constitutes such as salts, and from ion-suppressing substances. However, LC remains the primary bottleneck in almost all

LC/MS methods. This has led to a number of approaches to shorten the LC run times. Total run times of a few minutes are achieved without reducing column capacity by using short columns, small particle size packing materials, sharp gradients and high flow rates (Mutton, 1998; Cheng et al., 2001). Different versions of sample pooling prior to analysis are also widely used to increase throughput (Korfmacher et al., 2001).

DMPK studies in drug discovery

HTS identifies compounds on the basis of affinity for the selected target with little regard for drug-like properties. Many authors have documented the trend towards increasing lipophilicity and molecular weight in lead compounds originating from HTS (Lipinski, 2000).

Unless 'druggability' is addressed early in discovery, it may become extremely difficult to build it in without compromising affinity or selectivity for the primary target. Many of the problems relate to DMPK properties.

Drug discovery (see Chapter 4) progresses from hits to leads (lead identification), and from leads to drug candidates (lead optimization). In this chapter we describe how DMPK studies can be incorporated into the lead identification and lead optimization stages.

Different companies may use a different nomenclature, and may elect to perform particular DMPK studies earlier or later in the project than the programme described here. Until very recently, DMPK properties were not taken into account when evaluating hits. Pressure on DMPK resources meant that the later phases of drug development tended to be supported at the expense of early drug discovery projects. As discussed above, however, there is increasing recognition throughout the industry of the need to address DMPK problems as early as possible, and to remedy them if possible by chemical design, thus reducing the risk of meeting unsurmountable obstacles during development.

During lead identification one aim is to identify potential DMPK deficiencies, which then need to be resolved during lead optimization. As the project progresses, more detailed DMPK information is needed.

Early in lead optimization, as in late lead identification, parallel synthesis plays a dominant role and many compounds are being tested, and emphasis is put on in vitro screening. Early assessment of pharmaokinetic–pharmacodynamic (PK-PD) relationships is increasingly performed during this phase.

In mid-lead optimization, traditional medicinal chemistry complements parallel synthesis and in vivo studies complement in vitro experiments. To improve in vivo DMPK properties, it is important to understand the major factors (e.g. poor solubility, low permeability, metabolic weak points) that need to be changed.

Table 10.2
Desirable DMPK properties of lead compounds and drug candidates intended for oral use

Lead compound	Drug candidate
Complies with Lipinski's 'Rule of 5'	Sufficient aqueous solubility for intended formulation
Aqueous solubility	Predicted high oral bioavailability in man
High permeability and low active efflux in Caco-2 cell or similar assay	Scaled half-life compatible with intended frequency of dosing in man
Sufficient oral bioavailability in laboratory species to achieve measurable plasma concentration and significant pharmacological effect.	Linear pharmacokinetics over the therapeutic dose range
Good metabolic stability in presence of liver microsome preparation.	'Balanced' clearance, i.e. no reliance on a single route of elimination or a single metabolizing enzyme
Plasma half-life in laboratory species sufficient for pharmacodynamic and pharmacokinetic studies	No major metabolism by polymorphic enzymes
	No major active metabolite
	No reactive metabolites
	No inhibition or induction of drug-metabolizing enzymes at relevant concentrations
	PK–PD relationships understood in relevant animal models

Finally, in late lead optimization, when a short list of compounds with acceptable attributes is identified, more complete studies, together with mechanistic investigations, are carried out to understand PK-PD relationships as fully as possible, and predict PK parameters in man.

Desired DMPK profiles of leads and drug candidates

In the discussion that follows, we are assuming that the aim is to develop a drug for oral use in one or two daily doses. Needless to say, where drugs are developed for topical, intravenous or other routes of administration, or formulated for special delivery systems, DMPK profiling has to be adapted accordingly. For an anti-inflammatory skin cream, for example, low systemic absorption and rapid metabolic inactivation are desirable attributes, in contrast to the requirements of an oral drug.

The main DMPK characteristics typically required of lead compounds and drug candidates are summarized in Table 10.2.

As a first step at the lead identification stage, compliance with the Lipinski 'Rule of 5' criteria (see Chapter 9), which are based on computed, rather than measured properties, provides a useful filter. The same set of rules can be used as a broad guide for acceptable metabolic stability (Smith, 2001). Within a series of structurally related compounds, the likelihood of poor metabolic stability often increases drastically when logD >3.

At the lead identification stage emphasis is placed on 'optimizability', i.e. on the potential for improving properties such as metabolic stability, solubility or lipophilicity without compromising affinity for the target. During the lead identification phase, 6–9 months of iterative cycles between chemistry, in vitro pharmacology and DMPK are expected to result in compounds with acceptable profiles according to the criteria summarized in Table 10.2. Although the lead compound does not need to have a long half-life or oral bioavailability, it should reach detectable plasma concentrations for a sufficiently long period to allow in vivo testing in the relevant animal model (typically in rodents).

Throughout lead identification and lead optimization obtaining timely DMPK results is necessary to guide the chemistry strategy. DMPK departments, traditionally aligned with toxicology groups, are now closely linked with medicinal chemistry (Smith, 2001), ensuring rapid feedback of information. As DMPK screening generates target-independent data, information obtained in one project can be used in another.

In silico predictions of DMPK properties
Usefulness and limitations

Pharmaceutical companies are investing considerable time and effort in the development of in silico models of drug absorption, distribution, metabolism and excretion (ADME). Predictions can be 'human based', as data are now often obtained with human cells or subcellular fractions.

It is well recognized that ADME predictions are more difficult to establish than in vitro pharmacology structure–activity relationships (SAR) because of the many distinct mechanisms that determine the overall ADME characteristics of a compound (see above, Figure 10.1). For example, metabolic stability in liver microsomes can reflect the activity of a number of Phase I enzymes (encompassing both affinity and capacity factors), and permeability across Caco-2 monolayers can be the resultant of both passive diffusion and active transport. This complexity is a serious obstacle, and predictive models (see van der Waterbeemd and Gifford, 2003) remain far from perfect. The main approaches that are being used are:

- The *reductionist* approach, i.e. the development of computational models based on screens designed to isolate a specific component (e.g. artificial membrane screen for passive diffusion or inhibition assays based on a specific CYP isoform)
- The *restrictive* approach, i.e. the restriction of computational models to a family of chemical congeners, rather than molecules in general, on the assumption that the major driver of metabolic instability or other pharmacokinetic shortcomings will be similar for the whole family;
- The '*holistic*' approach, commonly referred to as *physiologically based pharmacokinetic modelling (PBPK)*. This is an ambitious attempt to put together the various individual components (intestinal permeability, active transport, metabolic degradation, renal excretion, protein binding etc.) in the setting of the whole animal, making allowance for physiological factors such as intestinal transit time, regional blood flow, tissue composition, tissue location of enzymes etc. The ultimate goal – not yet reached, though the prophets remain optimistic – is to be able to predict the time course of drug and metabolite concentrations in all relevant tissues under different dosage regimens.

Developing reliable computational models in general requires large coherent data sets to provide an empirical basis for further predictions. One of the main problems, currently, is that such data sets are too small, or too limited in terms of chemical diversity. The development of high-throughput assay methods is quickly expanding the avail-

Drug discovery

able data, but the reluctance of companies to reveal chemical structures impedes large-scale initiatives in the public domain.

Most computational ADME models tend to be *exclusionary* (i.e. they identify compounds that are unsuitable because of low solubility, poor permeability or metabolic instability). The justification for excluding compounds early on the basis of physicochemical properties is summarized in Figure 10.2, taken from the data of Wenlock et al. (2003), who compared the physicochemical properties of drugs at various stages of development and found that successful compounds at each stage had on average lower values of the Lipinski parameters, and fewer rotatable bonds, than did unsuccessful compounds.

Predictors of absorption and oral bioavailability

Although extremely useful to guide physicochemical properties, the Rule of 5 cannot be directly applied to predict oral bioavailability, and several authors have highlighted the importance of other descriptors (Chaturvedi et al., 2001). For example, in 1997, Palm and collaborators described the negative impact of polar surface area (PSA) on intestinal absorption. PSA is related to molecular hydrogen bonding capacity (Stenberg et al., 1999) and can be defined as the area occupied by nitrogen and oxygen atoms plus the hydrogen atoms attached to them (Stenberg et al., 2001). From data obtained on 20 compounds, Palm et al. suggested that a PSA >140 Å^2 resulted in poor oral absorption (<10%), whereas a PSA <60 Å^2 resulted in excellent absorption (>90%).

Oral bioavailability is determined by both absorption and first-pass metabolism, and is difficult to predict with accuracy from structural data alone.

A recent review of rat bioavailability data for more than 1100 compounds tested by SmithKlineBeecham showed that 65% of all compounds with fewer than seven rotatable bonds had an oral bioavailability of more than 20% (Veber et al., 2002). They found (Figure 10.3) that over a MW range of 220–770 Da bioavailability was indeed higher in the lower MW group (in agreement with Lipinski), but that it was also closely associated with

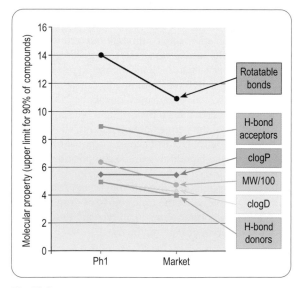

Fig. 10.2
Comparison of physicochemical properties of drugs entering Phase I and drugs eventually registered. (Data from Wenlock et al., 2003.)

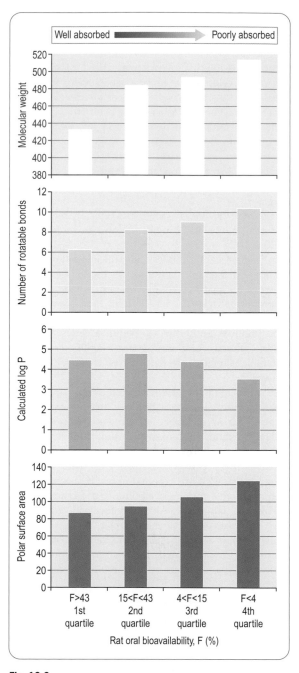

Fig. 10.3
Relationship between oral absorption and physicochemical properties. (Data from Veber et al., 2002.)

lower rotatable bond and hydrogen bond counts and lower PSA. Within a narrower MW range, i.e. in the 400–550 or >550 Da subsets, the relationship between bioavailability and the number of rotatable bonds was even more apparent. Hence the common belief of increased bioavailability with lower MW may stem from the fact that molecules with low MW (especially <400 Da) have reduced flexibility and fewer rotatable bonds. In view of the trend towards higher MW of HTS hits, the consideration of PSA and rotatable bond descriptors may prove useful in prioritizing compounds. Most of the compounds analysed by Veber et al. (2002) had cLogP values below 5 (the Lipinski limit), and compounds with much lower values were, contrary to expectations, actually less well absorbed.

One difficulty in predicting absorption is that transporters and drug metabolizing enzymes associated with enteric cells can play an important role, but cannot currently be predicted for novel molecules.

Predicted volume of distribution

Lombardo and colleagues (2002) recently published a model for predicting the steady-state volume of distribution (Vd_{ss}) for neutral and basic compounds in man, based on three easily measured properties, namely human plasma protein binding, experimental logD, and

pKa. The model was built from a training set of 64 reference compounds (literature data) and its accuracy was determined using a test set of 14 compounds. Predicted Vd_{ss} values were close to measured values (within a factor of 2) and as accurate as estimates from allometric scaling methods based on pharmacokinetic data in animals (Obach et al., 1997). The method has the obvious advantage of not relying on animal PK data and could be applicable to an early discovery setting when predicted Vd_{ss} is a necessary component of half-life predictions.

However, experimental logD and pK_a are not obtained routinely on all compounds. Lombardo et al. (2002) therefore tried using computed estimates of logD and found that, although the error was greater than with estimates based on measures logD values, the Vd_{ss} estimates still correlated well with actual values (Figure 10.4). The use of such models in early phases of drug discovery is likely to increase as in silico predictions of physicochemical properties and plasma protein binding become more accurate and widely available.

Experimental DMPK testing

The purpose of the work during the lead investigation phase is to determine the DMPK properties of potential

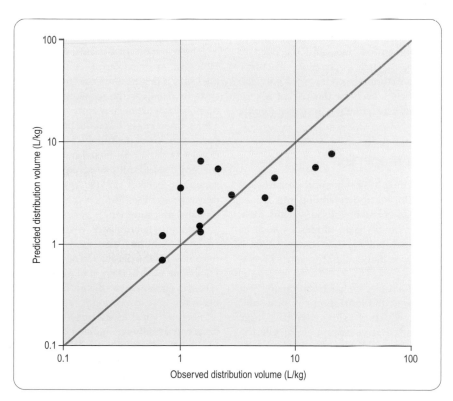

Fig. 10.4
Comparison of predicted and actual distribution volumes of development compounds. (Data from Lombardo et al., 2002.)

lead compound classes. It is important during this phase to show a correlation between the chemical characteristics of compounds and possible DMPK deficiencies, and to show that these deficiencies are not inherent to the pharmacophore. The high capacity of in vitro methods can be very useful during this phase, but it is also important to establish early on a correlation between in vitro and in vivo properties. In addition, monitoring for in vivo exposure is important for the interpretation of pharmacological experiments in whole animals in the lead identification and lead optimization phases. In this section, we describe some of the in vitro and in vivo methods used in DMPK evaluation.

Data handling

The inclusion of DMPK in the lead identification and lead optimization phases has resulted in a tremendous increase in experimental data. At the same time, short cycle times between synthesis of compounds and feedback of pharmacological and DMPK data are essential. This has placed new demands on data capture and handling, and created a need for improved data and knowledge management systems (Summer-Smith, 2001).

Various tools to handle large amounts of captured data have become available, such as ActivityBase (www.idbs.com), Assay Explorer (www.mdl.com) and RS[3] Discovery (www.accelrys.com). Building databases for DMPK data (and secondary screening data in general) has proved difficult owing to the complexity of the assays and the generated data, and the need to include other data objects such as chemical structures. Currently there are no complete commercial software solutions, but approaches such as the use of object-oriented programming are showing promise (Smith, 2002).

Physicochemical properties

A basic knowledge of the physicochemical properties of compounds is important for understanding interactions between chemical moieties and biological systems. Measurement and prediction of basic properties such as pK_a, lipophilicity and solubility is now routine (Avdeef, 2001), and this has necessitated a shift towards higher-throughput assays.

The charge state of a molecule has traditionally been assessed by determining the ionization constant, pK_a, using pH titration, which is slow, requires large amounts of compound, and is susceptible to interference by impurities. Using capillary electrophoresis (CE) for the determination of pK_a has the advantage of low sample consumption and insensitivity to impurities (Wan et al., 2002). Further, the coupling of CE to mass spectrometry (CE-MS) will allow for the parallel analysis of a large number of compounds.

Lipophilicity is probably the property that has the strongest influence on a wide array of DMPK properties. Absorption, protein binding, distribution and metabolic stability all tend to show a correlation with lipophilicity. Lipophilicity has traditionally been defined by the equilibrium partition coefficient, P, of a compound between water and octanol: P represents the partition coefficient of a non-ionizable compound. LogP >5 implies a partition coefficient exceeding 10^5, i.e. a highly lipophilic compound, which partitions strongly in favour of the octanol phase. Many relevant compounds are weak acids or bases, and for these P varies with pH; the lipophilicity of such compounds is generally measured at pH 7.4, and expressed as $logD_{(pH7,4)}$.

Although it is true that compounds with logP >5 rarely survive in development, the relationship between lipohilicity and PK properties is complex. High logP values are normally associated with high membrane permeability, which favours absorption, but also with low aqueous solubility (see below), which hinders absorption. In practice, absorption is usually poor if logP >5, but is not necessarily improved at lower logP values (see Figure 10.3). Because there are differences in the pH of different body compartments, the pH dependence of logD can markedly affect the absorption, renal excretion and distribution of compounds.

The determination of logP or logD by direct measurement in a two-phase system is slow and troublesome. Reversed-phase chromatography (Valkó et al., 1997) is much more convenient, allowing estimates of logP and logD based on column retention times.

The relevance of a partition measure such as logP to biological systems can of course be questioned. There are today a large number of 'more biologically relevant' systems used for the measure of lipophilicity, such as immobilized artificial membranes (IAM) (Pidgeon et al., 1995), liposomes (Lundahl and Beigi, 1997), and the parallel artificial membrane permeability assay, PAMPA (Kansy et al., 1998). Nevertheless, logP/log D remains the gold standard. Both can be estimated with reasonable precision on the basis of chemical structure (see www.acdlabs.com/products/phys_chem_lab/), but physical measurement is generally preferred.

Aqueous solubility is a central issue in drug discovery. Solubility is usually determined in 96-well plate format, with the dissolved concentration determined by LC-UV or LC-MS (Pan et al., 2001). Higher-throughput turbidimetric assays (Bevan and Lloyd, 2000), can be used, but give lower-quality results.

For biological assay purposes, adequate concentrations can usually be obtained by dissolving compounds in 10 mM dimethylsulfoxide (DMSO), subsequently diluted in buffered aqueous solutions. For in vivo experiments DMSO can produce troublesome vehicle effects, and it is not acceptable for human studies. Therefore, if compounds have low aqueous solubility, special formulations are likely to be needed.

Compounds with an aqueous solubility less than 50–100 µg/mL are usually poorly absorbed. If a drug discovery project aims at a target dose in man of 1 mg/kg, solubility should be at least 50 µg/mL (Curatolo, 1998; Horter and Dressman, 2001). Compounds with lower solubility will be problematic unless potency is extremely high. Low-solubility compounds can become useful drugs, but usually at the expense of extensive formulation work.

Only occasionally does a project strike lucky and identify lead compounds with very favourable physicochemical properties and good oral absorption. More often, preliminary formulation studies are needed to identify vehicles suitable for the desired route of administration, and many pharmaceutical companies now use a 'formulatability' score (based on the compatibility of the compound with commonly used co-solvents) in addition to aqueous solubility as a preliminary to in vivo studies. Usually a common vehicle is used for the early studies (e.g. pH3 buffer, 20% cyclodextrin or 25% polyethylene glycol), with generic formulations being identified for specific series. In addition to improving pharmacokinetic behaviour, early preformulation support (see Chapter 17) allows a greater confidence in the outcome of pharmacodynamic studies by making the action of the compound in vivo more predictable.

Membrane permeability

Passive diffusion

For most drugs passive diffusion across cell membranes is necessary to allow access to the target. Oral absorption,

penetration of the blood–brain barrier and access to intracellular sites of action all depend, in most cases, on the ability of compounds to diffuse across cell membranes, exceptions being compounds such as L-dopa, which cross membranes by active transport. Over the last 10 years assays that measure compound permeability across layers of cells such as Caco-2 and Madin–Derby canine kidney (MDCK) cells, have become routine in the pharmaceutical industry (Irvine et al., 1999). The cells are grown as monolayers on permeable filter supports, and drug transport is measured by applying compound on one side of the cell layer and measuring the rate at which it crosses to the other side. Test compounds are compared to standard marker compounds, such as those listed in the Biological Classification System (BCS) published by the FDA (www.fda.gov/cder/guidance/3618fnl.htm). This model is very simple and easy to describe mathematically, but is an oversimplification of the in vivo situation, where transport is a distributed process (i.e. a concentration gradient exists along the gastrointestinal tract as well as across the wall). In addition, the permeability number generated from these experiments is in reality a composite term, as compounds cross multiple biological membranes when permeating a cell layer. Finally, the contribution of active processes to the overall transport of compounds across these cells adds additional complexity to the system. Despite these caveats, Caco-2 cell permeability generally correlates well with oral absorption in humans (Figure 10.5).

Although permeability is routinely measured or calculated for many compounds during the lead identification process, relating this number to the cri-

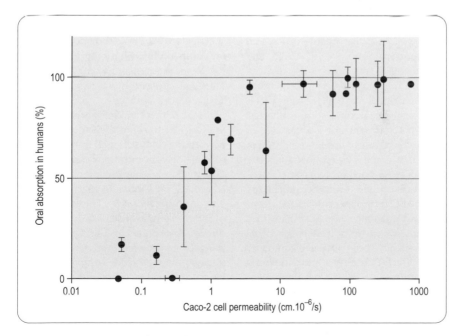

Fig. 10.5
Relationship between oral absorption in man and permeability of compounds through Caco-2 cell monolayers. (Data from Sternberg et al., 2001.)

teria a compound must meet to qualify as a potential drug candidate is not simple. This relationship is best understood for absorption, as there are human absorption data available to compare to in vitro permeability information. In addition, the in vitro permeability data can be put into context by calculating a maximum absorbable dose (MAD) of an oral formulation based on clinical potency, solubility, gastrointestinal tract transit time and permeability (Curatolo, 1998). This calculation can be used to rank series of compounds and identify problematic compounds/series. However, for permeability across other biological barriers, such as the blood–brain barrier, such analyses are less well developed, and designing molecules to optimize cell permeability remains a challenge for medicinal chemistry.

Active transport (transporters)

Specific transport proteins catalyse the movement of many water-soluble ions, nutrients, metabolites and drugs across cell membranes. It has been estimated that there are *at least* 2000 transporters in the human genome, most of which have yet to be cloned, and it is becoming clear that transporters play a significant role in ADME processes. Their relevance to drug discovery and development is reviewed by Ayrton and Morgan (2001). Screening compounds for their interactions with certain transporters that are known to modulate drug disposition is becoming widely practised in the pharmaceutical industry.

Several families of cloned transporters are known to play a role in drug disposition, including the ATP-binding cassette (ABC) family (e.g. *P-glycoprotein, MRP1* and *MRP2*); the organic anion transporting polypeptide family, (e.g. *OATP-C*); the organic cation and organic anion transporter families (e.g. *OAT3* and *OCT1*). The cloning of these transporters has allowed assay systems based on microinjected oocytes or transfected cells to be developed, in which transport is measured by the intracellular accumulation of the test compound. In vitro test systems include isolated cells or cell lines that represent the tissue of origin, or natural or transfected cell lines that express a certain transporter protein. Expression of transport proteins in cDNA-transfected *Xenopus laevis* oocytes is another potentially useful technique. For ABC transport proteins the determination of ATPase activity in microsomal systems may provide an alternative test system for transport activity. However, inconsistencies have been observed compared to cellular systems in which transport of the compound is measured directly (Polli et al., 2001). Commonly used efflux monolayer systems include the human cells Caco-2, HT-29 and T84, as well as cDNA-transfected MDCK and LLC-PK1 pig kidney cells. Caco-2 cell monolayers are currently the most commonly used in vitro technique. For nine out of 10 efflux proteins from the ABC transporter family investigated, Caco-2 cells have been reported to resemble human jejunum in transcript levels (Taipalensuu et al., 2001).

Large datasets detailing compound interactions with various transporters now exist within most pharmaceutical companies. However, at present, data of this sort are of limited value in predicting pharmacokinetic behaviour in humans, and so transporter assays are not used routinely in lead identification.

An area of increasing interest is that of drug–drug interactions mediated by transporters. In recent years, efflux transporters such as P-glycoprotein have been shown to be responsible for many such interactions. *Talinolol*, for example, which undergoes little metabolism, shows increased bioavailability when co-administered with *verapamil*, which is an inhibitor of P-glycoprotein-mediated transport. Various methods are used to profile the interaction potential of candidate drugs. A limited number of compounds may be tested during the lead identification phase, though most of this effort usually comes later in the lead optimization phase of the project.

The effect of compounds on the efflux of a substrate marker from cells (i.e. from the intracellular to the extracellular compartment) is easy to measure, but the results correlate poorly with interactions that occur in vivo. Measurement of effects on substrate transport across cell monolayers is a preferred technique.

As mentioned earlier, transporter involvement in humans cannot currently be accurately predicted from non-clinical studies. Predictions based on animal data could be flawed because some reports indicate that there are marked species differences in the tissue distribution of transporters and their substrate specificity. When predictions are made from cell-based systems such as Caco-2, active transport may be of no relevance for compounds with a high intrinsic permeability; furthermore, the transporter may be saturated at the high intestinal concentrations achieved during absorption. Thus, in the absence of good physiologically based pharmacokinetic models for the prediction of in vivo relevance of transporters, current best practices include performing bidirectional transport studies in Caco-2 cells, using concentrations corresponding to the clinical dosage dissolved in 250 mL or less (thereby achieving a concentration similar to that in the GI tract following oral dosing in humans). This approach gives some indication of the relevance of active transport contributions during absorption. In addition, interpretation of drug transport by isolated transporters in various expression systems should include comparison of transport characteristics of the test compounds with those of compounds for which transport processes are known to be clinically relevant (e.g. *digoxin, vinblastine, talinolol, fexofenadine* etc). The extent to which such studies are carried out in the lead optimization phase will vary, depending on a judgement of how important transporters are likely to be for the particular drug class being investigated.

CNS exposure

The blood–brain barrier (BBB) is a significant obstacle for compounds acting on CNS targets. The endothelial cells that comprise the BBB possess tight junctions and express the efflux transporter P-glycoprotein (Pgp), both of which play a major role in the barrier function of the BBB. Recently, in vitro cell models have been developed to assess BBB permeability and the transport of novel compounds. Primary culture models of endothelial cells grown in the presence or absence of astrocytes provide good models of BBB properties (Lundquist et al., 2002), but are too slow and costly for routine use. Instead, generic permeability models such as Caco-2 or MDCK cells are commonly used to predict BBB permeability, though their limitations need to be recognized. The astrocyte co-culture BBB model remains the model of choice for more detailed mechanistic studies. Several attempts have been made to develop in silico models for predicting BBB permeability from molecular descriptors (Clark, 2003), but such models are not yet sufficiently reliable for general use.

P-glycoprotein (Pgp) is the major efflux transporter at the BBB and can drastically reduce the access of drugs to the brain (de Lange et al., 1995). Therefore, screening of compounds for Pgp efflux has become routine practice in CNS drug discovery. Many different assay systems are in use, ranging from transport assays to competition assays with fluorescence detection. In addition, computational approaches that predict Pgp-mediated transport from chemical structure are available.

The *rate* and *extent* of CNS exposure are, strictly speaking, independent of each other (i.e. a drug may equilibrate rapidly but reach only a low concentration in the CNS, or reach a high concentration but only slowly). They depend on various drug properties, including BBB permeability, active transport, plasma and tissue binding, and partition into brain lipids, such that in vivo brain penetration kinetics are hard to predict on the basis of in vitro data. Nevertheless, adequate BBB permeability and the absence of a rapid efflux mechanism are generally required for drugs directed to CNS targets.

The relationship between the pharmacokinetic characteristics and pharmacological effects (PK/PD relationships) of CNS-active drugs is more complex than is the case with other drug classes. The brain is not a single pharmacokinetic 'compartment', and different anatomical brain regions may show different levels of drug exposure. Furthermore, the accumulation of drugs in brain lipids may produce high overall brain concentrations that do not reflect the effective drug concentration in the relevant biophase. To resolve complexities of this kind, it is important during the lead optimization phase to obtain information on the PK/PD relationship for the compounds under investigation. This will require correlating drug levels in the brain with a pharmacological response (a 'biomarker') that reflects as closely as possible the desired therapeutic effect. As discussed in Chapter 11, choosing the right animal model and biomarker for certain types of drug (e.g. antipsychotics and antidepressants) is often problematic.

Overall, it is fair to say that designing in appropriate CNS penetration properties early in the project still presents considerable difficulties, and unsatisfactory CNS penetration remains a common cause of failure.

Metabolic stability

The cytochrome P450 (CYP) superfamily consists of haem-containing monooxygenase enzymes that play an important role in the oxidative metabolism of endogenous substances, natural products and xenobiotics. More than 55 CYP genes (divided into families and subfamilies according to their sequence similarities) have been sequenced in humans (see http://drnelson.utmem.edu/CytochromeP450.html). Four human CYP families (CYP1–4) code for liver-expressed enzymes that metabolize foreign compounds as well as endogenous lipophilic substrates. The CYP2 family is the largest, accounting for approximately one-third of all CYPs found in humans.

A subset of CYPs, CYP1A2, CYP2C9, CYP2C19, CYP2D6 and CYP3A4, appear to account for the metabolism of most drugs (Rendic and Di Carlo, 1997). Their importance relates to their abundance (CYP3A4 is the major CYP in human liver; Waxman, 1999) or their preference for specific drug-like features. For example, CYP2D6 metabolizes a wide range of cardiac and psychotropic drugs with basic amine moieties (de Groot et al., 1999).

Because the liver is the main drug-metabolizing organ, for many drugs hepatic clearance is a major determinant of total clearance (*Cl*). The relationship between clearance and oral bioavailability is well established (Benet and Zia-Amirhosseini, 1995), and in general compounds with high hepatic clearance will have low oral bioavailability because of first-pass metabolism (Clarke and Jeffrey, 2001). Therefore, metabolic stability criteria generally have to be more stringent in a project seeking an orally active drug than in one seeking an injectable drug.

The in vitro preparations most commonly used for studying drug metabolism (Plant, 2004) are liver microsomes, a preparation known as the 'S9 fraction', and intact hepatocytes.

Liver microsomes

Liver microsomes are the simplest and most useful tools for determining metabolic stability during the early stages of drug discovery (Bertrand et al., 2000). They can be prepared from all animal species (including humans), contain high activities of all CYPs and a variety of other Phase I drug and Phase II drug metabolizing enzymes (e.g. conjugation enzymes, which require appropriate cofactors to be added to the incubation medium).

Microsomes are commercially available, and are stable for up to 5 years at –80°C.

S9 fraction

This consists of both microsomal and cytosolic fractions and includes a wide range of Phase I and Phase II enzymes, a broader range than microsomes, albeit at lower activity. A standard cocktail of cofactors needs to be added for these activities to be expressed. Enzyme induction does not occur.

Hepatocytes

Hepatocytes contain all liver enzymes and cofactors and preserve intact cell–cell communication systems. Availability of human liver tissue is often a problem, which is likely to improve with the development of cryopreservation methods (Li et al., 1999). Cryopreserved hepatocytes now retain almost all their drug metabolizing capacities and can be used to assess rates and routes of metabolism (Coleman et al., 2001), as well as modelling enzyme induction. Overall metabolic stability can be assessed by incubating compounds with human hepatocytes in suspension, but the characterization of metabolic routes may require longer incubation times and the use of monolayer cell cultures. The latter should be regarded as qualitative rather than quantitative studies, as the expression of most drug-metabolizing enzymes declines in monolayer cultures (Coleman et al., 2001). An alternative system giving the preservation of liver-specific functions (Ben-Ze'ev et al., 1988; Dunn et al., 1991) involves hepatocyte monolayers overlaid on extracellular matrix, which dramatically improves cell viability and allows the formation of functional bile canalicular networks (LeCluyse et al., 1994). Despite being labour intensive, this system allows the measurement of permeability and active transport in addition to the production of metabolites, and is becoming widely used in drug discovery.

The use of metabolic stability studies

In order to provide first estimates of metabolic stability with adequate throughput, most companies approximate intrinsic clearance (Cl_{int}) values by measuring the disappearance of the compound as a function of time, the substrate concentration (typically 0.5 or 1 µM) being well below the assumed Michaelis Menten constant (K_m) value. This allows a more accurate ranking of compounds than the percentage metabolic stability at a single time point (e.g. 60 min), as the incubation of higher concentrations (e.g. 10 or 100 µM) can lead to metabolic saturation and the overestimation of metabolic stability. Cl_{int} values are derived from the in vitro half-life (calculated from the exponential disappearance of the parent drug), taking into account the incubation volume and the amount of microsomal proteins per gram of liver (Obach, 1997, 1999).

Metabolic stability assays are generally automated on robotic workstations. Typically 50–100 compounds can be evaluated in one experiment. Incubations are carried out in 96- or 384-well plates, aliquots are collected at various time points (typically up to 30 min), quenched with an organic solvent (e.g. acetonitrile) and analysed by LC-MS. Peak areas corresponding to the parent drug are usually determined with a mass spectrometry detector operated in selected ion monitoring mode, obviating the need for lengthy LC separations. To increase throughput, incubation samples can be pooled before analysis (known as 'n in 1' analysis, where n can vary from 2 to 10, depending on chemical diversity). This is especially attractive when several discovery projects are run in parallel, as unrelated chemical series are less likely to have overlapping molecular weights.

In 2001, Clarke and Jeffrey evaluated the ability of metabolic stability measurements in rat liver microsomes to predict in vivo clearance in rats with a retrospective analysis of 1163 compounds from 48 chemistry programmes at SmithKlineBeecham. Overall, in vitro approaches were effective in selecting compounds with desirable pharmacokinetic properties, the in vivo clearance of approximately 64% of the compounds being adequately predicted. About 24% of the compounds had a higher in vivo clearance than predicted, which is not surprising as liver microsomes do not contain all metabolizing enzymes and cannot reflect extrahepatic metabolism. Although these 'false positives' would have been erroneously progressed to in vivo testing, they do not represent missed opportunities. For 13% of compounds in vitro tests overestimated the in vivo clearance; however, most of these were found to have undesirable physicochemical properties, CYP-inhibiting properties or short half-lives (e.g. because of restricted volumes of distribution due to high plasma protein binding), which made them unsuitable for development. This example illustrates the utility of in vitro screens such as metabolic stability measurements in microsomes, so long as they are not carried out in isolation but are followed up by complementary tests, in vitro or in vivo, which can be used to eliminate false positives or negatives.

As the project progresses through lead optimization rough estimates of Cl_{int} need to be refined to allow adequate predictions of in vivo clearance. Whereas early studies rely on parent drug disappearance for the estimation of an apparent K_m for overall metabolism, later studies will measure the formation of specific metabolite(s) for the determination of one or more K_m and V_{max} values. Incubation conditions need to be carefully chosen to ensure linearity of product formation with respect to time and substrate concentration, and the inclusion of an excess of necessary cofactors.

In recent years there has been a growing interest in the use of hepatocytes to predict quantitative pharmacokinetic parameters of drug transformation in man before the first clinical studies are undertaken (Cross and Bayliss, 2000).

Metabolic profiling

When metabolic stability testing reveals high Cl_{int} values the metabolites need to be identified (metabolic profiling) in order to discover the weak points in the parent molecule. Liver microsomes are well suited for this purpose in many cases. Incubating a few compounds with hepatocytes can help to validate the use of liver microsomes as the primary screen (if microsomal metabolism is predominant) or indicate the need to modify the assay (e.g. by the inclusion of specific cofactors). Metabolic stability and profiling in rat hepatocytes offer lower throughput but can be used if liver microsomes provide unsatisfactory results.

In the past, metabolite identification was a time-consuming activity, undertaken only for approved development compounds. However, recent technical advances have made it possible to incorporate it into the lead identification and optimization phases (Clarke et al., 2001). Fast gradient HPLC (Hop et al., 2002) and new technologies such as monolithic columns (Dear et al., 2001) allow short run times. However, the true bottleneck in metabolite identification is the interpretation of MS spectra. Software packages to facilitate this work are becoming available, and some, such as MetaboLynx from Micromass and Mass Frontier from Thermo-Finnigan, should soon allow semiautomated metabolite identification, thereby dramatically decreasing throughput times. Easy access to very accurate mass measurements (±0.005 Da), obtained by the use of hybrid tandem mass spectrometers equipped with orthogonal acceleration time-of-flight mass analysers, will greatly facilitate automated metabolite identification.

Reactive metabolites

Reactive metabolites can lead to failures in development, as their ability to react with DNA and proteins is often the cause of genotoxicity, organ-specific toxicities or other adverse drug reactions. Most importantly, idiosyncratic drug toxicities caused by reactive metabolites, which are likely to be missed in animal safety testing and human clinical trials, can result in the most expensive type of failure, namely withdrawal of a drug from the market. The seriousness of the problem requires that the issue be addressed before selection of a candidate drug.

When reactive metabolites are suspected, owing to theoretical 'structural alerts', metabolic profiling information or equivocal or positive genotoxicity data, microsomal incubations can be carried out in the presence of N-acetylcysteine or glutathione (GSH) in order to favour conjugate formation (a likely source of electrophilic metabolites), followed by LC-MS analysis. Linking the production of such metabolites to toxicity in vivo is generally difficult, but any hint of such metabolites will weigh heavily against a compound's being selected for clinical development.

Pharmacologically active metabolites

The products of Phase I and Phase II metabolism may possess pharmacological activity on the same target as the parent compound or on a different target, which can have an important effect on the pharmacodynamic response. This will not normally be a serious obstacle to development, but it can lead to discrepancies between in vitro and in vivo pharmacological tests, and will need to be taken into account if the compound is taken into development.

During early stages of a drug discovery project, pure samples of metabolites are not usually available for testing. It may be possible to obtain material for simple in vitro testing (e.g. binding assays) from microsomal incubations, followed by LC fractionation to determine how many active metabolites may be present. Detailed testing requires the synthesis and production of pure samples of the main metabolites, a labour-intensive process that will not normally be undertaken until late in the lead optimization phase.

CYP inhibition

Since CYP inhibition was identified as the cause of hundreds of life-threatening ventricular arrhythmias in patients treated with a combination of *terfenadine* and *ketoconazole* (Monahan et al., 1990), it has become a major concern as a cause of drug interactions (FDA Guidance for Industry, 1997).The various types of inhibitory interactions (e.g. reversible, quasi-irreversible, and irreversible or mechanism-based 'suicide inhibition') have been reviewed by Weaver (2001) and Lin and Lu (2001). Compounds that are metabolized by a specific CYP are potential inhibitors of that enzyme, but some drugs inhibit CYPs without themselves being substrates (for example, *quinidine* is a CYP3A4 substrate and a CYP2D6 inhibitor; Otton et al., 1988).

Earlier methods for measuring CYP inhibition were based on the co-incubation of test compounds and specific CYP substrates with human liver microsomes, followed by HPLC analysis to measure the reaction rate (Crespi and Stresser, 2000). Although successful, these methods were too slow to be used in an early drug discovery setting.

Automated, multiwell plate-based assays are now available for all major CYPs (CYP1A2, CYP2C9, CYP2C19, CYP2D6 and CYP3A4) and for some additional isoforms such as CYP2A6 and CYP2C8 (Crespi and Stresser, 2000; Miller et al., 2000, Stresser et al., 2000). Recombinant CYPs are incubated with standard substrates in the presence of the test compound. The metabolites generated are detected by fluorescence, enabling rapid data acquisition and high throughput (Kaplita et al., 2002). In the lead identification phase a simple high-throughput screen may be used, and compounds causing less than 50% inhibition of a given CYP at 10 μM are generally considered acceptable.

More detailed CYP inhibition tests are carried out routinely during lead optimization. If CYP inhibition has been identified as a major issue with a particular chemical series, automated CYP inhibition assays are likely to be run before permeability or metabolic screening assays. During lead optimization, data obtained with recombinant CYPs need to be confirmed with human liver microsomes.

Nowadays, a compound causing significant CYP inhibition (i.e. K_i <1 μM, or below the clinically relevant plasma concentration) is unlikely to be developed unless it is a 'first in class' molecule in an area of high medical need. Even then, its clinical development will be more costly and prolonged, as more clinical interaction studies with drugs that are likely to be co-prescribed will need to be undertaken.

For all CYPs except CYP3A4, the inhibitory potency of test compounds is independent of the substrate and assay method employed (Miller et al., 2000). In contrast, with CYP3A4 inhibition data for the recombinant enzyme can vary greatly (~300-fold), depending on the substrate being used (Stresser et al., 2000). Substrate-dependent effects warrant caution when interpreting screening data for CYP3A4 inhibition (Miller et al., 2000).

CYP induction

In contrast to CYP inhibition, for which in vitro methods are well established, CYP induction assays have lagged behind, mainly because of our incomplete understanding of the underlying mechanism(s). CYP induction was traditionally investigated in vivo, in conjunction with toxicology studies, by measuring the levels of specific CYP isoforms by ELISA or Western blot assays, or by measuring CYP activities (using probe substrates, such as testosterone) in livers or liver microsomes from chronically treated animals (Worboys and Carlile, 2001).

Nowadays, hepatocytes are increasingly used to evaluate induction. Several studies have shown the inducibility of CYP1A, CYP2B, CYP3A and CYP4A in cultured hepatocytes (Worboys and Carlile, 2001). Until recently, cells were typically cultured in the presence of the test compound for a defined period, and enzyme activity was determined by measuring the metabolism of a probe substrate. This technique was associated with false results caused by trapping of the test compound within the hepatocytes and competition with the probe substrate. To avoid this, CYP activity could be measured in microsomes prepared from the treated hepatocytes. The more sensitive technique of RT-PCR is now increasingly used to detect CYP induction in human or animal hepatocytes exposed to new compounds. Unfortunately,

throughput remains relatively low, and such assays cannot be used for screening of large numbers of compounds. Moreover, when human hepatocytes are used, interindividual donor variation in their response to inducers is considerable, necessitating the use of several preparations to determine an 'average' response. The limited availability of high-quality donor tissue means that induction studies with human hepatocytes are usually limited to tests on a few compounds at a late stage of the project (Luo et al., 2002).

CYP 3A induction

CYP3A enzymes account for many drug interactions (Thummel and Wilkinson, 1998). They are the most abundant CYP isoforms in human liver and small intestine (Shimada et al., 1994); they metabolize many structurally diverse substrates (Kuehl et al., 2001), and are readily inducible by numerous steroids, antibiotics and other pharmacological agents. This has stimulated the search for new in vitro assays of CYP induction (Lehmann et al., 1998).

The human *pregnane X receptor* (PXR, also known as SXR or PAR) plays a key role in regulating the expression of specific CYP enzymes, particularly CYP3A. PXR also plays a key role in the regulation of drug efflux, by activating the expression of genes encoding efflux transporters (Synold et al., 2001; see later).

Assays for PXR activation can therefore be used to test for CYP3A4 induction. Recently, several laboratories have developed PXR reporter gene assays for this purpose (Lehmann et al., 1998; Moore et al., 2000). These assays correlate well with induction studies in cultured hepatocytes and have several advantages (El-Sankary et al., 2001; Luo et al., 2002). They use inexpensive human-derived cell lines and are amenable to automation and high-throughput screening in plate format (Luo et al., 2002), and may provide a means of assessing CYP3A4 induction potential at an early stage.

Crystal structure data have revealed that PXR possesses a highly hydrophobic and flexible ligand-binding pocket (Watkins et al., 2001), allowing a wide range of molecular structures to bind in multiple orientations. Using literature data derived from 12 ligands, Ekins and Erickson (2002) have recently proposed a pharmacophore for human PXR ligands (one H-bond acceptor and four hydrophobic regions). Although this model needs to be refined and validated, it may eventually be possible to model the important structural features, allowing ligands to interact with PXR (Ekins and Schuetz, 2002).

The results from PXR reporter gene assays need to be confirmed in vivo (e.g. by measuring CYP levels in liver tissue samples following chronic treatment), and this is usually done later in the project in conjunction with multiple dose toxicity studies.

Species differences in the induction response are well known (Kocarek et al., 1995; Waxman, 1999). For example, *pregnenolone 16α-carbonitrile* is an effective inducer of CYP3A in rats but not in humans, whereas the reverse is true for *rifampicin*, possibly because of species differences in the PXR ligand-binding domain[1] (Barwick et al., 1996; Waxman, 1999; LeCluyse, 2001; Watkins et al., 2001).

Because of these species differences, results from animal studies need to be compared with data from human hepatocytes, either freshly isolated or cryopreserved. Clinical relevance can be assessed by obtaining comparison with clinically important inducers (e.g. rifampicin) and by evaluating the concentration dependence of the induction response. If the effect occurs only at concentrations well above those expected to occur clinically, it is unlikely that induction will be a serious problem. As with CYP inhibition studies, results from induction studies are used to plan future drug–drug interaction investigations.

Enzyme identification

The identification of the enzymes responsible for metabolizing a new compound is necessary to assess the risk of drug–drug interactions and the potential variability in drug response, as many drug-metabolizing enzymes show high interindividual variability or are polymorphic[2].

Although CYP3A4 does not appear to be polymorphic, it is highly inducible and susceptible to environmental conditions and is a major cause of drug–drug interactions. CYP3A5, another member of the same subfamily, is polymorphic, and because it can represent more than 50% of total hepatic CYP3A it may be an important genetic contributor to interindividual and interracial differences in drug metabolism. Obviously, drugs that are metabolized almost exclusively by a single enzyme, particularly if it is polymorphic, are more likely to show pharmacodynamic variability, and nowadays such a drug will only be selected for development if it fulfils an urgent medical need.

Various in vitro preparations of human liver can be used to identify the major enzymes implicated in the metabolism of a given drug, including microsomes,

cytoplasmic fractions, S9 fractions (containing both microsomal and cytosolic components), liver slices or hepatocytes. In addition, heterologous expression systems (e.g. recombinant human CYPs or conjugating enzymes) can provide useful confirmatory evidence of the involvement of specific isoforms. Test compounds can also be incubated in the presence of a panel of characterized human liver microsomes (available commercially), and correlations between the metabolism of the test compound and that of marker substrates will help to identify the important isoforms.

These investigations are usually carried out late in the lead optimization phase, or at the time of drug candidate selection. Regulatory authorities will request in vitro data identifying all major metabolizing enzymes, as detailed metabolic information is important for optimal clinical management (Glue and Clement, 1999). It offers a basis for the explanation and prediction of drug interactions, provides guidelines for dose selection in particular patient groups, and may account for unexpected toxicity, lack of efficacy, or variability in the clinical response.

In vivo pharmacokinetic evaluations

During the lead identification phase, in vivo pharmacokinetic studies are important to assess the predictiveness of in vitro experiments (microsomes or hepatocytes) and to detect any non-hepatic clearance mechanisms. These studies are typically carried out for selected compounds representing different chemical classes, including reference compounds against which NCEs will be benchmarked. The purpose is to flag any project-specific issues that would need to be addressed during lead optimization.

Early PK evaluations are run in a standardized fashion, with standard protocols that allow direct comparisons between compounds (e.g. same dose, dose volume, vehicle, number of animals, fasted or fed, body weight). Most often, data are obtained in rats, as many pharmacological tests are performed on that species, thereby allowing the preliminary assessment of PK-PD correlations. Mice can also be used, but have the disadvantage that only one plasma sample can be obtained per animal.

'Cassette pharmacokinetics', also called the '*n*-in-1' approach, where a mixture of test compounds (typically 5–10) is administered to one animal, can be used as a first step in determining in vivo pharmacokinetic profiles, with MS analysis providing the necessary sensitivity and selectivity needed to measure plasma concentration of multiple compounds simultaneously. In vitro metabolic profiling information can be used to anticipate the main metabolites, and the cassette composition can be optimized for efficient MS separation by algorithms based on mass differences between the compounds and their likely metabolites. The compounds are usually given

---

[1]In humans, natural PXR allelic variants appear rare (Hustert et al., 2001; Kuehl et al., 2001), indicating a limited contribution of PXR protein variants to human variation in PXR induction of genes (Ekins and Schuetz, 2002).

[2]Genes are considered polymorphic if one or more genetic variants (allelic variants) exists stably in the population (Evans and Relling, 1999), typically in more than 1% of a defined population. Among cytochromes, CYP2D6, CYP2C9, CYP2C19, CYP2A6, CYP1A1 and CYP2E1 fall into this category (Ingelman-Sundberg et al., 1999; Brockmoller et al., 2000). For full details see http://www.imm.ki.se/CYPalleles.

intravenously, and doses have to be kept low to minimize toxicity and drug–drug interactions. Oral administration can be used, but the chances of significant drug–drug interactions are higher and bioavailability estimates are not reliable. The results of cassette-dosing experiments generally agree well with those of single-dose studies (Berman et al., 1997).

In early lead optimization the DMPK testing protocol used during lead identification is generally continued, with increasing emphasis on in vivo studies. By taking a systematic approach to DMPK testing the aim is to establish relationships between chemical structure and key pharmacokinetic parameters, which can be used to generate in silico predictions and simulations of physiologically based pharmacokinetics or absorption processes. For example, provided solubility, pK_a and permeability measurements are available, some models are able to simulate the time course of drug distribution between various intestinal compartments and plasma. In addition to providing valuable data on development compounds in case mechanistic questions should arise later, these physiologically based pharmacokinetic models can also help during the lead optimization phase. For example, the influence of hepatic clearance on pharmacokinetic parameters or bioavailability can be simulated to investigate how much improvement in a particular parameter is necessary to meet transition criteria. The use of such approaches during the lead optimization phase paves the way for a more comprehensive pharmacokinetic–pharmacodynamic comparison of a few compounds in contention for drug candidate nomination.

During the lead optimization phase the goal is to combine all desired attributes (see Table 10.1) into one compound, the drug candidate, intended for preclinical development (see Chapter 15). A preliminary shortlist of three or four compounds will often be identified and subjected to further testing before the final selection of drug candidate is made. The point at which a compound is designated as a drug candidate and moves from discovery into development varies between companies. In some cases, as described here, a considerable amount of in vivo DMPK data is obtained before this transition point is reached, whereas other companies postpone most of this work until later. The tendency is to perform in vivo DMPK studies earlier in the discovery cycle than hitherto.

Further DMPK studies, performed either during the lead optimization phase or soon after the transition to early development, will include measurements in a second species, normally dogs, to provide data applicable to the toxicology programme. In vivo PK profiles will be obtained at different dose levels, to detect any pharmacokinetic non-linearity at therapeutically relevant doses. For compounds intended for oral use bioavailability is an important issue, and different formulations will be tested over a range of doses. During the early stages of lead optimization a typical cut-off for rat/mouse oral bioavailability would be about 20%, so as to include potentially interesting leads. For drug candidate nomination a higher level is usually required, with particular attention given to the likelihood that bioavailability can be increased by suitable formulation.

PK-PD correlations

As we have seen, pharmacokinetic profiling is an essential part of drug discovery, but it is only recently that linking systemic drug concentrations with pharmacodynamic endpoints has been integrated into the discovery process. Although there has been good progress in identifying the molecular factors that govern in vivo drug disposition, it is often difficult to relate this information to the magnitude and time course of the pharmacodynamic response. The problem can be considered in two stages: predicting the time course of drug concentrations in different tissues and organs; and predicting the clinically relevant pharmacodynamic response, on the basis of the expected pattern of drug disposition.

Physiologically based pharmacokinetic (PBPK) modelling

The first stage of the problem is addressed by the emerging discipline of *PBPK modelling* (Derendorf et al., 2000; Grass and Sinko, 2002; Theil et al., 2003), which aims to take into account a range of physiological variables, including, for example, transit time, alteration of pH during gastrointestinal transit, blood flow distribution among peripheral organs and tissues (liver, kidney, body fat, brain etc.), plasma protein and tissue binding. As in compartmental pharmacokinetic analysis, PBPK modelling treats the body as a series of distinct compartments, each characterized by volume, tissue/plasma partition coefficient, and inflow and outflow terms based on physiological and pharmacokinetic measurements. In this way the individual components responsible for drug absorption, disposition and clearance can be combined to produce an overall pharmacokinetic model that more accurately reflects the in vivo situation. PBPK modelling is highly dependent upon obtaining multiple parameters from in vitro and in vivo experiments, but it can nevertheless be a useful tool, particularly if nonlinear kinetics or non-metabolic routes of elimination are involved. For example, clearance that is primarily mediated by an uptake transporter in the liver can be modelled on the basis of in vitro data obtained from the species-specific transporter expressed in cultured cells. PBPK modelling is used to place the molecular and cellular mechanisms that have been identified and analysed in a realistic physiological context, so as to predict whole-animal pharmacokinetics. Still at an early and imprecise stage, PBPK modelling is proving to be a useful approach, and its value in drug discovery will undoubtedly grow as the models and software evolve. One of the main difficulties is that of translating animal data to humans, which remains a minefield of uncertainty despite years of effort in devising accurate *allometric scaling* algorithms (see below).

Pharmacokinetic/pharmacodynamic (PKPD) modelling

The second aspect of the problem is to predict the pharmacodynamic response, once the drug disposition is fully understood. This can be straightforward. For example, changes in heart rate follow quickly and directly the plasma concentration of a β-adrenoceptor agonist. But in other cases many processes intervene between the interaction of a drug molecule with its molecular target and the production of a response. The therapeutic effect of antidepressant drugs, for example, occurs only after several weeks, reflecting delayed adaptive responses to the primary disturbance of transmitter function that the drug produces. The relationship between the extent and the time course of the therapeutic effect and the pharmacokinetic properties of the drug is often far from clear. For antipsychotic drugs it has been suggested that the balance between the therapeutic effect and the main side effect (disturbance of motor function) depends on the kinetics of the drug–receptor interaction (Kapur and Seeman, 2001), in particular the dissociation rate – a property that will not be revealed by measurements of pharmacokinetics or receptor occupancy. Of course, not all examples are as complex, and there are successful examples of PKPD modelling (Meibohm and Derendorf, 2002); nevertheless, it will remain a particularly challenging problem until we have a better understanding of the chain of events that causes the binding of a drug to its target to produce a pharmacological effect leading to therapeutic benefit.

With the increasing emphasis on chronic disease, and treatments aimed at preventing or retarding disease processes, the link between what is easily measured in the laboratory and clinical response becomes more tortuous. Consequently, identifying a measurable biological endpoint that can translate into clinical benefit becomes more difficult. However, it is becoming increasingly clear that building such PKPD understanding during the drug discovery process is important, as it shifts the emphasis of DMPK towards understanding, and improving upon, the determinants of in vivo efficacy, rather than focusing solely on in vivo disposition.

Scaling to man

Two main approaches are used to predict human PK from animal data, namely *allometric scaling* and *physiologically based pharmacokinetic (PBPK) modelling* (see above).

Allometric scaling (Obach et al., 1997) is based on empirical relationships between body size and the structural and functional capacities of organs (Juergens, 1991). Attempts to define the rules relating physiological variables to body size among species have a long and chequered history. Many physiological variables, such as heart rate, metabolic rate etc, and also drug clearance, show interspecies differences that generally fit the relationship:

$$Y = \alpha W^\beta$$

where Y is the variable in question, W is body weight, and α and β are arbitrary constants, which are not the same for all physiological variables. By measuring Y for a range of species, α and β can be estimated. The relationship is not usually exact, and man is usually the largest species studied, and so extrapolating measurements of, say, drug clearance from laboratory animals to man on this allometric basis is often inaccurate. Introducing further scaling factors, such as maximum lifespan and relative brain weight, has been claimed to improve the accuracy of allometric scaling of animal-derived pharmacokinetic variables to man (Mahmood, 1999), but the value of this type of empirical approach has also been strongly criticized (Bonate and Howard, 2000).

Estimating important pharmacokinetic variables, such as clearance or volume of distribution of unbound drug, in man necessitates definition of the equation relating these parameters to body weight in four or five species. Plasma half-life in humans can then be estimated. Renal clearance can be similarly predicted (Chaturvedi et al., 2001). Predictions of volume of distribution can be improved by allowing for the fraction bound to plasma proteins (Obach et al., 1997). However, hepatic clearance predictions have been less successful because large interspecies differences in metabolism can confound allometric scaling (Ito et al., 1998). As species-specific metabolism can be revealed by in vitro studies in liver microsomes and hepatocytes, the latter can be used judiciously to select the best species for preclinical PK studies.

An alternative approach to empirical allometric scaling is to use physiologically based PK modelling to predict what will happen in man. Human liver microsome or hepatocyte incubations can be used to derive an in vitro metabolism parameter, i.e. the in vitro *intrinsic clearance* (Cl_{int}), which can be used to predict in vivo hepatic clearance (Cl_H). On the basis of physiological parameters (hepatic blood flow, liver weight, microsomal yield etc.), in vitro Cl_{int} can then be scaled to in vivo clearance, provided that certain assumptions are made, namely: (1) that metabolism is the predominant contributor to clearance; (2) that the liver is the major clearance organ; (3) (if microsome data are used) that oxidative microsomal metabolism is the predominant route of metabolism; and (4) that metabolic rates and enzyme activities measured in vitro are representative of those operating in vivo (Obach et al., 1997). In practice, scaling from human hepatocyte data can be complicated by the high interindividual variability in Cl_{int} values derived from different donor preparations (Shibata et al., 2002).

Obach et al. (1997) reviewed several approaches to predicting PK parameters in man and reported that estimates based on animal PK parameters were associated with mean errors ranging from about 1.6-fold to three-fold. Most DMPK experts agree that scaling procedures are considered successful when predicted clearance values are within a factor of 2 of actual clearance values (Lavé et al., 1999). An obvious explanation for discrepancies between predicted and measured values is the fact that in vivo, clearance also depends on non-hepatic (e.g. renal) processes.

Whereas all pharmaceutical companies routinely use these scaling methods to predict human PK, efforts in medicinal chemistry to reduce metabolic clearance are leading to more compounds that are cleared by non-metabolic routes, such as active biliary, intestinal or renal secretion. Not only does reliance on such elimination routes increase the chance of transporter-mediated drug–drug interactions, but in addition the errors associated with allometric scaling to man increase, leading to greater application of PBPK modelling.

Predicting toxicity

The focus of this chapter has been on the approaches being used to incorporate DMPK studies early in the drug discovery process, so as to reduce the risk of compounds failing in development for reasons of poor pharmacokinetics. At the beginning of the chapter, a second common reason for failure was noted, namely toxicity, and similar efforts are being made to identify problem compounds as early as possible in drug discovery. The problem is inherently more difficult than predicting efficacy or pharmacokinetics, because the mechanisms of toxicity are more diverse. Whereas efficacy, in the ideal case, boils down to action at a single identified target, and pharmacokinetics depends mainly on well-characterized mechanisms as discussed above, toxicity can take many forms and can result from any number of mechanisms, and new examples are constantly emerging.

Nevertheless, certain common patterns of toxicity, such as genotoxicity, cardiac dysrhythmias, hepatotoxicity etc, are well understood mechanistically, and can be more or less predictable on the basis of in silico and in vitro screening approaches.

Computational prediction of toxicity (Barratt and Rodford, 2001; van der Waterbeemd and Gifford, 2003) relies mainly on the empirical association of certain chemical structures or groups with particular types of toxicity (e.g. mutagenicity and carcinogenicity, where large datasets exist), and several commercial software packages are available for screening virtual compound libraries.

A simple battery of in vitro toxicology screening assays with sufficient throughput for inclusion at the lead optimization stage has been described by Atterwill and Wing (2002). It includes high-throughput assays for genotoxicity and cytotoxicity (see Chapter 16), and medium-throughput cell-based assays predictive of immunotoxicity, reproductive toxicity (including embryo-toxicity), endocrine disruption (estrogenic and andro-genic effects), hepatotoxicity and neurotoxicity. Other cell-based assays predictive of skin and corneal irritancy – generally more relevant to environmental and industrial chemicals, rather than pharmaceuticals – are also available (Davila et al., 1998).

Currently, routine toxicity screening at the lead optimization stage of drug discovery is largely confined to assessing genotoxicity and cytotoxicity. However, just as with DMPK studies, there is interest in performing more in vitro toxicology screening at the lead identification and optimization stages of the project, rather than assessing toxicity only after the decision to develop the compound, following the protocols outlined in Chapter 16. As this happens, toxicology departments will become more involved in the iterative process of lead optimization, and in solving, rather than merely identifying, toxicological problems.

Future prospects

The role of DMPK scientists in drug discovery has radically changed in recent years. In addition to providing more traditional DMPK data and interpretation, scientists now participate actively in project teams, where they ensure that DMPK considerations are fully incorporated into project plans and decisions. This integration will go further, as the greater molecular understanding of DMPK mechanisms further shifts the chemical focus towards molecules that are not only potent and selective for a particular target, but also possess appropriate DMPK properties. The success of these approaches has already resulted in increasing pressure on DMPK experts, and they will continue to develop novel tools that will help them provide better, more accurate advice and guidance to project teams. Virtual (in silico) screening will play an increasing role. In addition, drug design will take into account structural data on drug-metabolizing enzymes and drug transporters. Bioanalytical technologies, which are central to DMPK measurements, are also evolving such that faster method development coupled with automation technologies and non-LCMS techniques will allow the analysis of hundreds of samples per day. Finally, the incorporation of drug delivery technologies that are designed based on the interplay of DMPK information, physiology and formulation will allow greater exploitation of targets that currently cannot be reached because of unfavourable pharmacokinetics. Extrapolation of animal data to man is likely to remain a problem. Empirical allometric scaling, which starts from the assumption that larger mammals are simply scaled-up versions of smaller ones, may have run its course, but replacing it with an approach that takes into account species differences at the molecular, cellular and physiological levels is still some way off. One thing of which we can be confident is that the first trials of a drug candidate in man will continue to spring pharmacokinetic surprises.

References

Atterwill CK, Wing MG (2002) In vitro preclinical lead optimization technologies (PLOTs) in pharmaceutical development. Toxicology Letters 127: 143–151.

Avdeef A (2001) Physicochemical profiling (solubility, permeability and charge state. Current Topics in Medicinal Chemistry 1: 277–351.

Ayrton A, Morgan P (2001) Role of transport proteins in drug absorption, distribution and excretion. Xenobiotica 31: 469–497.

Barratt M D, Rodford R A 2001 The computational prediction of toxicity. Current Opinion in Chemical Biology 5: 383–388.

Barwick JL, Quattrochi LC, Mills AS, Potenza C, Tukey RH, Guzelian PS (1996) Trans-species gene transfer for analysis of glucocorticoid-inducible transcriptional activation of transiently expressed human CYP3A4 and rabbit CYP3A6 in primary cultures of adult rat and rabbit hepatocytes. Molecular Pharmacology 50: 10–16.

Benet LZ, Zia-Amirhosseini (1995) Basic principles of pharmacokinetics. Toxicologic Pathology 23: 115–123.

Ben-Ze'ev A, Robinson GS, Bucher NL, Farmer SR (1988) Cell–cell and cell–matrix interactions differentially regulate the expression of hepatic and cytoskeletal genes in primary cultures of rat hepatocytes. Proceedings of the National Academy of Sciences of the USA 85: 2161–2165.

Berman J, Halm K, Adkison K, Shaffer J (1997) Simultaneous pharmacokinetic screening of a mixture of compounds in the dog using API LC/MS/MS analysis for increased throughput. Journal of Medicinal Chemistry 40: 827–829.

Bertrand M, Jackson P, Walther B (2000) Rapid assessment of drug metabolism in the drug discovery process. European Journal of Pharmaceutical Science 11(Suppl. 2): S61–S72.

Bevan CD, Lloyd RS (2000) A high-throughput screening method for the determination of aqueous drug solubility using laser nephelometry in microtitre plates. Analytical Chemistry 72: 1781–1787.

Bonate PL, Howard D (2000) Critique of allometric scaling: does the emperor have clothes? Journal of Clinical Pharmacology 40: 335–340.

Brockmoller J, Kirchheiner J, Meisel C, Roots I (2000) Pharmacogenetic diagnostic of cytochrome P450 polymorphisms in clinical drug development and in drug treatment. Pharmacogenomics 1: 125–151.

Cech NB, Enke CG (2001) Practical applications of some recent studies in electrospray ionization fundamentals. Mass Spectrometry Reviews 20: 362–387.

Chaturvedi PR, Decker CJ, Odinecs A (2001) Prediction of pharmacokinetic properties using experimental approaches during early discovery. Current Opinion in Chemistry and Biology 5: 452–463.

Cheng YF, Lu Z, Uwe N (2001) Ultrafast liquid chromatagraphy/ultraviolet and liquid chromatography/tandem mass spectrometric analysis. Rapid Communications in Mass Spectrometry 15: 141–151.

Clark DE (2003) In silico prediction of blood–brain barrier permeation. Drug Discovery Today 8: 927–933.

Clarke NJ, Rindgren D, Korfmacher WA, Cox KA (2001) Systematic LC/MS metabolite identification in drug discovery. Analytical Chemistry 430A–439A.

Clarke SE, Jeffrey P (2001) Utility of metabolic stability screening: comparison of in vitro and in vivo clearance. Xenobiotica 31: 591–598.

Coleman RA, Bowen WP, Baines IA, Woodrooffe AJ, Brown AM (2001) Use of human tissue in ADME and safety profiling of development candidates. Drug Discovery Today 6: 1116–1126.

Crespi CL, Stresser DM (2000) Fluorometric screening for metabolism-based drug–drug interactions. Journal of Pharmacological and Toxicological Methods 44: 325–331.

Cross DM, Bayliss MK (2000) A commentary on the use of hepatocytes in drug metabolism studies during drug discovery and development. Drug Metabolism Reviews 32: 219–240.

Curatolo W (1998) Physical chemical properties of oral drug candidates in the discovery and exploratory development settings. Pharmacologic Science and Technology Today 1: 387–393.

Davila JC, Rodriguez RJ, Melchert RB, Acosta D (1998) Predictive value of in vitro model systems in toxicology. Annual Review of Pharmacology and Toxicology 38: 63–96.

Dear G, Plumb R, Mallett D (2001) Use of monolithic silica columns to increase analytical throughput for metabolite idenitfication by liquid chromatography/tandem mass spectrometry. Rapid Communications in Mass Spectrometry 15: 152–158.

de Groot MJ, Ackland MJ, Horne VA, Alex AA, Jones BC (1999) A novel approach to predicting P450 mediated drug metabolism. CYP2D6 catalyzed N-dealkylation reactions and qualitative metabolite predictions using a combined protein and pharmacophore model for CYP2D6. Journal of Medicinal Chemistry 42: 4062–4070.

de Lange EC, Hesseling MB, Danhof M, de Boer AG, Breimer DD (1995) The use of intracerebral microdialysis to determine changes in blood–brain barrier transport characteristics. Pharmaceutical Research 12: 129–133.

Derendorf H, Lesko LJ, Chaikin P et al. (2000) Pharmacokinetic/pharmacodynamic modeling in drug research and development. Journal of Clinical Pharmacology 40: 1399–1418.

Dunn JCY, Tompkins RG, Yarmush ML (1991) Long-term in vitro function of adult hepatocytes in a collagen sandwich configuration. Biotechnology Progress 7: 237–245.

Ekins S, Erickson JA (2002) A pharmacophore for human pregnane X receptor ligands. Drug Metabolism and Disposition 30: 96–99.

Ekins A, Schuetz E (2002) The PXR crystal structure: the end of the beginning. Trends in Pharmacologic Science 23: 49–50.

El-Sankary W, Gordon Gibson G, Ayrton A, Plant N (2001) Use of a reporter gene assay to predict and rank the potency and efficacy of CYP3A4 inducers. Drug Metabolism and Disposition 29: 1499–1504.

Evans WE, Relling MV (1999) Pharmacogenomics: translating functional genomics into rational therapeutics. Science 286: 487–491.

FDA Guidance for Industry: April 1997 Drug metabolism/drug interaction studies in the drug development process: studies in vitro. http//www.fda.gov/cder/guidance/clin3.pdf.

Glue P, Clement RP (1999) Cytochrome P450 enzymes and drug metabolism – basic concepts and methods of assessment. Cell and Molecular Neurobiology 19: 309–323.

Grass GM, Sinko PJ (2002) Physiologically based pharmacokinetic simulation modelling. Advanced Drug Delivery Reviews 54: 433–451.

Hop, CE, Tiller PR, Romanyshyn L (2002) In vitro metabolite identification using fast gradient high performance liquid chromatography combined with tandem mass spectrometry. Rapid Communications in Mass Spectrometry 16: 212–219.

Horter D, Dressman JB (2001) Influence of physicochemical properties on dissolution of drugs in the gastrointestinal tract. Advanced Drug Delivery Reviews 46: 75–87.

Hustert E, Zibat A, Presecan-Siedel E (2001) Natural protein variants of pregnane X receptor with altered transactivation activity toward CYP3A4. Drug Metabolism and Disposition 29: 1454–1459.

Ingelman-Sundberg M, Oscarson M, McLellan RA (1999) Polymorphic human cytochrome P450 enzymes: an opportunity for individualized drug treatment. Trends in Pharmacologic Science 20: 342–349.

Irvine JD, Takahashi L, Lockhart K et al. (1999) MDCK (Madin–Darby canine kidney) cells: a tool for membrane permeability screening. Journal of Pharmaceutical Sciences 88: 28–33.

Ito K, Iwastubo T, Kanamitsu S, Nakajima Y, Sugiyama Y (1998) Quantitative prediction of in vivo drug clearance and drug interactions from in vitro data on metabolism together with binding and transport. Annual Review of Pharmacology and Toxicology 38: 461–499.

Juergens KD (1991) Allometry as a tool for extrapolation of biological variables. Communications in Biochemistry and Physiology 100C: 287–290.

Kansy M, Senner F, Gubernator K (1998) Physicochemical high throughput screening: parallel artifical membrane permeability assay in the description of passive absorption processes. Journal of Medicinal Chemistry 41: 1007–1010.

Kaplita PV, Magolda RL, Homon CA (2002) Employing high-throughput automation to better characterize early discovery candidates. PharmaGenomics Jan–Feb: 34–39.

Kapur S, Seeman P (2001) Does the dissociation from the dopamine D_2 receptor explain the action of atypical antipsychotics? A new hypothesis. American Journal of Psychiatry 158: 360–369.

Kennedy T (1997) Managing the drug discovery/development interface. Drug Discovery Today 2: 436–444.

Kocarek TA, Schuetz EG, Strom SC, Fisher RA, Guzelian PS (1995) Comparative analysis of cytochrome P4503A induction in primary cultures of rat, rabbit, and human hepatocytes. Drug Metabolism and Disposition 23: 415–421.

Korfmacher WA, Cox KA, Ng KJ et al. (2001) Cassette-accelerated rapid rat screen: a systematic procedure for the dosing and liquid chromatography/atmospheric pressure ionization tandem mass spectrometric analysis of new chemical entities as part of new drug discovery. Rapid Communications in Mass Spectrometry 15: 335–340.

Kuehl P, Zhang J, Lin Y et al. (2001) Sequence diversity in CYP3A promoters and characterisation of the genetic basis of polymorphic CYP3A5 expression. Nature Genetics 27: 383–391.

Lavé T, Coassolo P, Reigner B (1999) Prediction of hepatic metabolic clearance based on interspecies allometric scaling techniques and in vitro–in vivo correlations. Clinical Pharmacokinetics 36: 211–231.

LeCluyse EL (2001) Pregnane X receptor: molecular basis for species differences in CYP3A induction by xenobiotics. Chemico-Biological Interactions 134: 283–289.

LeCluyse EL, Audus KL, Hochman JH (1994) Formation of extensive canalicular networks by rat hepatocytes cultured in collagen sandwich configuration. American Journal of Physiology 266 (Cell Physiol 35): C1764–C1774.

Lehmann JM, McKee DD, Watson MA, Willson TM, Moore JT, Kliewer SA (1998) The human orphan nuclear receptor PXR is activated by compounds that regulate CYP3A4 gene expression and cause drug interactions. Journal of Clinical Investigation 102: 1016–1023.

Li AP, Gorycki PD, Hengstler JG et al. (1999) Present status of the application of cryopreserved hepatocytes in the evaluation of xenobiotics: consensus of an international expert panel. Chemico-Biological Interactions 121: 117–123.

Lin JH, Lu AY (2001) Interindividual variability in inhibition and induction of cytochrome P450 enzymes. Annual Review of Pharmacology and Toxicology 41: 535–567.

Lipinski CA (2000) Drug-like properties and the causes of poor solubility and poor permeability. Journal of Pharmacologic and Toxicologic Methods 44: 235–249.

Lombardo F, Obach RS, Shalaeva MY, Gao F (2002) Prediction of volume of distribution values in humans for neutral and basic drugs using physicochemical measurements and plasma protein binding data. Journal of Medicinal Chemistry 45: 2867–2876.

Lundahl P, Beigi F (1997) Immobilized liposome chromatography of drugs for model analysis of drug–membrane interactions. Advanced Drug Delivery Reviews 23: 221–227.

Lundquist S, Renftel M, Brillault J, Fenart L, Cecchelli R, Dehouck MP (2002) Prediction of drug transport through the blood–brain barrier in vivo: a comparison between two in vitro cell models. Pharmaceutical Research 19: 976–981.

Luo G, Cunningham M, Kim S et al. (2002) CYP3A4 induction by drugs: correlation between a pregnane X receptor reporter gene assay and CYP3A4 expression in human hepatocytes. Drug Metabolism and Disposition 30: 795–804.

Mahmood I (1999) Prediction of clearance, volume of distribution and half-life by allometric scaling and by use of plasma concentrations predicted from pharmacokinetic constants: a comparative study. Journal of Pharmaceutics and Pharmacology 51: 905–910.

Meibohm B, Derendorf H (2002) Pharmacokinetic/pharmacodynamic studies in drug product development. Journal of Pharmaceutical Science 9: 18–31.

Miller VP, Stresser DM, Blanchard AP, Turner S, Crespi CL (2000) Fluorometric high-throughput screening for inhibitors of cytochrome P450. Annals of the New York Academy of Science 919: 26–32.

Monahan BP, Ferguson CL, Killeavy ES, Lloyd BK, Troy J, Cantilena LR Jr (1990) Torsades de pointes occurring in association with terfenadine use [comment]. Journal of the American Medical Association 264: 2788–2790.

Moore LB, Parks DJ, Jones SA et al. (2000) Orphan nuclear receptors constitutive androstane receptor and pregnane X receptor share xenobiotic and steroid ligands. Journal of Biological Chemistry 275: 15122–15127.

Mutton IM (1998) Use of short columns and high flow rates for rapid gradient reversed-phase chromatography. Chromatographia 47: 291–298.

Obach RS (1997) Nonspecific binding to microsomes: impact on scale-up of in vitro intrinsic clearance to hepatic clearance as assessed through examination of warfarin, imipramine, and propranolol. Drug Metabolism and Disposition 25: 1359–1369.

Obach RS (1999) Prediction of human clearance of twenty-nine drugs from hepatic microsomal intrinsic clearance data: an examination of in vitro half-life approach and nonspecific binding to microsomes. Drug Metabolism and Disposition 27: 1350–1359.

Obach RS, Baxter JG, Liston TE et al. (1997) The prediction of human pharmacokinetic parameters from preclinical and in vitro metabolism data. Journal of Pharmacology and Experimental Therapeutics 283: 46–58

Otton SV, Brinn RU, Gram LF (1988) In vitro evidence against the oxidation of quinidine by the sparteine/debrisoquine monooxygenase of human liver. Drug Metabolism and Disposition 16: 15–17.

Palm K, Stenberg P, Luthman K, Artursson P (1997) Polar molecular surface properties predict the intestinal absorption of drugs in humans. Pharmaceutical Research 14: 568–571.

Pan L, Ho Q, Tsutsui K, Takahashi L (2001) Comparison of chromatographic and spectroscopic methods used to rank compounds for aqueous solubility. Journal of Pharmaceutical Science 90: 521–529.

Pidgeon C, Ong S, Liu H et al. (1995) IAM chromatography: an in vitro screen for predicting drug membrane permeability. Journal of Medicinal Chemistry 38: 590–594.

Plant N (2004) Strategies for using in vitro screens in drug metabolism. Drug Discovery Today 9: 328–336.

Plumb RS, Dear GJ, Mallett DN, Highton DM, Pleasance S, Biddlecombe RA (2001) Quantitative analysis of pharmaceuticals in fluids using high-performance liquid chromatography coupled to mass spectrometry: a review. Xenobiotica 31: 599–617.

Polli JW, Wring SA, Humphreys JE et al. (2001) Rational use of in vitro P-glycoprotein assays in drug discovery. Journal of Pharmacology and Experimental Therapy 299: 620–628.

Prentiss RA, Lis Y, Walker SR (1988) Pharmaceutical innovation by the seven UK-owned pharmaceutical companies. British Journal of Clinical Pharmacology 25: 387–396.

PriceWaterhouseCoopers (1997) Pharma 2005. An industrial revolution in R&D.

Rendic S, Di Carlo FJ (1997) Human cytochrome P450 enzymes: a status report summarising their reactions, substrates, inducers and inhibitors. Drug Metabolism and Disposition 29: 413–580.

Rodrigues D (1997) Preclinical drug metabolism in the age of high-throughput screening: an industrial perspective. Pharmaceutical Research 14: 1504–1510.

Shibata Y, Takahashi H, Chiba M, Ishii Y (2002) Prediction of hepatic clearance and availability by cryopreserved hepatocytes: an application of serum incubation method. Drug Metabolism and Disposition 30: 892–896.

Shimada T, Yamazake H, Mimura M, Inui Y, Guengerich FP (1994) Interindividual variations in human liver cytochrome P450 enzymes involved in the oxidation of drugs, carcinogens and toxic chemicals: studies with liver microsomes of 30 Japanese and 30 Caucasians. Journal of Pharmacology and Experimental Therapy 270: 414–423.

Smith DA (2001) The long, hard road: drug metabolism in the lifetime of the DMDG. Xenobiotica 31: 459–467.

Smith PM (2002) Component architecture in drug discovery informatics. Current Opinion in Drug Discovery and Development 5: 361–366.

Stenberg P, Luthman K, Artursson P (1999) Prediction of membrane permeability to peptides from calculated dynamic molecular surface properties. Pharmaceutical Research 16: 205–212.

Stenberg P, Norinder U, Luthman K, Artursson P (2001) Experimental and computational screening models for the prediction of intestinal drug absorption. Journal of Medicinal Chemistry 44: 1927–1937.

Stresser DM, Blanchard AP, Turner SD et al. (2000) Substrate-dependent modulation of CYP3A4 catalytic activity: analysis of 27 test compounds with four fluorometric substrates. Drug Metabolism and Disposition 28: 1440–1448.

Summer-Smith M (2001) Beginning to manage drug discovery and development knowledge. Current Opinion in Drug Discovery and Development 4: 319–324.

Synold TW, Dussault I, Forman BM (2001) The orphan nuclear receptor SXR coordinately regulates drug metabolism and efflux. Nature Medicine 7: 584–590.

Taipalensuu J, Tornblom H, Lindberg G et al. (2001) Correlation of gene expression of ten drug efflux proteins of the ATP-binding cassette transporter family in normal human jejunum and in human intestinal epithelial Caco-2 cell monolayers. Journal of Pharmacology and Experimental Therapy 299: 164–170.

Theil F-P, Guentert TW, Haddad S, Poulin P (2003) Utility of physiologically based pharmacokinetic models to drug development and rational drug discovery candidate selection. Toxicology Letters 138: 29–49.

Thummel KE, Wilkinson GR (1998) In vitro and in vivo drug interactions involving human CYP3A. Annual Review of Pharmacology and Toxicology 38: 389–430.

Valkó K, Bevan C, Reynolds D (1997) Chromatographic hydrophobicity index by fast-gradient RP-HPLC: a high-throughput alternative to logP/logD. Analytical Chemistry 69: 2022–2029.

van der Waterbeemd H, Gifford E (2003) ADMET in silico modelling: towards prediction paradise. Nature Reviews Drug Discovery 2: 192–204.

Veber DF, Johnson SR, Cheng HY, Smith BR, Ward KW, Kopple KD (2002) Molecular properties that influence the oral bioavailability of drug candidates. Journal of Medicinal Chemistry 45: 2615–1623.

Wan H, Holmén A, Någård M, Lindberg W (2002) Rapid screening of pKa values of pharmaceuticals by pressure-assisted capillary electrophoresis combined with short-end injection. Journal of Chromatography A 979: 369–377.

Watkins RE, Wisely GB, Moore LB et al. (2001) The human nuclear xenobiotic receptor PXR : structural determinants of directed promiscuity. Science 292: 2392–2333.

Waxman DJ (1999) P450 gene induction by structurally diverse xenochemicals: central role of nuclear receptors CAR, PXR and PPAR. Archives of Biochemistry and Biophysics 369: 11–23.

Weaver RJ (2001) Assessment of drug–drug interactions: concepts and approaches. Xenobiotica 31: 499–538.

Wenlock MC, Austin RP, Barton P, Davis AM, Leeson PD (2003) A comparison of the molecular property profiles of development and marketed oral drugs. Journal of Medicinal Chemistry 46: 1250–1256.

Worboys PD, Carlile DJ (2001) Implications and consequences of enzyme induction on preclinical and clinical drug development. Xenobiotica 31: 539–556.

11 Pharmacology: its role in drug discovery

H P Rang

Introduction

Pharmacology as an academic discipline, loosely defined as the study of the effects of chemical substances on living systems, is so broad in its sweep that it encompasses all aspects of drug discovery, ranging from the molecular details of the interaction between the drug molecule and its target to the economic and social consequences of placing a new therapeutic agent on the market. In this chapter we consider the more limited scope of 'classical' pharmacology, in relation to drug discovery. Typically, when a molecular target has been selected, and lead compounds have been identified which act on it selectively, and which are judged to have 'drug-like' chemical attributes (including suitable pharmacokinetic properties), the next stage is a detailed pharmacological evaluation. This means investigation of the effects, usually of a small number of compounds, on a range of test systems, up to and including whole animals, to determine which, if any, is the most suitable for further development (i.e. for nomination as a drug candidate). Pharmacological evaluation typically involves:

- **Selectivity screening**, consisting of in vitro tests on a broad range of possible drug targets to determine whether the compound is sufficiently selective for the chosen target to merit further investigation;
- **Pharmacological profiling**, aimed at evaluating in isolated tissues or normal animals the range of effects of the test compound that might be relevant in the clinical situation. Some authorities distinguish between *primary pharmacodynamic studies*, concerning effects related to the selected therapeutic target (i.e. therapeutically relevant effects), and *secondary pharmacodynamic studies*, on effects not related to the target (i.e. side effects). At the laboratory level the two are often not clearly distinguishable, and the borderline between secondary pharmacodynamic and safety pharmacology studies (see below) is also uncertain. Nevertheless, for the purposes of formal documentation, the distinction may be useful;
- **Testing in animal models of disease** to determine whether the compound is likely to produce therapeutic benefit;
- **Safety pharmacology**, consisting of a series of standardized animal tests aimed at revealing

Drug discovery

undesirable side effects, which may be unrelated to the primary action of the drug. This topic is discussed in Chapter 16.

The pharmacological evaluation of lead compounds does not in general follow a clearly defined path, and often it has no clearcut endpoint but will vary greatly in its extent, depending on the nature of the compound, the questions that need to be addressed and the inclinations of the project team. Directing this phase of the drug discovery project efficiently, and keeping it focused on the overall objective of putting a compound into development, is one of the trickier management

tasks. It often happens that unexpected, scientifically interesting data are obtained which beg for further investigation even though they may be peripheral to the main aims of the project. From the scientists' perspective, the prospect of opening up a new avenue of research is highly alluring, whether the work contributes directly to the drug discovery aims or not. In this context, project managers need to bear in mind the question: Who needs the data and why? – a question which may seem irritatingly silly to a scientist in academia, but totally obvious to the commercial mind. The same principles apply, of course, to all parts of a drug discovery and development project, but it tends to be at

Table 11.1
Characteristics of pharmacological test systems

Attribute \ Test system	Molecular/ Cellular assays	In vitro pharmacology	Whole animal pharmacology (normal animals)	Whole animal disease models
Throughput	High (thousands/day)	Moderate (ca. 10/day)	Low (<10/day)	Generally low or very low, depending on nature of model
Quantitative precision	Good	Good, but may be subject to environmental and physiological variation	Relatively poor, due to uncontrolled pharmacokinetic and physiological factors	As for whole animal pharmacology, plus added variability of disease model phenotype
Cost	Low	Fairly low depending on number and cost of animals needed	High, depending on number and cost of animals needed	High, depending on number and cost of animals needed
Flexibility of experimental design	Generally inflexible. Washout effects, repeat dose effects etc. difficult to study	Highly adaptable	Adaptable, but limitations imposed by pharmacokinetics.	
Suitability for chronic experiments	Unsuitable	Unsuitable	Depends on model. Suitable if repeated non-invasive readouts are feasible. Possible, but expensive for one-off terminal readouts	As for whole animal, provided disease phenotype remains stable
Species dependence	Often performed on human cell lines or cloned human targets	Rarely possible with human tissues	Animal studies may not be applicable to humans	Animal studies may not be applicable to human
Usefulness for predicting therapeutic efficacy	OK for me-too drugs. Poor for drugs acting through novel mechanisms	OK for me-too drugs. Poor for drugs acting through novel mechanisms	As above	Variable, depending on characteristics of model
Usefulness for predicting side effects	Useful if broad selectivity screen is performed	Sometimes useful	Generally useful as basis for 'safety pharmacology' screening.	Usually not informative

the stage of pharmacological evaluation that conflicts first arise between scientific aspiration and commercial need.

An important principle in pharmacological evaluation is the use of a *hierarchy* of test methods, covering the range from the most reductionist tests on isolated molecular targets to much more elaborate tests of integrated physiological function. Establishing and validating such a series of tests appropriate to the particular target and indication being addressed is one of the most important functions of pharmacologists in the drug discovery team. In general, assays become more complicated, slow and expensive, and more demanding of specialist skills as one moves up this hierarchy.

The strengths and weaknesses of these test systems are summarized in Table 11.1.

Pharmacological characterization of a candidate compound often has to take into account active metabolites, based on information from drug metabolism and pharmacokinetics (DMPK) studies (see Chapter 10). If a major active metabolite is identified, it will be necessary to synthesize and test it in the same way as the parent compound in order to determine which effects (both wanted an unwanted) relate to each. Particular problems may arise if the metabolic fate of the compound shows marked species differences, making it difficult to predict from animal studies what will happen in humans.

Although most of the work involved in pharmacological characterization of a candidate drug takes place before clinical studies begin, it does not normally end there. Both ongoing toxicological studies and early trials in man may reveal effects that need to be investigated pharmacologically, and so the discovery team needs to remain actively involved and able to perform experiments well into the phase of clinical development. They cannot simply wave the compound goodbye once the discovery phase is completed.

Screening for selectivity

The selectivity of a compound for the chosen molecular target needs to be assessed at an early stage. Compounds selected for their potency, for example on a given amine receptor, protease, kinase, transporter or ion channel, are very likely to bind also to related – or even unrelated – molecular targets, and thereby cause unwanted side effects. Selectivity is therefore as important as potency in choosing potential development candidates, and a 'selectivity screen' is usually included early in the project. The range of targets included in such a screen depends very much on the type of compound and the intended clinical indication. Ligands for monoamine receptors and transporters form a large and important group of drugs, and several contract research organizations (e.g. CEREP, MDL) offer a battery of assays – mainly binding assays, but also a range of functional assays – designed to detect affinity for a wide range of receptors, transporters and channels. In the field of monoamine receptors, for example, it is usually important to avoid compounds that block or activate peripheral muscarinic receptors, adrenergic receptors or histamine (particularly H_1) receptors, because of the side effects that are associated with these actions, and a standard selectivity test battery allows such problems to be discovered early. Recently, several psychotropic and anti-infective drugs have been withdrawn because of sudden cardiac deaths, probably associated with their ability to block a particular type of potassium channel (known as the *hERG channel*; see Chapter 16) in myocardial cells. This activity can be detected by electrophysiological measurements on isolated myocardial cells, and such a test is now usually performed at an early stage of development of drugs of the classes implicated in this type of adverse reaction.

Interpretation of binding assays

Binding assays, generally with membrane preparations made from intact tissues or receptor-expressing cell lines, are widely used in drug discovery projects because of their simplicity and ease of automation. Detailed technical manuals describing the methods used for performing and analysing drug binding experiments are available (Keen, 1999; Vogel, 2002). Generally, the aim of the assay is to determine the dissociation constant, K_D, of the test compound, as a measure of its affinity for the receptor. In most cases, the assay (often called a *displacement assay*) measures the ability of the test compound to inhibit the binding of a high-affinity radioligand which combines selectively with the receptor in question, correction being made for 'non-specific' binding of the radioligand.

In the simplest theoretical case, where the radioligand and the test compound bind reversibly and competitively to a homogeneous population of binding sites, the effect of the test ligand on the amount of the radioligand specifically bound is described by the simple mass–action equation:

$$B/B_{max} = ([A]/K_A)/([A]/K_A + [L]/K_L + 1) \qquad (1)$$

where B = the amount of radioligand bound, after correcting for non-specific binding, B_{max} = the maximal amount of radioligand bound, i.e. when sites are saturated, [A] = radioligand concentration, K_A = dissociation constant for the radioligand, [L] = test ligand concentration, and K_L = dissociation constant for the test ligand.

By testing several concentrations of L at a single concentration of A, the concentration, $[L]_{50}$, needed for 50%

inhibition of binding can be estimated. By rearranging Equation 1, K_L is given by:

$$K_L = [L]_{50}/([A]/K_A + 1) \qquad (2)$$

This is often known as the Cheng–Prusoff equation, and is widely used to calculate K_L when $[L]_{50}$, $[A]$ and K_A are known. It is important to realize that the Cheng–Prusoff equation applies only (a) at equilibrium, (b) when the interaction between A and L is strictly competitive, and

(c) when neither ligand binds cooperatively. However, an $[L]_{50}$ value can be measured for any test compound that inhibits the binding of the radioligand by whatever mechanism, irrespective of whether equilibrium has been reached. Applying the Cheng–Prusoff equation if these conditions are not met can yield estimates of K_L that are quite meaningless, and so it should strictly be used only if the conditions have been shown experimentally to be satisfied – a fairly laborious process.

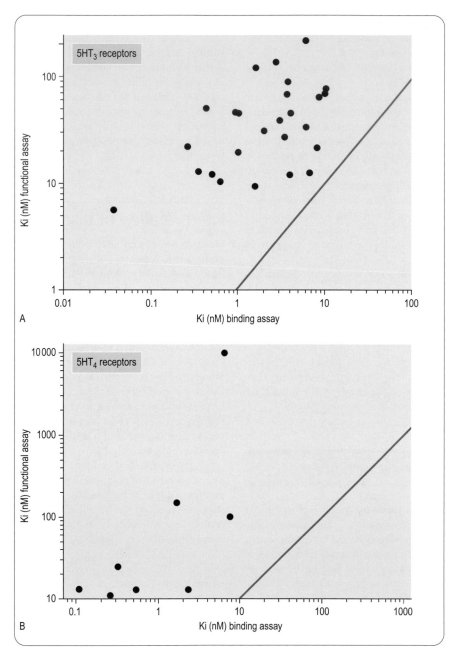

Fig. 11.1
Correlation of binding and functional data for 5HT receptor ligands. (A) $5HT_3$ receptors (data from Heidempergher et al., 1997). (B) $5HT_4$ receptors (data from Yang et al., 1997).

Nevertheless, 'Cheng–Prusoff' estimates of ligand affinity constants are often quoted without such checks having been performed. In most cases it would be more satisfactory to use the experimentally determined $[L]_{50}$ value as an operational measure of potency. A further important caveat that applies to binding studies is that they are often performed under conditions of low ionic strength, in which the sodium and calcium concentrations are much lower than the physiological range. This is done for technical reasons, as low $[Na^+]$ commonly increases both the affinity and the B_{max} of the radio-ligand, and omitting $[Ca^{2+}]$ avoids clumping of the membrane fragments. Partly for this reason, ligand affinities estimated from binding studies are often considerably higher than estimates obtained from functional assays (Hall, 1992), although the effect is not consistent, presumably because ionic bonding, which will be favoured by the low ionic strength medium, contributes unequally to the binding of different ligands. Consequently, the correlation between data from binding assays and functional assays is often rather poor (see below). Figure 11.1 shows data obtained independently on $5HT_3$ and $5HT_4$ receptors; in both cases the estimated K_D values for binding are on average about 10 times lower than estimates from functional assays, and the correlation is very poor.

Pharmacological profiling

Pharmacological profiling aims to determine the pharmacodynamic effects of the new compound – or more often of a small family of compounds – on in vitro model systems, e.g. cell lines or isolated tissues, normal animals, and animal models of disease. The last of these is particularly important, as it is intended to give the first real pointer to therapeutic efficacy as distinct from pharmacodynamic activity. It is valuable to assess the activity of the compounds in a series of assays representing increasingly complex levels of organization. The choice of test systems depends, of course, on the nature of the target. For example, characterization of a novel antagonist of a typical G-protein-coupled receptor might involve:

- Ligand-binding assay on membrane fragments from a cell line expressing the cloned receptor;
- Inhibition of agonist activity in a cell line, based on a functional readout (e.g. raised intracellular calcium);
- Antagonism of a selective agonist in an isolated tissue (e.g. smooth muscle, cardiac muscle). Such assays will normally be performed with non-human tissue, and so interspecies differences in the receptor need to be taken into account;

- Antagonism of the response (e.g. bronchoconstriction, vasoconstriction, increased heart rate) to a selective receptor agonist in vivo. Prior knowledge about species specificity of the agonist and antagonist is important at this stage.

Pharmacological profiling is designed as a hypothesis-driven programme of work, based on the knowledge previously gained about the activity of the compound on its specific target or targets. In this respect it differs from safety pharmacology (see below), which is an open-minded exercise designed to detect unforeseen effects. The aim of pharmacological profiling is to answer the following questions:

- Do the molecular and cellular effects measured in screening assays actually give rise to the predicted pharmacological effects in intact tissues and whole animals?
- Does the compound produce effects in intact tissues or whole animals not associated with actions on its principal molecular target?
- Is there correspondence between the potency of the compound at the molecular level, the tissue level and the whole animal level?
- Do the in vivo potency and duration of action match up with the pharmacokinetic properties of the compound?
- What happens if the drug is given continuously or repeatedly to an animal over the course of days or weeks? Does it lose its effectiveness, or reveal effects not seen with acute administration? Is there any kind of 'rebound' after effect when it is stopped?

In vitro profiling

Measurements on isolated tissues

Studies on isolated tissues have been a mainstay of pharmacological methodology ever since the introduction of the isolated organ bath by Magnus early in the 20th century. The technique is extremely versatile and applicable to studies on smooth muscle (e.g. gastrointestinal tract, airways, blood vessels, urinary tract, uterus, biliary tract etc.) as well as cardiac and striated muscle, secretory epithelia, endocrine glands, brain slices, liver slices, and many other functional systems. In most cases the tissue is removed from a freshly killed or anaesthetized animal and suspended in a chamber containing warmed oxygenated physiological salt solution. With smooth muscle preparations the readout is usually mechanical (i.e. tension, recorded with a simple strain gauge). For other types of preparation, various electrophysiological or biochemical readouts are often used. Vogel (2002) and Enna et al. (2002) give details of a comprehensive range of standard pharmacological assay methods, including technical instructions.

Studies of this kind have the advantage that they are performed on intact normal tissues, as distinct from isolated enzymes or other proteins. The recognition molecules, signal transduction machinery and the mechanical or biochemical readout are assumed to be a reasonable approximation to the normal functioning of the tissue. There is abundant evidence to show that tissue responses to GPCR activation, for example, depend on many factors, including the level of expression of the receptor, the type and abundance of the G proteins present in the cell, the presence of associated proteins such as receptor activity-modifying proteins (RAMPs; see Morfis et al., 2003), the state of phosphorylation of various constituent proteins in the signal transduction cascade, and so on. For compounds acting on intracellular targets, functional activity depends on permeation through the membrane, as well as affinity for the target. For these reasons – and probably also for others that are not understood – the results of assays on isolated tissues often differ significantly from results found with primary screening assays. The discrepancy may simply be a quantitative one, such that the potency of the ligand does not agree in the two systems, or it may be more basic. For example, the *pharmacological efficacy* of a receptor ligand, i.e. the property that determines whether it is a full agonist, a partial agonist, or an antagonist, often depends on the type of assay used (Kenakin, 1999), and this may have an important bearing on the selection of possible development compounds. Examples that illustrate the poor correlation that may exist between measurements of target affinity in cell-free assay systems, and functional activity in intact cell systems, are shown in Figures 11.1 and 11.2. Figure 11.1 shows the relationship between binding and functional assay data for $5HT_3$ and $5HT_4$ receptor antagonists. In both cases, binding assays overestimate the potency in functional assays by a factor of about 10 (see above), but more importantly, the correlation is poor, despite the fact that the receptors are extracellular, and so membrane penetration is not a factor. Figure 11.2 shows data on tyrosine kinase inhibitors, in which activity against the isolated enzyme is plotted against inhibition of tyrosine phosphorylation in intact cells, and inhibition of cell proliferation for a large series of compounds. Differences in membrane penetration can account for part of the discrepancy between enzyme and cell-based data, but the correlation between intracellular kinase inhibition and blocking of cell proliferation is also weak, which must reflect other factors.

It is worth noting that these examples come from very successful drug discovery projects. The quantitative discrepancies that we have emphasized, though worrying to pharmacologists, should not therefore be a serious distraction in the context of a drug discovery project.

A very wide range of physiological responses can be addressed by studies on isolated tissues, including measurements of membrane excitability, synaptic function, muscle contraction, cell motility, secretion and release of mediators, transmembrane ion fluxes, vascular resis-

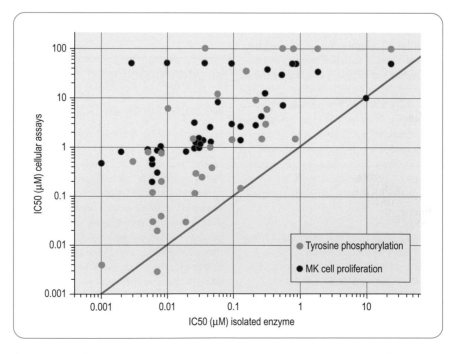

Fig. 11.2
Correlation of cellular activity of EGFR receptor kinase inhibitors with enzyme inhibition. (Data from Traxler et al., 1997.)

tance and permeability, and epithelial transport and permeability. This versatility and the relative technical simplicity of many such methods are useful attributes for drug discovery. Additional advantages are that concentration–effect relationships can be accurately measured, and the design of the experiments is highly flexible, allowing rates of onset and recovery of drug effects to be determined, as well as measurements of synergy and antagonism by other compounds, desensitization effects etc.

The main shortcomings of isolated tissue pharmacology are (a) that tissues normally have to be obtained from small laboratory animals, rather than humans or other primates; and (b) that preparations rarely survive for more than a day, so that only short-term experiments are feasible.

In vivo profiling

As already mentioned, experiments on animals have several drawbacks. They are generally time-consuming, technically demanding and expensive. They are subject to considerable ethical and legal constraints, and in some countries face vigorous public opposition. For all these reasons, the number of experiments is kept to a bare minimum, and experimental variability is consequently often a problem. Animal experiments must therefore be used very selectively and must be carefully planned and designed so as to produce the information needed as efficiently as possible. In the past, before target-directed approaches were the norm, routine in vivo testing was often used as a screen at a very early stage in the drug discovery process, and many important drugs (e.g. *thiazide diuretics, benzodiazepines, ciclosporin*) were discovered on the basis of their effects in vivo. Nowadays, the use of in vivo methods is much more limited, and will probably decline further in response to the pressures on time and costs, as alternative in vitro and in silico methods are developed, and as public attitudes to animal experimentation harden. An additional difficulty is the decreasing number of pharmacologists trained to perform in vivo studies[1].

Imaging technologies (Rudin and Weissleder, 2003) are increasingly being used for pharmacological studies on whole animals. Useful techniques include *magnetic resonance imaging (MRI), ultrasound imaging, X-ray densitometry tomography, positron emission tomography (PET)* and others. They are proving highly versatile for both structural measurements (e.g. cardiac hypertrophy, tumour growth) and functional measurements (e.g. blood flow, tissue oxygenation). Used in conjunction with radioactive probes, PET can be used for studies on receptors

and other targets in vivo. Many of these techniques can also be applied to humans, providing an important bridge between animal and human pharmacology. Apart from the special facilities and equipment needed, currently the main drawback of imaging techniques is the time taken to capture the data, during which the animal must stay still, usually necessitating anaesthesia. With MRI and PET, which are currently the most versatile imaging techniques, data capture normally takes a few minutes, so they cannot be used for quick 'snapshots' of rapidly changing events.

A particularly important role for in vivo experiments is to evaluate the effects of long-term drug administration on the intact organism. 'Adaptive' and 'rebound' effects (e.g. tolerance, dependence, rebound hypertension, delayed endocrine effects etc.) are often produced when drugs are given continuously for days or weeks. Generally, such effects, which involve complex physiological interactions, are evident in the intact functioning organism but are not predictable from in vitro experiments.

The programme of in vivo profiling studies for characterization of a candidate drug depends very much on the drug target and therapeutic indication. A comprehensive catalogue of established in vivo assay methods appropriate to different types of pharmacological effect is given by Vogel (2002). Charting the appropriate course through the plethora of possible studies that might be performed to characterize a particular drug can be difficult.

A typical example of pharmacological profiling is summarized in Box 11.1. The studies were carried out as part of the recent development of a cardiovascular drug, *beraprost* (Melini and Goa, 2002). Beraprost is a stable analogue of prostaglandin I_2 (PGI_2) which acts on PGI_2 receptors of platelets and blood vessels, thereby inhibiting platelet aggregation (and hence thrombosis) and dilating blood vessels. It is directed at two therapeutic targets, namely *occlusive peripheral vascular disease* and *pulmonary hypertension* (a serious complication of various types of cardiovascular disease, drug treatment or infectious diseases), resulting in hypertrophy and often contractile failure of the right ventricle. The animal studies were therefore directed at measuring changes (reduction in blood flow, histological changes in vessel wall) associated with peripheral vascular disease, and with pulmonary hypertension. As these are progressive chronic conditions, it was important to establish that long-term systemic administration of beraprost was effective in retarding the development of the experimental lesions, as well as monitoring the acute pharmacodynamic effects of the drug.

---

[1]The rapid growth in the use of transgenic animals to study the functional role of individual gene products has recently brought in vivo physiology and pharmacology back into fashion, however.

Species differences

It is important to take species differences into account at all stages of pharmacological profiling. For projects

> ➤ **Box 11.1 Pharmacological profiling of beraprost**
>
> *In vitro studies*
>
> Binding to PGI_2 receptors of platelets from various species, including human.
> PGI_2 agonist activity (cAMP formation) in platelets
> Dilatation of arteries and arterioles in vitro, taken from various species
> Increased red cell deformability (hence reduced blood viscosity and increased blood flow) in blood taken from hypercholesterolaemic rabbits
>
> *In vivo studies*
>
> Increased peripheral blood flow in various vascular regions (dogs)
> Cutaneous vasodilatation (rat)
> Reduced pulmonary hypertension in rat model of drug-induced pulmonary hypertension (measured by reduction of right ventricular hypertrophy)
> Reduced tissue destruction (gangrene) of rat tail induced by ergotamine/epinephrine infusion
> Reduction of vascular occlusion resulting from intra-arterial sodium laureate infusion in rats
> Reduction of vascular occlusion and thrombosis following electrical stimulation of femoral artery in anaesthetized dogs and rabbits
> Reduction of vascular damage occurring several weeks after cardiac allografts in immunosuppressed rats

based on a defined molecular target – nowadays the majority – the initial screening assay will normally involve the human isoform. The same target in different species will generally differ in its pharmacological specificity; commonly, there will be fairly small quantitative differences, which can be allowed for in interpreting pharmacological data in experimental animals, but occasionally the differences are large, so that a given class of compounds is active in one species but not in another. An example is shown in Figure 11.3, which compares the activities of a series of bradykinin receptor antagonists on cloned human and rat receptors. The complete lack of correlation means that, for these compounds, tests of functional activity in the rat cannot be used to predict activity in man.

Species differences are, in fact, a major complicating factor at all stages of drug discovery and preclinical development. The physiology of disease processes such as inflammation, septic shock, obesity, atherosclerosis etc. differs markedly in different species. Most importantly (see Chapter 10), drug metabolism often differs, affecting the duration of action, as well as the pattern of metabolites, which can in turn affect the observed pharmacology and toxicity.

Species differences are, of course, one of the main arguments used by animal rights activists in opposing the use of animals for the purpose of drug discovery. Their claim – misleading when examined critically (see Research Defense Society website) – is that animal data

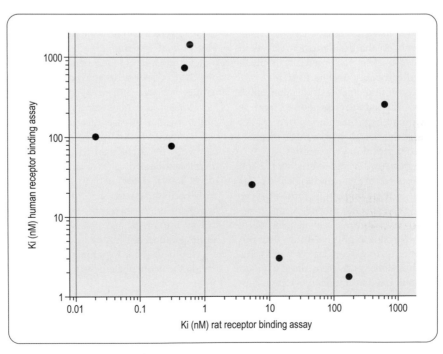

Fig. 11.3
Species differences in bradykinin B$_2$ receptors. (Data from Dziadulewicz et al., 2002.)

actually represent disinformation in this context. While being aware of the pitfalls, we should not lose sight of the fact that non-human data, including in vivo experiments, have actually been an essential part of every major drug discovery project to date. The growing use of transgenic animal models will undoubtedly lead to an increase, rather than a decrease, in animal experimentation.

Animal models of disease

The animal models discussed earlier were used to investigate the pharmacodynamic effects of the drug and to answer the question: How do the effects observed at the molecular and cellular levels of organization translate into physiological effects in the whole animal?

The next, crucial, question is: Can these physiological effects result in therapeutic benefit? Animal experiments can never answer this conclusively – only clinical trials can do that – but the use of animal models of human disease provides a valuable link in the chain of evidence, and there is strong pressure on drug discovery teams to produce data of this sort as a basis for the important decision to test a new compound in man. Despite the immense range and diversity of animal models that have been described, this is often the most problematic aspect of a drug discovery project, particularly where a novel target or mechanism is involved, so that there is no mechanistic precedent among established drugs. The magnitude of the difficulties varies considerably among different therapeutic areas. Many inflammatory conditions, for example, are straightforward to model in animals, as are some cancers. Animal models of hypertension generally predict very well the ability of compounds to lower blood pressure in man. Endocrine disorders involving over- or undersecretion of particular hormones can also be simply modelled in animals. Psychiatric disorders are much more difficult, as the symptoms that characterize them are not observable in animals. In most therapeutic areas there are certain disorders, such as migraine, temporal lobe epilepsy, asthma or irritable bowel syndrome, for which animal models, if they exist at all, are far from satisfactory in predicting clinical efficacy.

Here we consider, with a few selected examples, the main experimental approaches to generating animal models, and the criteria against which their 'validity' as models of human disease need to be assessed.

Types of animal model

Animal models of disease can be divided broadly into acute and chronic physiological and pharmacological models, and genetic models.

Acute physiological and pharmacological models are intended to mimic certain aspects of the clinical disorder. There are many examples, including:

- Seizures induced by electrical stimulation of the brain as a model for epilepsy (see below);
- Histamine-induced bronchoconstriction as a model for asthma;
- The hotplate test for analgesic drugs as a model for pain;
- Injection of lipopolysaccharide (LPS) and cytokines as a model for septic shock;
- The elevated maze test as a model for testing anxiolytic drugs.

Chronic physiological or pharmacological models involve the use of drugs or physical interventions to induce an ongoing abnormality similar to the clinical condition. Examples include:

- The use of alloxan to inhibit insulin secretion as a model for Type I diabetes;
- Procedures for inducing brain or coronary ischaemia as models for stroke and ischaemic heart disease;
- 'Kindling' and other procedures for inducing ongoing seizures as models for epilepsy;
- Self-administration of opiates, nicotine or other drugs as a model for drug-dependence;
- Cholesterol-fed rabbits as a model for hypercholesterolaemia and atherosclerosis;
- Immunization with myelin basic protein as a model for multiple sclerosis;
- Administration of the neurotoxin MPTP, causing degeneration of basal ganglia neurons as a model of Parkinson's disease;
- Transplantation of malignant cells into immunodeficient animals to produce progressive tumours as a model for certain types of cancer.

Details of these and many other examples of physiological and pharmacological models can be found in Vogel (2002). As discussed above, species differences need to be taken into account in the selection of animal models, and in the interpretation of results. In *septic shock*, for example, rodents show a much larger elevation of nitric oxide (NO) metabolites than do humans, and respond well to NO synthesis inhibitors, which humans do not. Rodents and rabbits transgenically engineered to favour cholesterol deposition nevertheless develop atherosclerosis only when fed high-cholesterol diets, whereas humans often do so even on low-cholesterol diets. Genetically obese mice are deficient in the hormone *leptin* and lose weight when treated with it, whereas obese humans frequently have high circulating leptin concentrations and do not respond to treatment with it. It is often not clear whether such discrepancies reflect inherent species differences, or simply failure of the model to replicate satisfactorily the human disease state (see Validity Criteria below).

Genetic models

There are many examples of spontaneously occurring animal strains that show abnormalities resembling human disease. In addition, much effort is going into producing transgenic strains with deletion or over-expression of specific genes, which exhibit disease-like phenotypes.

Long before genetic mapping became possible, it was realized that certain inbred strains of laboratory animal were prone to particular disorders, examples being spontaneously hypertensive rats, seizure-prone dogs, rats insensitive to antidiuretic hormone (a model for diabetes insipidus), obese mice, and mouse strains exhibiting a range of specific neurological deficits. Many such strains have been characterized (see Jackson Laboratory website, www.jaxmice.jax.org) and are commercially available, and are widely used as models for testing drugs.

The development of transgenic technology has allowed inbred strains to be produced that over- or under-express particular genes. In the simplest types, the gene abnormality is present throughout the animal's life, from early development onwards, and throughout the body. More recent technical developments allow much more control over the timing and location of the transgene effect. For reviews of transgenic technology and its uses in drug discovery, see Polites (1996), Rudolph and Moehler (1999), Törnell and Snaith (2002) and Pinkert (2002).

The genetic analysis of disease-prone animal strains, or of human families affected by certain diseases, has in many cases revealed the particular mutation or mutations responsible (see Chapters 6 and 7), thus pointing the way to new transgenic models. Several diseases associated with single-gene mutations, such as *cystic fibrosis* and *Duchenne muscular dystrophy*, have been replicated in transgenic mouse strains. Analysis of the obese mouse strain led to the identification of the leptin gene, which is mutated in the *ob/ob* mouse strain, causing the production of an inactive form of the hormone and overeating by the mouse. Transgenic animals closely resembling *ob/ob* mice have been produced by targeted inactivation of the gene for leptin or its receptor. Another example is the discovery that a rare familial type of Alzheimer's disease is associated with mutations of the amyloid precursor protein (APP). Transgenic mice expressing this mutation show amyloid plaque formation characteristic of the human disease. This and other transgenic models of Alzheimer's disease (Yamada and Nabeshima, 2000) represent an important tool for drug discovery, as there had hitherto been no animal model reflecting the pathogenesis of this disorder.

The number of transgenic animal models, mainly mouse, that have been produced is already large and is growing rapidly. Creating and validating a new disease model is, however, a slow business. Although the methodology for generating transgenic mice is now reliable and relatively straightforward, it is both time-consuming and labour-intensive. The first generation of transgenic animals are normally hybrids, as different strains are used for the donor and the recipient, and it is necessary to breed several generations by repeated back-crossings to create animals with a uniform genetic background. This takes 1–2 years, and is essential for consistent results. Analysis of the phenotypic changes resulting from the transgene can also be difficult and time-consuming, as the effects may be numerous and subtle, as well as being slow to develop as the animal matures. Despite these difficulties, there is no doubt that transgenic disease models will play an increasing part in drug testing, and many biotechnology companies have moved into the business of developing and providing them for this purpose. The fields in which transgenic models have so far had the most impact are cancer, atherosclerosis and neurodegenerative diseases, but their importance as drug discovery tools will certainly extend to all areas.

Producing transgenic rat strains proved impossible until recently, as embryonic stem (ES) cells cannot be obtained from rats. Success in producing gene knockout strains by an alternative method has now been achieved (Zan et al., 2003), and it is likely that the use of transgenic rats will increase, this being the favoured species for pharmacological and physiological studies in many laboratories.

The choice of model

Apart from resource limitations, regulatory constraints on animal experimentation, and other operational factors, what governs the choice of disease model?

As discussed in Chapter 2, naturally occurring diseases produce a variety of structural biochemical abnormalities, and these are often displayed separately in animal models. For example, human allergic asthma involves (a) an immune response; (b) increased airways resistance; (c) bronchial hyperreactivity; (d) lung inflammation; and (e) structural remodelling of the airways. Animal models, mainly based on guinea pigs, whose airways behave similarly to those of humans, can replicate each of these features, but no single model reproduces the whole spectrum. The choice of animal model for drug discovery purposes therefore depends on the therapeutic effect that is being sought. In the case of asthma, existing bronchodilator drugs effectively target the increased airways resistance, and steroids reduce the inflammation, and so it is the other components for which new drugs are particularly being sought.

A similar need for a range of animal models covering a range of therapeutic targets applies in many disease areas.

Validity criteria

Obviously an animal model produced in a laboratory can never replicate exactly a spontaneous human disease state, so on what basis can we assess its 'validity' in the context of drug discovery?

Three types of validity criteria were originally proposed by Willner (1984) in connection with animals models of depression. These are:

- Face validity
- Construct validity
- Predictive validity.

Face validity refers to the accuracy with which the model reproduces the phenomena (symptoms, clinical signs and pathological changes) characterizing the human disease.

Construct validity refers to the theoretical rationale on which the model is based, i.e. the extent to which the aetiology of the human disease is reflected in the model. A transgenic animal model in which a human disease-producing mutation is replicated will have, in general, good construct validity, even if the manifestations of the human disorder are not well reproduced (i.e. it has poor face validity).

Predictive validity refers to the extent to which the effect of manipulations (e.g. drug treatment) in the model is predictive of effects in the human disorder. It is the most pragmatic of the three and the most directly relevant to the issue of predicting therapeutic efficacy, but also the most limited in its applicability, for two main reasons. First, data on therapeutic efficacy are often sparse or non-existent, because no truly effective drugs are known (e.g. for Alzheimer's disease, septic shock). Second, the model may focus on a specific pharmacological mechanism, thus successfully predicting the efficacy of drugs that work by that mechanism but failing with drugs that might prove effective through other mechanisms. The knowledge that the first generation of antipsychotic drugs act as dopamine receptor antagonists enabled new drugs to be identified by animal tests reflecting dopamine antagonism, but these tests cannot be relied upon to recognize possible 'breakthrough' compounds that might be effective by other mechanisms. Thus, predictive validity, relying as it does on existing therapeutic knowledge, may not be a good basis for judging animal models where the drug discovery team's aim is to produce a mechanistically novel drug. The basis on which predictive validity is judged carries an inevitable bias, as the drugs that proceed to clinical trials will normally have proved effective in the model, whereas drugs that are ineffective in the model are unlikely to have been developed. As a result, there are many examples of tests giving 'false positive' expectations but very few false negatives, giving rise to a commonly held view that conclusions from pharmacological tests tend to be overoptimistic.

Some examples

We conclude this discussion of the very broad field of animal models of disease by considering three disease areas, namely epilepsy, psychiatric disorders and stroke. Epilepsy-like seizures can be produced in laboratory animals in many different ways. Many models have been described and used successfully to discover new antiepileptic drugs (AEDs). Although the models may lack construct validity and are weak on face validity, their predictive validity has proved to be very good. With models of psychiatric disorders, face validity and construct validity are very uncertain, as human symptoms are not generally observable in animals and because we are largely ignorant of the cause and pathophysiology of these disorders; nevertheless, the predictive validity of available models of depression, anxiety and schizophrenia has proved to be good, and such models have proved their worth in drug discovery. In contrast, the many available models of stroke are generally convincing in terms of construct and face validity, but have proved very unreliable as predictors of clinical efficacy. Researchers in this field are ruefully aware that despite many impressive effects in laboratory animals, clinical successes have been negligible.

Epilepsy models

The development of antiepileptic drugs, from the pioneering work of Merritt and Putnam, who in 1937 developed phenytoin, to the present day, has been highly dependent on animal models involving experimentally induced seizures, with relatively little reliance on knowledge of the underlying physiological, cellular or molecular basis of the human disorder. Although existing drugs have significant limitations, they have brought major benefits to sufferers from this common and disabling condition – testimony to the usefulness of animal models in drug discovery.

Human epilepsy is a chronic condition with many underlying causes, including head injury, infections, tumours and genetic factors. Epileptic seizures in humans take many forms, depending mainly on where the neural discharge begins and how it spreads.

Some of the widely used animal models used in drug discovery are summarized in Table 11.2. The earliest models, namely the *maximal electroshock (MES) test* and the *pentylenetetrazol-induced seizure (PTZ) test*, which are based on acutely induced seizures in normal animals, are still commonly used. They model the seizure, but without distinguishing its localization and spread, and do not address either the chronicity of human epilepsy or its aetiology (i.e. they score low on face validity and construct validity). But, importantly, their predictive validity for conventional antiepileptic drugs in man is very good, and the drugs developed on this basis, taken regularly to reduce the frequency of seizures or eliminate them altogether, are of proven therapeutic value.

Table 11.2
Epilepsy and epileptogenesis models

Model	Procedure	Face validity	Construct validity	Predictive validity
Acute seizure models				No acute seizure models show 'treatment-resistance' to conventional anti-epileptic drugs, though this occurs in ~30% of human cases
Maximal electroshock model	Acute seizures evoked by whole-brain stimulation. Measure: proportion of mice responding with seizures	Weak. No spontaneous seizures. No neuropathological changes	Weak. Production of seizures not related to epileptogenesis	Good. Predictive of activity of drugs against partial seizures and generalized tonic–clonic seizures (with some false positives). Poor prediction of drugs effective in absence seizures
Pentylenetetrazole (PTZ)-induced seizure model	Seizures induced by s.c. injection of the convulsant drug PTZ. Measure: proportion of mice responding with seizures	As above	As above.	Quite good as predictor of efficacy in absence seizures. Unreliable for other clinical types
Epileptogenesis models				
Kindling model	Weak electrical stimulation of amygdala repeated over several days. Evoked full-blown seizures develop gradually	Moderate, though spontaneous seizures are rarely produced. Histological, electrophysiological and biochemical changes similar to human epilepsy	Uncertain	Moderate, but model is generally more drug-responsive than human epilepsy
Post-seizure models	Various procedures (e.g. injection of kainate, lithium or other agents into brain, sustained stimulation of amygdala or other pathways) evoke sustained seizures, with ongoing spontaneous seizures appearing days or weeks later Can be used to test drug effects on fully kindled seizures, or on the kindling process	Good. Spontaneous seizures, latent period after initial trigger. Replicates histological and other changes, including neurodegeneration	Probably good for some clinical forms of epilepsy	As MES for anti-seizure drugs. Uncertain for antiepileptogenic drugs, of which there are no proven clinical examples
Surgical procedures	Cortical undercutting. Isolated region of cortex gradually develops spontaneous seizure activity	Good as model of post-traumatic epilepsy. Replicates histological and other changes	Probably good for post-traumatic epilepsy	As above

Following on from these acute seizure models, attempts have been made to replicate the processes by which human epilepsy develops and continues as a chronic condition with spontaneous seizures, i.e. to model *epileptogenesis* (Löscher, 2002; White, 2002) by the use of models that show greater construct and face validity. This has been accomplished in a variety of ways (see Table 11.2), in the hope that such models would be helpful in developing drugs capable of preventing epilepsy. Such models have thrown considerable light on the pathogenesis of epilepsy, but have not so far contributed significantly to the development of improved antiepileptic drugs. Because there are currently no drugs known to prevent epilepsy from progressing, the predictive validity of epileptogenesis models remains uncertain.

Psychiatric disorders

Animal models of psychiatric disorders are in general problematic, because in many cases the disorders are defined by symptoms and behavioural changes unique to humans, rather than by measurable physiological, biochemical or structural abnormalities. This is true in conditions such as schizophrenia, Tourette's syndrome and autism, making face validity difficult to achieve. Depressive symptoms, in contrast, can be reproduced to some extent in animal models (Willner and Mitchell, 2002), and face validity is therefore stronger. The aetiology of most psychiatric conditions is largely unknown[2], making construct validity questionable.

Models are therefore chosen largely on the basis of predictive validity, and suffer from the shortcomings mentioned above. Nonetheless, models for some disorders, particularly depression, have proved very valuable in the discovery of new drugs. Other disorders, such as autism and Tourette's syndrome, have proved impossible to model so far, whereas models for others, such as schizophrenia (Lipska and Weinberger, 2000; Moser et al., 2000), have been described but are of doubtful validity. The best prediction of antipsychotic drug efficacy comes from pharmacodynamic models reflecting blockade of dopamine and other monoamine receptors, rather than from putative disease models, with the result that drug discovery has so far failed to break out of this mechanistic straitjacket.

Stroke

Many experimental procedures have been devised to produce acute cerebral ischaemia in laboratory animals, resulting in long-lasting neurological deficits that resemble the sequelae of strokes in humans (Small and Buchan, 2000). Interest in this area has been intense, reflecting the fact that strokes are among the commonest causes of death and disability in developed countries, and that there are currently no drugs that significantly improve the recovery process. Studies with animal models have greatly advanced our understanding of the pathophysiological events. Stroke is no longer seen as simple anoxic death of neurons, but rather as a complex series of events involving neuronal depolarization, acti-

vation of ion channels, release of excitatory transmitters, disturbed calcium homeostasis leading to calcium overload, release of inflammatory mediators and nitric oxide, generation of reactive oxygen species, disturbance of the blood–brain barrier and cerebral oedema (Dirnagl et al., 1999). Glial cells, as well as neurons, play an important role in the process. Irreversible loss of neurons takes place gradually as this cascade builds up, leading to the hope that intervention after the primary event – usually thrombosis – could be beneficial. Moreover, the biochemical and cellular events involve well-understood signalling mechanisms, offering many potential drug targets, such as calcium channels, glutamate receptors, scavenging of reactive oxygen species, and many others. Ten years ago, on the basis of various animal models with apparently good construct and face validity and a range of accessible drug targets, the stage seemed to be set for major therapeutic advances. Drugs of many types, including glutamate antagonists, calcium and sodium channel blocking drugs, antiinflammatory drugs, free radical scavengers and others, produced convincing degrees of neuroprotection in animal models, even when given up to several hours after the ischaemic event. Many clinical trials were undertaken (de Keyser et al., 1999), with uniformly negative results. The only drug currently known to have a beneficial – albeit small – effect is the biopharmaceutical 'clot-buster' tissue plasminogen activator (TPA), widely used to treat heart attacks. Stroke models thus represent approaches that have revealed much about pathophysiology and have stimulated intense efforts in drug discovery, but whose predictive validity has proved to be extremely poor, as the drug sensitivity of the animal models seems to be much greater than that of the human condition. Surprisingly, it appears that whole-brain ischaemia models show better predictive validity (i.e. poor drug responsiveness) than focal ischaemia models, even though the latter are more similar to human strokes.

GLP compliance in pharmacological studies

Good laboratory practice (GLP) comprises adherence to a set of formal, internationally agreed guidelines established by regulatory authorities, aimed at ensuring the reliability of results obtained in the laboratory. The rules (see *The GLP Pocketbook*, 1999; EEC directives 87/18/EEC, 88/320/EEC, available online: pharmacos.eudra.org/F2/eudralex/vol-7/A/7AG4a.pdf) cover all stages of an experimental study, from planning and experimental design to documentation, reporting and archiving. They require, among other things, the assignment of specific GLP-compliant laboratories,

---

[2]Many psychiatric disorders have a strong genetic component in their aetiology, and much effort has gone into identifying particular susceptibility genes. Success has so far been very limited, but the expectation is that, in future, success in this area will enable improved transgenic animal models to be developed.

certification of staff training to agreed standards, certified instrument calibration, written standard operating procedures covering all parts of the work, specified standards of experimental records, reports, notebooks and archives, and much else. Standards are thoroughly and regularly monitored by an official inspectorate, which can halt studies or require changes in laboratory practice if the standards are thought not to be adequately enforced. Adherence to GLP standards carries a substantial administrative overhead and increases both the time and cost of laboratory studies, as well as limiting their flexibility.

The regulations are designed primarily to minimize the risk of errors in studies that relate to safety. They are therefore not generally applied to pharmacological profiling as described in this chapter. They are obligatory for toxicological studies that are required in submissions for regulatory approval. Though not formally required for safety pharmacology studies, most companies and contract research organizations choose to do such work under GLP conditions.

References

Current protocols in pharmacology. New York: John Wiley and Sons. [Published as looseleaf binder and CD-ROM, and regularly updated.)

De Keyser J, Sulter G, Luiten PG (1999) Clinical trials with neuroprotective drugs in ischaemic stroke: are we doing the right thing? Trends in Neurosciences 22: 535–540.

Dirnagl U, Iadecola C, Moskowitz MA (1999) Pathobiology of ischaemic stroke: an integrated view. Trends in Neurosciences 22: 391–397.

Dziadulewicz EK, Ritchie TJ, Hallett A et al. (2002) Nonpeptide bradykinin B$_2$ receptor antagonists: conversion of rodent-selective bradyzide analogues into potent orally active human bradykinin B$_2$ receptor antagonists. Journal of Medicinal Chemistry 45: 2160–2172.

Enna S, Farkany J W, Kenakin T, Williams M, Porsolt RD, Sullivan JP (eds) (2002)

Hall JM (1992) Bradykinin receptors: pharmacological properties and biological roles. Pharmacology and Therapeutics 56: 131–190.

Heidempergher F, Pillan A, Pinciroli V et al. (1997) Phenylimidazolidin-2-one derivatives as selective 5-HT3 receptor antagonists and refinement of the pharmacophore model for 5-HT3 receptor binding. Journal of Medicinal Chemistry 40: 3369–3380.

Holker M H, van Deursen J (2002) Transgenic mouse methods and protocols. Totowa, NJ: Humana Press.

Keen M (ed) (1999) Receptor binding techniques. Totowa, NJ: Humana Press.

Kenakin T (1999) The measurement of efficacy in the drug discovery agonists selection process. Journal of Pharmacologic and Toxicologic Methods 42: 177–187.

Lipska BK, Weinberger DR (2000) To model a psychiatric disorder in animals: schizophrenia as a reality test. Neuropsychopharmacology 23: 223–239.

Löscher W (2002) Animal models of epilepsy for the development of antiepileptogenic and disease-modifying drugs. A comparison of the pharmacology of kindling and post-status epilepticus models of temporal lobe epilepsy, Epilepsy Research 50: 105–123.

Melini EB, Goa KL (2002) Beraprost: a review of its pharmacology and therapeutic efficacy in the treatment of peripheral arterial disease and pulmonary hypertension. Drugs 62: 107–133.

Morfis M, Christopoulos A, Sexton PM (2003) RAMPs: 5 years on, where to now? Trends in Pharmacological Sciences 24: 596–601.

Moser PC, Hitchcock JH, Lister S, Moran PM (2000) The pharmacology of latent inhibition as an animal model of schizophrenia. Brain Research Reviews 33: 275–307.

Pinkert CA (2002) Transgenic animal technology, 2nd edn. San Diego, CA: Academic Press.

Polites HG (1996) Transgenic model applications to drug discovery. International Journal of Experimental Pathology 77: 257–262.

Research Defense Society website: www.rds-online.org.uk/ethics/arclaims – a reasoned rebuttal of the view put forward by opponents of animal experimentation that the use of such experiments in drug discovery is at best unnecessary, if not positively misleading.

Rudin M, Weissleder R (2003) Molecular imaging in drug discovery and development. Nature Reviews Drug Discovery 2: 122–131.

Rudolph U, Moehler H (1999) Genetically modified animals in pharmacological research: future trends. European Journal of Pharmacology 375: 327–337.

Small DL, Buchan AM (2000) Stroke: animal models. British Medical Bulletin 56: 307–317.

The GLP Pocketbook, 1999. London: MCA Publications. Contains the *Good Laboratory Practice (GLP) Regulations 1999* and the *Guide to the GLP Regulations*.

Törnell J, Snaith M (2002) Transgenic systems in drug discovery: from target identification to humanized mice. Drug Discovery Today 7: 461–470.

Traxler P, Bold G, Frei J et al. (1997) Use of a pharmacophore model for the design of EGF-R tyrosine kinase inhibitors: 4-(phenylamino)pyrazolo[3,4-d]pyrimidines. Journal of Medicinal Chemistry 40: 3601–3616.

Vogel WH (ed) (2002) Drug discovery and evaluation: pharmacological assays. Heidelberg: Springer-Verlag.

White HS (2002) Animal models of epileptogenesis. Neurology 59: S7–S14.

Willner P (1984) The validity of animal models of depression. Psychopharmacology 83: 1–16.

Willner P, Mitchell PJ (2002) The validity of animal models of predisposition to depression. Behavioural Pharmacology 13: 169–188.

Yamada K, Nabeshima T (2000) Animal models of Alzheimer's disease and evaluation of anti-dementia drugs. Pharmacology and Therapeutics 88: 93–113.

Yang D, Soulier J-L, Sicsic S et al. (1997) New esters of 4-amino-5-chloro-2-methoxybenzoic acid as potent agonists and antagonists for 5-HT4 receptors. Journal of Medicinal Chemistry 40: 608–621.

Zan Y, Haag JD, Chen KS et al. (2003) Production of knockout rats using ENU mutagenesis and a yeast-based screening assay. Nature Biotechnology 21: 645–51

12 Biopharmaceuticals

H LeVine

Introduction

The term 'biopharmaceutical' was originally coined to define therapeutic proteins produced by genetic engineering, rather than by extraction from normal biological sources. Its meaning has broadened with time, and the term now encompasses nucleic acids as well as proteins, vaccines as well as therapeutic agents, and even cell-based therapies. In this chapter we describe the nature of biopharmaceuticals, and the similarities and differences in discovery and development between biopharmaceuticals and conventional small-molecule therapeutic agents. The usual starting point for biopharmaceuticals is a naturally occurring peptide, protein or nucleic acid. The 'target' is thus identified at the outset, and the process of target identification and validation, which is a major and often difficult step in the discovery of conventional therapeutics (see Chapter 6), is much less of an issue for biopharmaceuticals. Equally, the process of lead finding and optimization (Chapters 7, 8, 9) is generally unnecessary, or at least streamlined, because Nature has already done the job. Even if it is desirable to alter the properties of the naturally occurring biomolecule, the chemical options will be much more limited than they are for purely synthetic compounds. In general, then, biopharmaceuticals require less investment in discovery technologies than do conventional drugs. Toxicity associated with reactive metabolites – a common cause of development failure with synthetic compounds – is uncommon with biopharmaceuticals. On the other hand, they generally require greater investment in two main areas, namely *production methods* and *formulation.* Production methods rely on harnessing biological systems to do the work of synthesis, and the problems of yield, consistency and quality control are more complex than they are for organic synthesis. Formulation problems arise commonly because biomolecules tend to be large and unstable, and considerable ingenuity is often needed to improve their pharmacokinetic properties, and to target their distribution in the body to where their actions are required.

It is beyond the scope of this book to give more than a brief account of the very diverse and rapidly developing field of biopharmaceuticals. More detail can be found in textbooks (Buckel, 2001; Ho and Gibaldi, 2003; Walsh, 2003). As the field of biopharmaceuticals moves on from being mainly concerned with making key hormones, antibodies and other signalling molecules available as therapeutic agents, efforts – many of them highly ingenious – are being made to produce therapeutic effects in other ways. These include, for example, using antisense nucleic acids, ribozymes or RNAi (see below and Chapter 6) to reduce gene expression, the use of catalytic antibodies to control chemical reactions in specific cells or tissues, and the development of 'DNA vaccines'. So far, very few of these more complex 'second-generation' biopharmaceutical ideas have got beyond the experimental stage, but there is little doubt that the therapeutic strategies of the future will be based on more sophisticated ways of affecting biological control mechanisms than the simple 'ligand → target → effect' pharmacological principle on which most conventional drugs are based.

Recombinant DNA technology – the engine driving biotechnology

The discovery of enzymes for manipulating and engineering DNA – the bacterial restriction endonucleases, polynucleotide ligase and DNA polymerase – and the invention of the enabling technologies of DNA sequencing and copying of DNA sequences by using the polymerase chain reaction (PCR), allowed rapid determination of the amino acid sequence of a protein from its mRNA message. Versatile systems for introducing nucleic acids into target cells or tissues and for the control of host nucleic acid metabolism brought the potential for correction of genetic defects and for new therapeutic products for disorders poorly served by conventional small-molecule drugs. The importance of these discoveries for the biological sciences was indicated by the many Nobel Prizes awarded for related work. No less critical was the impact that these reagents and technologies had on applied science, especially in the pharmaceutical industry. The business opportunities afforded by biotechnology spawned thousands of startup companies and profoundly changed the relationship between academia and industry. The mainstream pharmaceutical industry, with its 20th-century focus on small-molecule therapeutic agents, did not immediately embrace the new methodologies except as research tools in the hands of some discovery scientists. Entrepreneurs in biotechnology startup firms eventually brought technology platforms and products to large pharmaceutical companies as services or as products for full-scale development. This alliance allowed each party to concentrate on the part they did best.

Biotechnology products were naturally attractive to the small startup companies. Because the protein or nucleic acid itself was the product, it was unnecessary to have medicinal chemists synthesize large collections of organic small-molecule compounds to screen for activity. A small energetic company with the right molecule could come up with a profitable, and very useful product. The niche markets available for many of the initial protein or nucleic acid products were sufficient to support a small research-based company with a high profit-margin therapeutic agent.

The early days of protein therapeutics

Along with plant-derived natural products, proteins and peptides were some of the first therapeutic agents produced by the fledgling pharmaceutical industry in the latter half of the 19th century, before synthetic chemistry became established as a means of making drugs. Long before antibiotics were discovered, serum from immune animals or humans was successfully used to treat a variety of infectious diseases. Serotherapy was the accepted treatment for *Haemophilus influenzae* meningitis, measles, diphtheria, tetanus, hepatitis A and B, poliovirus, cytomegalovirus and lobar pneumonia. Antisera raised in animals were used to provide passive protection from diphtheria and tetanus infection.

Extracts of tissues provided hormones, many of which were polypeptides. After its discovery in 1921, insulin extracted from animal pancreas replaced a starvation regimen for treating diabetes. The size of the diabetic population, and the activity in humans of the hormone isolated from pancreas of pigs and cows, permitted early commercial success. Generally, however, the low yield of many hormones and growth factors from human or animal sources made industrial scale isolation difficult and often uneconomic. Nevertheless, several such hormones were developed commercially, including *follicle-stimulating hormone* (FSH) extracted from human urine and used to treat infertility, *glucagon* extracted from pig pancreas to treat hypoglycaemia, and *growth hormone*, extracted from human pituitary to treat growth disorders. Some enzymes, such as *glucocerebrosidase*, extracted from human placenta and used to treat an inherited lipid storage disease (Gaucher's disease), and *urokinase*, a thrombolytic agent extracted from human urine, were also developed as commercial products.

Some serious problems emerged when proteins extracted from human or animal tissues were developed for therapeutic use. In particular:

● Repeated dosage of non-human proteins generated an immune response in some patients against the foreign sequences, which differed by several amino acids from the human sequence. Such immune responses could cause illnesses such as serum sickness, or loss of efficacy of the protein.

- Human tissue was in short supply and was subject to potential contamination with infectious agents. Growth hormone extracted from human cadaver pituitary glands was contaminated with prions that cause Creutzfeld–Jakob disease, a dementing brain-wasting disease similar to bovine spongiform encephalitis (BSE) and sheep scrapie. Human blood plasma-derived products have been tainted with hepatitis B virus and HIV.
- Many agents (e.g. cytokines) cannot be extracted in sufficient quantities to be used therapeutically.
- Batch-to-batch variability was considerable, requiring standardization by bioassay in many cases.

The recombinant DNA revolution and the subsequent development of biotechnology resolved many of these issues. Many vaccines and antisera, however, are still prepared from blood products or infectious organisms, rather than by recombinant DNA methods.

Currently available classes of biopharmaceuticals

The major classes of biopharmaceuticals currently on the market include hormones, cytokines, growth factors, antibodies, enzymes, vaccines and nucleotide-based agents. Examples of therapeutic proteins, including antibodies, enzymes, and other proteins approved for clinical use, are presented in Table 12.1. Others not included in the compilation include therapeutic preparations such as serum albumin, haemoglobin and collagen, which are not drugs in the conventional sense.

In addition to the 'mainstream' biopharmaceuticals considered here are numerous speciality products for niche markets that are under investigation or in development by small 'boutique' companies.

Growth factors and cytokines

The production, differentiation and survival of the various types of blood cell are tightly regulated by an interacting network of hormones, cytokines and growth factors. Species-specific activities of many of these chemical mediators, and their very low abundance, highlighted the need for biopharmaceutical products.

The most common uses of haemopoietic factors are for the treatment of various types of neutropenia, where specific white cell levels are depressed as a result of infection, immune disorders, recovery from chemotherapy, or reaction to various drug regimens. They are especially useful in aiding recovery from the dose-limiting side effects of cancer chemotherapy. *Granulocyte colony-stimulating factor (G-CSF)* and *granulocyte–macrophage colony-stimulating factor (GM-CSF)* are used for this purpose to improve patient quality of life and allow the continuation of chemotherapy.

Erythropoietin (EPO), normally produced by the kidney to stimulate the production of red blood cells, is the most successful biotechnology product so far marketed. EPO boosts red cell counts and reduces transfusion requirements for patients rendered anaemic by cancer chemotherapy or renal disease. Various forms of EPO with clearance profiles – and hence duration of action – modified by linkage with polyethylene glycol (PEGylation) or alteration of its glycosylation (see below and Chapter 17) are also available. Off-label use of EPO by athletes to improve performance has caused controversy.

Interferons are a complex group of proteins that augment immune effector cell function. *Interferon-α* was the first recombinant biotherapeutic agent approved by the FDA for cancer treatment. Recombinant interferons have been approved for melanoma, hepatitis C, Karposi's sarcoma, T-cell lymphoma, chronic myelogenous leukaemia, multiple sclerosis and severe malignant osteopetrosis. Mechanism-based side effects have thus far restricted their utility to these severe disorders.

Hormones

Hormone replacement or augmentation is a commonly accepted medical practice in certain diseases of deficiency or misregulation. *Insulin* isolated from biological sources is administered to diabetics to control blood glucose levels. Immunological reaction to non-human (porcine or bovine) insulin preparations, which occur in a significant number of patients, are avoided by recombinant products incorporating parts of the human insulin sequence. A variety of human insulin and glucagon preparations are now on the market.

Human growth hormone (somatotropin) was originally developed for treating paediatric growth failure and Turner's syndrome. Originally, growth hormone was extracted from human pituitary tissue post mortem, but this material carried a significant risk of transmitting Creutzfeld–Jakob disease, a fatal neurodegenerative condition now known to be transmitted by a prion, an abnormal protein found in affected brain tissue, whose existence was unsuspected when human-derived growth hormone was introduced as a therapeutic agent. The production of human growth hormone by recombinant methods rather than extraction avoids this serious problem as well as providing a much more abundant

Drug discovery

Table 12.1
Examples of approved therapeutic proteins produced by recombinant technology

Product	Trade name	Date approved	Indications
Blood clotting factors and plasminogen activators			
Human factor VIII	Kogenate, Recombinate	1992	Haemophilia A
Human factor IX	Benefix	1997	Haemophilia B
Human tissue plasminogen activator (tPA)	Activase Ecokinase	1987	Heart attacks, stroke
Haemopoietic factors			
Erythropoietin	Epogen, Procrit	1989	Anaemia
Granulocyte–macrophage colony-stimulating factor (GM-CSF)	Leukine	1991	Neutropenia
Hormones			
Human insulin	Humulin, Novolin, Protropin	1982	Diabetes mellitus
Human glucagons	Glucagen	1998	Hypoglycaemia
Human growth hormone	Humatrope, Nutropin	1987	Growth hormone deficiency
Human thyroid-stimulating hormone (TSH)	Thyrogen	1998	Thyroid deficiency
Human follicle-stimulating hormone (FSH)	Gonal F, Follistim	1995	Infertility
Interferons and interleukins			
Human interferon-α	Intron A, Viraferon	1986	Hepatitis B and C
Human interferon-β	Betaferon	1995	Multiple sclerosis
Human interferon-γ	Actimmune	1990	Chronic inflammatory disease
Modified human interleukin-2	Proleukin	1992	Renal carcinoma
Modified human interleukin-11	Neumega	1997	Thrombocytopenia
Monoclonal antibodies			
Abciximab (against platelet GPIIb/IIIa)	ReoPro	1994	Blood clot prevention
Trastuzumab (against human EGF receptor)	Herceptin	1998	Breast cancer
Infliximab (against TNF-α)	Remicade	1998	Crohn's disease, arthritis
Rituximab (against CD20 lymphocyte antigen)	Rituxan	1997	Non-Hodgkin's lymphoma
Others			
Hirudin	Revasc, Refludan	1998	Prevention of thrombosis
Human β-cerebrosidase	Cerezyme	1994	Gaucher's disease (lipid storage disorder)
DNase	Pulmozyme	1993	Cystic fibrosis

source. Growth hormone has acquired notoriety since the potential for misuse to produce taller and stronger athletes was realized.

Human gonadotrophin-releasing hormones have been extensively used in fertility management as well as in treating endometriosis and precocious puberty.

Originally isolated from urine, there are now numerous recombinant products on the market.

Coagulation factors

Coagulation factors are a group of plasma proteins required for proper haemostasis. Deficiencies are associated with genetic lesions and occur as complications of viral infections such as hepatitis C and HIV. They were initially treated with plasma-derived concentrates, which carried a significant risk of viral and prion contamination. *Recombinant factor VIII* (Recombinate, Kogenate) and *factor IX* (BeneFix) avoid this risk and are now widely used.

Antithrombotic factors

To reduce blood coagulation, when conventional heparin or warfarin therapy is contraindicated, recombinant *thrombin inhibitors* (Leprudin, Bivalirudin) and *antiplatelet gpIIb/IIIa antagonists* (Eptifibatide) are now available. In conditions such as stroke, coronary thrombosis and pulmonary embolism early treatment with thrombolytic agents to relieve the vascular block is highly beneficial. *Streptokinase* and *urokinase* are proteases that process plasminogen to plasmin, activating its thrombolytic activity to dissolve fibrin clots. Newer products include *tissue plasminogen activator* (tPA) and TNKase, which catalyse the same reaction but in a fibrin-dependent fashion, so that plasmin production is concentrated in the region of the clot. These proteins are also less immunogenic than the bacterial streptokinase, which is important in cases where repeated administration of the thrombolytic agent is required.

Another regulator of coagulation is the serine protease *protein C*. The activated form of protein C breaks down the clotting factors Va and VIIIa and plasminogen activator inhibitor-1, tipping the balance in the favour of thrombolysis. These enzymes are important biopharmaceutical products that have no small-molecule counterpart.

Therapeutic antibodies

Monoclonal antibodies

A breakthrough in high-quality reproducible and scalable production of antibodies came with the development by Kohler and Milstein in 1975 of monoclonal antibodies. Fusion of primed T cells from an immunized mouse with an immortalized mouse myeloma (B-cell) line that secretes immunoglobulin light chains provided a cell culture system that could produce unlimited quantities of antibody with defined specificity. Single cell clones secreted antibody against a single epitope of the antigen. The initial immunization could, for toxic or scarce immunogens, be replaced by in vitro stimulation of isolated mouse thymocytes for fusion with the myeloma cells.

The technology for antibody production has now gone mouseless. It has moved into the realm of molecular biology, in which bacteriophages, gene libraries in plasmids and bacterial hosts are engineered to produce either whole antibodies or derivatives of antibodies with desired properties. 'Humanizing' the antibodies, or replacing the rodent constant domains with human sequences (chimerization), limits hypersensitivity reactions to foreign protein. Chimerization increases the half-life of the antibodies in human plasma up to sixfold and improves their function within the human immune network. The human Fc domain reacts with Fc receptors on human cells more avidly. Chimeric antibodies with human constant regions also interact optimally with human complement proteins, and are thus more effective in destroying target cells in patients than are their rodent counterpart.

Antibody selection by phage display

Phage display technology (Benhar, 2001) is a useful way to identify monoclonal antibodies that bind to therapeutically relevant antigens. Phages are viruses that replicate in bacteria, *Escherichia coli* being the organism of choice in most cases. For antibody selection (Figure 12.1) a large DNA library, encoding millions of different antibodies or antigen-binding domains, is incorporated into phage DNA, so that each phage particle encodes a single antibody. The mixed phage population is added to *E. coli* cultures, where the phage replicates, each phage particle expressing copies of a single antibody on its surface. The phage suspension is applied to plates coated with the antigen of interest ('panning') and those phage particles that express antibodies recognized by the antigen stick to the plates. The adherent phages are isolated, allowing the antibody-encoding DNA to be identified and used to produce further antibody as required.

Uses of antibodies as therapeutic agents

Cancer immunotherapy
Although high-affinity mouse monoclonal antibodies to target antigens can be reproducibly produced in industrial quantities, and bind to specific human targets, they generally function poorly in recruiting human effector functions. The therapeutic potency of these antibodies can be enhanced by taking advantage of the targeting

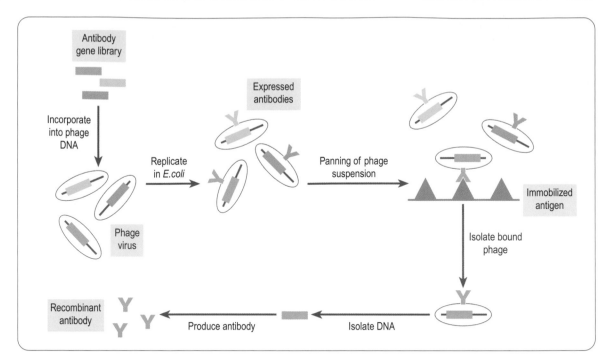

Fig. 12.1
Antibody selection by phage display technique.

selectivity of antibodies (see Chapter 17) for the purposes of drug delivery. Linking other agents, such as cytotoxic drugs, biological toxins, radioisotopes or enzymes to activate prodrugs to targeting antibodies enhances their delivery to the target cells and reduces side effects by directing the toxic agents to the tumour and minimizing clearance. Bispecific antibodies with one H-L chain pair directed against a target cell antigen and the other against a soluble effector such as a complement component, or against a cell surface marker of an effector cell type, have also been developed to bring the components of the reaction together. A number of these are in clinical trials for a variety of different malignancies, but have in general proved less successful than had been expected on the basis of animal studies.

Antibody use in transplantation and immunomodulation

The major obstacle in the transplantation of cells, tissues or organs is the body's recognition of foreign material. A strong immune response to rid the body of the non-self antigens leads to rejection of the transplant. Selective immunological suppression can ablate components of the antitransplant response. Fab fragments of antibodies to a number of surface antigens on T-cells are used to partially block T-cell responses to donor cells. Fab fragments are required because the Fc portion of the complete antibody targets the cell for destruction, resulting in unwanted complete immunosuppression.

Even human antibodies face disadvantages as therapeutics. Because of their size (MW ~150 kDa), their ability

to penetrate into tissues, such as solid tumours, is limited. Engineered versions lacking the Fc region, which is largely responsible for hypersensitivity responses of patients treated with monoclonal antibodies, have replaced the (Fab)$_2$ fragments generated by proteolysis from the intact antibody. Single sFv chains containing the H and L variable regions are the smallest antibodies containing a high-affinity antigen-combining site. Still in the experimental stage, 'di-antibodies' with two H-L units connected by a 15-amino acid linker (Gly$_4$Ser)$_3$ peptide have greatly increased affinity for antigen.

Catalytic antibodies

Antibodies can be used to enhance the chemical reactivity of molecules to which they bind. Such catalytic antibodies ('abzymes') created with transition state analogs as immunogens specifically enhance substrate hydrolysis by factors of 10^2–10^5 over the rate in their absence, and this principle has been applied to the development of therapeutic agents (Tellier, 2002). Both esterase and amidase activities have been reported. Catalytic turnover of substrates by abzymes is low in comparison to true enzymes, as high-affinity binding impedes the release of products. Attempts to improve catalytic efficiency and to identify therapeutic uses for catalytic antibodies have engrossed both academic and biotech startup laboratories. Targets being approached with these antibodies include cocaine overdose and drug addiction, bacterial endotoxin, and anticancer monoclonal antibody conjugated with a catalytic antibody designed to activate a cytotoxic prodrug. Attempts are also being made to develop proteolytic antibodies containing a catalytic triad analogous to that of serine proteases, designed to cleave gp120 (for treatment of HIV), IgE (for treatment of allergy), or epidermal growth factor receptor (for treatment of cancer).

Therapeutic enzymes

Enzymes can be useful therapeutic agents as replacements for endogenous sources of activity that are deficient as a result of disease or genetic mutation. Because enzymes are large proteins they generally do not pass through cellular membranes, and do not penetrate into tissues from the bloodstream unless assisted by some delivery system. Lysosomal hydrolases such as cerebrosidase and glucosidase have targeting signals that allow them to be taken up by cells and delivered to the lysosome. Genetic lysosomal storage diseases (Gaucher's, Tay–Sachs) are treated by enzyme replacement therapy. However, penetration of the enzymes into the nervous system, where the most severe effects of the disease are expressed, is poor. Cystic fibrosis, a genetic disorder characterized by deficits in salt secretion, is treated with digestive enzyme supplements and an inhaled DNase preparation (Dornase-α) to reduce the extracellular viscosity of the mucous layer in the lung to ease breathing. All of these are produced as recombinant proteins.

Vaccines

Using the immune system to protect the body against certain organisms or conditions is a powerful way to provide long-term protection against disease. Unlike with small-molecule pharmaceuticals, which are administered when needed, once immunity is present subsequent exposure to the stimulus automatically activates the response. Most current vaccines are against disease-causing organisms such as bacteria, viruses and parasites. More complex conditions where the antigens are not so well defined are also being addressed by immunization. Vaccines are being tested for cancer, neurodegenerative diseases, contraception, heart disease, autoimmune diseases, and alcohol and drug addiction (Rousseau et al., 2001; BSI Vaccine Immunology Group, 2002; Biaggi et al., 2002, Kantak, 2003). Immune induction is complex. Pioneering experiments with attenuation of disease organisms showed that illness was not required for immunity. The goal in immunization is to retain enough of the disease-causing trait of an antigen to confer protection without causing the disease. For infectious agents, various methods of killing or weakening the organism by drying or exposure to inactivating agents still dominate manu-

facturing processes. Isolation of antigens from the organisms, or modifying their toxins, can be used in some cases. Vaccine production of isolated antigen 'subunit' vaccines benefits from protein engineering.

Novel approaches to presenting antigens are expected to have an impact on vaccination. An example is the *phage display* technique (Benhar, 2001), described earlier as a technique for antibody selection. The same approach can be used to provide the protein antigen in a display framework that enhances its immunogenicity and reduces the requirement for immune adjuvants (of which there are few approved for human use). Viruses encoding multiple antigens ('vaccinomes') can also be employed.

Genetic vaccination (Liu, 2003) employs a DNA plasmid containing the antigen-encoding gene, which is delivered to the host tissue by direct injection of DNA, or by more exotic techniques such as attaching the DNA to microparticles which are shot into tissues at high speed by a 'gene gun', or introduced by other transfection methods (Capecchi et al., 2004; Locher et al., 2004; Manoj et al., 2004). When the DNA is transcribed, the mRNA translated and the protein expressed in the host tissue, eukaryotic sequences will undergo appropriate post-translational modification, which does not occur with conventional protein vaccines. In general, partial sequences of pathogen-derived proteins are fully immunogenic, despite lacking the toxicity of full-length transcripts. The first human trial for a genetic vaccine against HIV took place in 1995, and others quickly followed, including hepatitis, influenza, melanoma, malaria, cytomegalovirus, non-Hodgkin's lymphoma, and breast, prostate and colorectal tumours. Initial results have been promising, but currently (2004) vaccines against hepatitis A and B are the only recombinant vaccines that are commercially available. Single or multiple proteins from an organism can be included, and proteins that interfere with the immune response (common in many infectious agents) excluded.

Gene therapy

The development and present status of gene therapy are discussed in Chapter 3. Here we focus on the technical problems of gene delivery and achieving expression levels sufficient to produce clinical benefit, which are still major obstacles.

Introduction of genetic material into cells

Nucleic acid polymers are large, highly charged polyanions at physiologic pH. The mechanism by which such cumbersome hydrophilic molecules traverse multiple membrane lipid bilayers in cells is poorly understood, although a variety of empirical techniques for getting DNA into cells have been devised by molecular biologists. Eukaryotic cells use many strategies to distinguish between self and foreign DNA to which they are continually exposed. Some mechanisms apparently interfere with the incorporation and expression of engineered genes in gene therapy and other DNA transfer applications. Despite advances in technology, expression of foreign genes in cells or animals in the right place, at the right moment, in the right amount, for a long enough time remains difficult. Doing so in a clinical situation where so many more of the variables are uncontrollable is yet more challenging. The high expectations of gene therapies, which conceptually seemed so straightforward when the first trials were started, have run aground on the shoals of cellular genetic regulatory mechanisms. Effective gene therapy awaits the selective circumventing of these biological controls to deliver precise genetic corrections.

Delivery of nucleic acids

A potential gene therapy requires three major components: the payload to accomplish the mission, a targeting system to direct the vehicle and its payload to the correct body compartment in the correct cell population, and finally gene regulatory element(s), such as promoters/enhancers, to control the time and place of expression of the payload sequence(s). Table 12.2 compares the properties of some gene therapy vectors that have been used in clinical trials.

To be clinically useful, a vehicle must elude host immunological or toxicological responses, must persist in the body, and must avoid sequestration in non-target organs such as the liver or kidney. Ideally, for clinical use one would want the ability to modulate or remove the genetic modification in case of adverse effects – the

equivalent of discontinuing administration of a traditional drug. In practice, major difficulties are experienced in obtaining sufficient expression of the desired product for long enough to measure a positive clinical outcome.

Strategies for nucleic acid-mediated intervention

There are several points of attack for nucleic acid therapeutics. Most diseases are not due to an identified gene mutation, but rather reflect secondary cellular malfunction, often in response to events entirely external to the cell being targeted. Overexpressing proteins or fragments, either normal or mutated so as to compete with the normal protein for participation in cellular functions – known as the 'dominant negative' strategy – is a commonly used approach.

RNA metabolism can be modulated in many different ways, including:

- Antisense RNA
- RNA decoys for viral RNA-binding proteins
- Specific mRNA-stabilizing proteins
- Interference with mRNA splicing to induce exon skipping or to correct abnormal splicing
- Sequence-specific cleavage by catalytic RNAs such as hammerhead and hairpin ribozymes. Bacterial introns that code for a multifunctional reverse transcriptase/RNA splicing/DNA endonuclease/integrase protein can be altered to target specific DNA sequences.

Transcription of DNA into mRNA can also be controlled either through transcription factors or through antisense oligonucleotide triplex formation. Direct interference with genomic DNA through quadruplex formation is another strategy. These oligonucleotide sequences can be provided by biologically derived

Table 12.2
Gene therapy vectors

	Naked DNA	Liposome-encapsulated DNA	Adenovirus	Adenoassociated virus (AAV)	Retrovirus
Genetic material (max size insert)	DNA or RNA ($\geq$50 kb)	DNA ($\geq$50 kb)	DNA (7.5 kb)	DNA (5 kb)	RNA (8 kb)
Efficiency	Low	Low	Very high	Medium	High (low in vivo)
Transform non-dividing cells	Possibly, weak integration	Possibly, weak integration	Yes, transient expression, non-integrating	Yes, site-specific integration	No, transient integration
Safety issues	None, good safety profile	None, good safety profile	Viral recombination, immune reactions	Viral recombination, immune reactions	Viral recombination, tumorogenesis

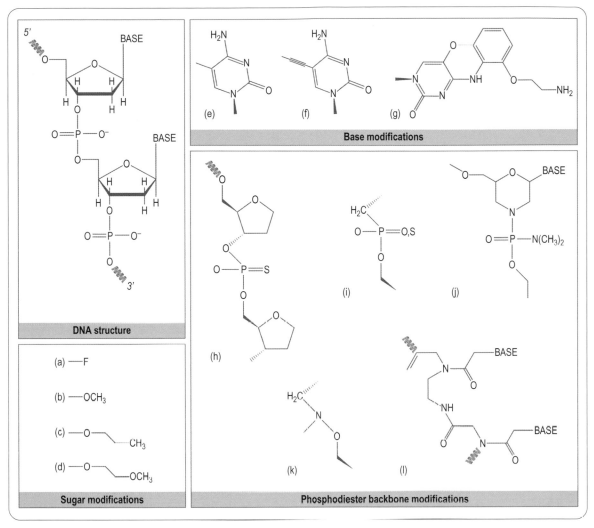

Fig. 12.2
Chemical modification of nucleotides. Key for modifications: Sugar modifications: (a) fluoro-, (b) methoxy-, (c) methoxyethyl-, (d) propoxy-. Base modifications: (e) 5-methyl cytosine, (f) 5-propyne cytosine, (g) tricyclic cytosine. Phosphodiester backbone modifications: (h) phosphorothioate, (i) mopholino-, (j) methylene- (on PDF), (k) methylene-methylimino, (l) peptide nucleic acid (PNA).

vector systems or by chemical synthesis. Short double- and single-strand oligonucleotide sequences are readily taken up by cells. Produced as single strands by auto-mated solid-phase chemical synthesis, these short, single-stranded 8–20-nucleotide sequences can be chem-ically modified on the base, sugar, or phosphate linker to enhance their stability against nuclease degradation and cellular penetration (Figure 12.2).

Table 12.3 lists a number of clinical trials with anti-sense oligonucleotides that are at different stages of completion.

RNA interference – gene silencing by RNAi

RNAi is a technique for reducing the expression of or silencing specific genes. Its usefulness as an experimental tool is discussed in Chapter 6, and it also has consider-able potential as a means of silencing genes for thera-peutic purposes. It is similar to antisense modulation of mRNA, but extends further into the command and control of cellular nucleic acids. Short double-stranded RNA (21–23 nucleotides) is used to silence homologous gene activity. Specific *RNA-induced silencing complexes* (RISC) guide multiple activities that target mRNA for degradation, block translation, or block gene transcrip-tion by methylation of chromatin (Denli and Hannon, 2003).

Examples of genes that have been targeted by RNAi include:

- Viruses such as HIV-1, poliovirus, respiratory syncytial virus and hepatitis C;
- Oncogenes and tumour suppressors such as Ras, bcl-abl, p53, p53bp and p73Dn;

Table 12.3
Clinical trials with antisense oligonucleotides

Agent	Target	Indication	Company
ISIS 2302	ICAM-1	Crohn's disease, ulcerative colitis, rheumatoid arthritis, psoriasis, renal transplant	ISIS Pharmaceuticals/Boehringer Ingelheim
ISIS 2105*	HPV 6 and 11 E2 gene product	Genital warts	ISIS Pharmaceuticals
ISIS 2922 (Formivirsen)	CMV IE2 gene	CMV retinitis	ISIS Pharmaceuticals
GEM 132	CMV UL36 gene	CMV retinitis	Hybridon
CGP 64128A/ ISIS 2531	Protein kinase C-α	Miscellaneous cancers	Novartis/ISIS Pharmaceuticals
CGP 69846A/ ISIS 5132	c-*raf* kinase	Miscellaneous cancers	Novartis/ISIS Pharmaceuticals
GEM 91*	HIV gag protein	AIDS	Hybridon
Genta 3139	Bcl-2 protein	Non-Hodgkin's lymphoma	Genta
LR3280	c-*myc*	Restenosis	Lynx Therapeutics
OL(1)p53	P53	Haemopoetic malignancy	University of Nebraska/Lynx Therapeutics
	c-*myb*	Chronic myelogenous leukaemia	University of Pennsylvania/Lynx Therapeutics

* Trials terminated.
Source: Bennett CF, Dean NM, Monia BP (1998) In: Harvey A L (ed) Advances in drug discovery techniques. Chichester: John Wiley; 174.

- Cell surface receptors for HIV-1- CD4, CCR5 and CXCR4, and the IL2 receptor α CD25 (Dykxhoorn et al., 2003).

Although RNAi is highly efficient as a gene-silencing technique under laboratory conditions, most of the difficulties with antisense or expression technology still remain to be overcome. Nevertheless, RNAi will probably dominate the next wave of gene therapeutics moving into clinical trials.

Comparing the discovery processes for biopharmaceuticals and small molecule therapeutics

The approach to discovering new protein/peptide therapeutics differs in many ways from the drug discovery approach for synthetic compounds described in other chapters in this section.

Protein/peptide drug discovery usually starts with known biomolecules, which it may be desirable to trim down to smaller domains with desired activities. Alternatively, native proteins are often optimized for desirable properties by mutation or other kinds of modification. These modifications can also provide the basis for patent protection. Unlike small-molecule synthesis, where the possibilities are virtually limitless, there is a finite number of natural proteins and a limited range of feasible modifications that may be introduced to improve their biological properties. The race to protect important proteins as starting points for therapeutics is critical for the future application of biotechnology.

The production of biotechnology-based therapeutics also involves technologies and facilities quite different from those used for producing synthetic compounds.

Manufacture of biopharmaceuticals

Expression systems

Full-size proteins, including a number of hormones, growth factors and mediators, are produced recom-

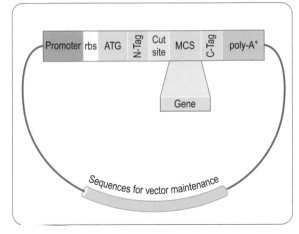

Fig. 12.3
Generic vector for protein expression. The cDNA for the protein to be expressed is cloned into restriction sites in the multiple cloning site (MCS) of an expression vector which contains appropriate sequences for maintenance in the chosen host cell. Expression of the gene is controlled by inducible promoter. A ribosome-binding site (rbs) optimized for maximum expression directs translation, beginning at the ATG initiation codon. Either N-terminal or C-terminal tags (N-, C-Tag) can be used to aid in purification or stabilization of the protein, and a protease cut site may be used to remove the tag after purification. A translation terminator codon is followed (in eukaryotic cells) by a poly-A+ tail to stabilize the mRNA.

machinery to produce mRNA from the inserted cDNA sequence, with appropriate initiation and termination codons and a ribosome-binding site. A polyA+ tail is added to eukaryotic expression systems to stabilize the mRNA. mRNA transcription, and hence protein production, is controlled by an induction element, so that protein is produced only when required. This is important, as some expressed proteins are toxic to growing and dividing host cells. Other sequences, such as protein export signal peptides, hexahistidine tags, immunologic epitopes, or fusion with protein partners such as glutathione S-transferase, thioredoxin, maltose-binding protein or IgG Fc, facilitate secretion or provide handles for the detection/purification of the expressed protein. Purification tags are particularly useful in eukaryotic expression systems, which express exogenous proteins at lower levels than do bacterial systems, where the expressed protein can be 10–50% of the total cellular protein. The tags are designed to be removed from the protein once it has been purified.

Bacterial protein expression, usually in *Escherichia coli*, is the system of choice for high expression levels of many proteins, and because scale-up technology is well developed. However, not every protein is amenable to bacterial expression. Proteins that contain disulfide bonds or are comprised of multiple subunits are problematic, as are proteins containing critical carbohydrate, lipid or other post-translational modifications. In some cases the enzymes responsible for post-translational modification, such as fatty acylation, can be co-transfected with the desired protein. Highly expressed proteins are frequently produced as insoluble inclusion bodies in the bacterial cytoplasm or periplasmic space. Active proteins must be recovered from these inclusion bodies after denaturation and in vitro refolding. Intrinsic membrane-bound proteins can pose additional problems.

binantly by inserting the cDNA version of the mRNA sequence coding for the protein of interest into specially designed plasmid vectors that orchestrate the expression of the desired protein product in the cell type of choice (Figure 12.3). The characteristics of different expression systems are compared in Table 12.4.

These vectors contain a selection marker to maintain the vector in the host cell along with regulatory DNA sequences that direct the host cell transcriptional

Table 12.4
Comparison of protein expression systems

Property			Similarity to human situation		
	E. coli	Yeast	*Aspergillus*	Insect	Mammalian cell culture
Folding	Some	Some	Some	Yes	Yes
Subunit assembly	No	Yes	?	Yes	Yes
Secretion	Some	Yes	Yes	Yes	Yes
Modifications: *					
acetylation	Yes	Yes	Probably	Probably	Yes
myristoylation	No	Yes	?	Yes	Yes
phosphorylation	No	Yes	?	Yes	Yes
glycosylation	No	Incomplete	Incomplete	Incomplete	Yes
* Co-transfection of appropriate enzymes into cells expressing the protein of interest can provide post-translational modifications.					

Eukaryotic microbial systems include *Saccharomycetes cerevisiae* and *Picha pastoralis* – yeasts that perform many mammalian post-translational modifications, including partial glycosylation. Insect cells, notably from *Spodoptera frugiperda* (Sf9), are infected with engineered baculovirus expression vectors carrying the protein of interest. This is a particularly efficient system for membrane protein expression. Many G-protein-coupled receptors, a large class of integral membrane proteins that includes many targets for currently marketed drugs, are often produced in these cells for use in screening assays for receptor ligands.

Cultured mammalian cells are used to express proteins on a research or production scale where faithful post-translational modification is required. Favourites include fibroblasts, anchorage-independent lymphocytes, Chinese hamster ovary (CHO) cells, and human embryonic kidney (HEK) cells. Mammalian cells grow more slowly and are more fastidious than the bacteria, yeasts or insect cells, and are therefore more expensive for production. Human cells are used in situations where there is some mammalian species dependence of bound carbohydrate. This can be particularly important for growth factors and the large glycoprotein hormones, as their glycosylation modulates the activity and stability of the protein product in vivo. Potential contaminating human pathogens in the human cell lines used for expression must be controlled. So must non-primate mammalian pathogens, as the possibility of transfer to humans cannot be ignored.

The use of transgenic animals and plants as 'factories' for genetically engineered proteins is discussed below.

Engineering proteins

Nature has devoted millions of years to optimizing protein structures for their biological roles. The natural configuration may not, however, be optimal for pharmaceutical applications. Recombinant DNA methods can be used to re-engineer the protein structure so as to better fulfil the requirements for a pharmaceutical agent.

Site-directed mutagenesis

Changes in the sequence of a protein at the level of a single amino acid can change the biochemical activity or the stability of the protein. It can also affect interactions with other proteins, and the coupling of those interactions to biological function. Stabilizing proteins to better withstand the rigours of industrial production and formulation is commercially important. Microorganisms adapted to extreme environments have evolved modified forms of enzymes and other functional proteins,

such as increased disulfide (cystine) content and more extensive core interactions, to withstand high temperatures. Similar tricks are used to stabilize enzymes for use at elevated temperatures, such as in industrial reactors, or in the home washing machine with enzyme-containing detergents. Other mutations alter the response of the protein to environmental conditions such as pH and ionic strength. Mutations to add or remove glycosylation signal sequences or to increase resistance to proteolytic enzymes may be introduced to alter immunogenicity or improve stability in body fluids. Protein activation by conformational changes due to phosphorylation, binding of protein partners or other signals may sometimes be mimicked by amino acid changes in the protein. The solubility of a protein can often be improved, as can the ability to form well-ordered crystals suitable for X-ray structure determination.

Fused or truncated proteins

Sometimes the full-size form of a protein or peptide is too difficult or expensive to produce or deliver to the target. Domains of proteins can often be stripped to their essentials, so that they retain the required characteristics of activity or targeting specificity. They may require fusion with a partner for proper folding or stability, the partner being removed as part of purification.

Ligands and receptor-binding domains can be attached to the active biomolecule in order to target it to specific sites. Pathogens and infectious agents, in addition to appropriating intracellular targeting motifs, have evolved protein sequences that enable them to penetrate the cell membrane to access the machinery for their propagation. Some of these sequences can be incorporated into biopharmaceuticals in order to deliver peptides and proteins into cells. Hydrophobic portions of Kaposi fibroblast growth factor, Grb2 SH2 domain, and human integrin α and β subunits have been employed in this way as cell-penetrating agents. The fusion sequence (1–23) of HIV-1 gp41 has been used to deliver synthetic antisense oligonucleotides and plasmid DNA into cells. Amphipathic sequences containing periodic arrangements of polar and hydrophobic residues, such as those found in the fusion peptide of the influenza haemagglutinin-2 protein, promote fusion with cell membranes and the delivery of associated agents. Polycationic sequences in penetratin (residues 43–58 from the Antp protein), HIV-1 tat protein (47–57), and the HIV-1 transcription factor VP22 (267–300), permeabilize membranes and increase the uptake of associated material.

Protein production

Although relatively small quantities of highly potent biologicals are normally required, production often presents problems. Only synthetic peptides and oligo-nucleotides and their derivatives can be produced by a scalable chemical synthesis. The others require large-scale fermentation or cell culture. The proteins and nucleic acids are then isolated and purified from the cells or media. Biotechnological process development is a complex field (Sofer and Zabriskie, 2000; Buckel, 2001). High-level production of recombinant proteins can result in heterogeneity because of the misincorporation of amino acids such as norvaline into the product, depending on the culture conditions, the nutrient composition of the medium and the producing organism. Post-translational modifications depend on the cultured organism and the subcellular localization of the protein. In cultured eukaryotic cells proteins undergo many kinds of post-translational modification, including glycosylation, sulfation, phosphorylation, lipidation, acetylation, γ-carboxylation and proteolytic processing. These and other modifications increase the heterogeneity of the product, affecting its biological half-life, immunogenicity and activity. The most homogeneous preparation consistent with retention of the important biological properties is standardized for production and a reproducible analytical profile is established. Nevertheless, protein products are invariably less homogeneous in composition than synthetic compounds, and the quality criteria for approval of clinical materials have to be adjusted to take account of this.

Formulation and storage conditions are critical because the protein primary amino acid sequences naturally display a variety of chemical instabilities. A major degradation route of protein products is through unfolding of the polypeptide chain and aggregation. Proteins have a finite half-life in an organism, governed partly by built-in chemical and conformational instabilities. Adsorption to surfaces of glass or plastic containers, particulates and air–liquid interfaces is often a cause of product loss.

The chemical reactivity of the various amino acid residues contributes to protein loss and heterogeneity. Succinimide formation, isomerization and racemization, as well as peptide bond cleavage, tend to occur at aspartate residues, to an extent that depends somewhat on the surrounding amino acid sequence. Examples include hACTH, soluble CD4, OKT-3 monoclonal antibody, hGH-releasing factor, IL-1β and hEGF. Oxidation, particularly at methionine residues, is catalysed by transition metal ions, pH, light, and various oxygen free radicals. Examples are relaxin A, hIGF-I and enkephalin analogs. Disulfide exchange (cysteine/cystine) can generate inappropriate folding or intermolecular bond formation, thereby promoting aggregation and precipitation of protein. Examples are interferon, and the acidic and basic forms of FGF. β-Elimination at cystine, cysteine, serine and threonine leads to dehydroalanine formation and reaction with nucleophilic side chains. Anhydride formation between the α amino group on a

protein and the C terminus is a major degradation pathway for insulin stored between pH3 and pH5. Sometimes peroxides contaminate the excipients and stabilizing agents, such as the polyethylene glycols or the surfactants Polysorbate 20 and Polysorbate 80 used in product formulation (see Chapter 17).

The first therapeutic proteins produced on an industrial scale were antibodies, which initially relied on immunization of large animals such as horses. Monoclonal technology paved the way for the production of murine antibodies in cell culture. With the ability to produce human antibody proteins and derivatives through molecular biological manipulation, the organism used to manufacture the protein is chosen on the basis of economics and requirements for post-translational modification. The characteristics of some commonly used organisms for protein production are summarized in Table 12.4.

Eukaryotic and prokaryotic microorganisms and eukaryotic cells in culture are the most common source of therapeutic proteins. Prokaryotic expression is generally the first choice, whereas higher organisms produce protein products that are most similar to human material and thus are more likely to be biologically active and pharmacokinetically stable. The production of proteins on a commercial scale by eukaryotic cell culture is, however, extremely expensive. The cells grow slowly (18–24 hours doubling time, compared with about 20 minutes for bacteria) and most require a serum source or expensive growth factor/hormone cocktails in the culture medium.

'Pharming' of protein expression in whole animals or plants is used for large-scale production of proteins for some therapeutics and for industrial applications. Transgenic farm animals – goats, cows, sheep and rabbits – have been engineered to secrete human proteins into their milk (van Berkel et al., 2002). Annual milk yields range from about 8 L (rabbit) to 8–10 000 L (cow). Expression levels of from 1 to 15 g of product per litre of milk have been achieved in favourable instances, allowing small herds of transgenic animals to do the work of large fermentation facilities. Currently (2004) no biopharmaceuticals made in this way are available, but many are under development by specialized biotechnology companies (Table 12.5), and 30 or more such products are expected to be registered in the next decade.

Plants can be directed to concentrate antibodies and other proteins in their leaves, seeds or fruit (Giddings et al., 2000; Daniell et al., 2001; Powledge, 2001; Streatfield and Howard, 2003), and are beginning to be used for the commercial production of antibodies and vaccines. Monoclonal antibodies expressed in plants – 'plantibodies' – have been produced in maize, tobacco and soybeans. Antibodies produced against *Streptococcus mutans*, the main cause of tooth decay in humans, have demonstrated efficacy against dental caries. Other

Table 12.5
Biopharmaceuticals produced in transgenic farm animals. (These products are in development; none have yet reached the market)

Protein	Indication	Host
Antithrombin III	Inflammation	Goat
α_1-Antitrypsin	Inflammation, inherited deficiency	Cow, goat, sheep
α-Glucosidase	Glycogen storage disease type II	Rabbit
h-Chorionic gonadotrophin	Infertility	Cow, goat
Factor VIII	Haemophilia	Pig
Factor IX	Haemophilia	Pig
Factor XI	Haemophilia	Sheep
Fibrinogen	Burns, surgery	Pig, sheep
Lactoferrin	GI bacterial infection	Cow
Monoclonal antibody	Colon cancer	Goat
Protein C	Deficiency, adjunct to tPA	Pig, sheep
Serum albumin	Surgery, burns, shock	Cow, goat
Tissue plasminogen activator (tPA)	Infarction, stroke	Goat

proteins, such as mouse and human interferon, human growth hormone, haemoglobin, human serum albumin and human epidermal growth factor, are also being targeted. Vaccine production for both animals and humans appears to be a most promising application of 'pharming'. By splicing the gene for the antigen into a modified plant virus (cowpea mosaic virus), companies such as Agricultural Genetics (Cambridge, UK) have produced effective vaccines for animals against mink enterovirus, HIV-1 and foot and mouth disease, obtaining up to 200 doses of vaccine from a single cowpea (black-eyed pea) leaf. Other companies are pursuing vaccines for hepatitis A and B, cold and wart viruses and *Plasmodium* (malaria). Splicing the antigen genes directly into the plant genome has been successful for hepatitis B, Norwalk, cholera and rabies virus vaccines.

Feeding antigen-producing plants to animals has shown promise for inducing immune protection (Judge et al., 2004), despite the differences in the type of immune response from oral exposure and the standard humoral administration. The oral route would be ideal for human vaccines, particularly in countries where refrigeration is uncertain. Although antigen expressed in potato for use in humans was effective in animals, the cooking required for human consumption of the vegetable destroyed the immunogenicity of the antigen. Current efforts are developing the technology for human foods that are eaten raw and which are suitable for tropical climates, such as tomato and banana (Korban et al., 2002).

There are many developments in plant-derived biopharmaceuticals for human use, but none has yet become commercially available. Widespread environmental and other concerns about transgenic crop productions are a significant impediment.

Pharmacokinetic, toxicological and drug-delivery issues with proteins and peptides

The main source of the bias against biologicals (proteins) as therapeutic agents in major pharmaceutical companies comes from the difficulties in delivering these expensive, large, highly charged molecules to the target in sufficient concentrations for long enough to achieve pharmacologic effects. The complexities faced in taking small molecules through preclinical development into clinical trials are compounded with biologicals. More detailed expositions of pharmacokinetics, toxicology and the delivery of therapeutic proteins are available (Frokjaer and Hovgaard, 2000; Sofer and Zabriskie, 2000; Ho and Gibaldi, 2003; Walsh, 2003).

Figure 12.4 illustrates the pathways that govern the distribution and elimination of a pharmacological agent. Factors that assume particular importance for biopharmaceuticals are (a) the choice of formulation and route of administration so as to achieve consistent absorption, (b) control of distribution by targeting to the required site of action, and (c) protection against rapid inactivation or elimination.

exocytosis at the apical membrane. However, much of the protein is degraded by the lysosomal system during transit.

Formulations have been devised to optimize the stability and delivery of protein and peptide therapeutics (Frokjaer and Hovgaard, 2000). Protection from proteolysis is a major concern for many routes of administration. Various entrapment and encapsulation technologies have been applied to the problem (see Chapter 17). The greater the protection, though, the less rapidly the protein is released from the preparation. Hydrogels, hydrophilic polymers formed around the protein, avoid proteolysis but limit absorption. Microcapsule and microsphere formulations are made by enclosing the active compound within a cavity surrounded by a semipermeable membrane or within a solid matrix. The surface area for absorption is much greater than that provided by hydrogel or solid matrix formulations.

A variety of penetration-enhancing protocols have been applied to increase the rate and amount of protein absorption. These include surfactants (sodium dodecyl sulfate, polyoxyethylene fatty acyl ethers), polymers (polyacrylic acid, chitosan derivatives), certain synthetic peptides (occulin-related peptides), bile salts (sodium deoxycholate, sodium glycocholate, sodium taurocholate), fatty acids (oleic acid, caprylic acid, acyl carnitines, acylcholines, diglycerides), and chelating agents (EDTA, citric acid, salicylates, N-amino acyl β-diketones).

The nasal mucosal route of administration is emerging as an acceptable and reasonably effective method of drug delivery. Some peptide drugs, such as *nafarelin, oxytocin, lypressin, calcitonin* and *desmopressin,* are effective as nasal sprays, although the fraction absorbed in humans is generally low (≤10%). Pulmonary administration is surprisingly effective when ~3 μm particles of the therapeutic are dispersed deep in the lung. The vast alveolar surface area and blood supply allow even macromolecules to be absorbed.

Transdermal delivery across the stratum corneum, the outermost, least-permeable skin layer, is being increasingly used for proteins and other drugs. Transport of drug molecules across the skin is facilitated by transient disruption of epithelial barrier function

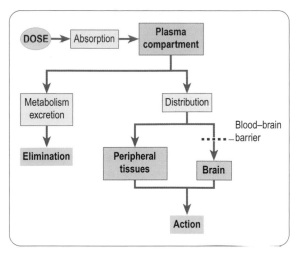

Fig 12.4
Simplified scheme showing the processes involved in drug absorption, distribution and elimination. Pink boxes, body compartments; grey boxes, transfer processes.

Absorption of protein/peptide therapeutics

Mucosal delivery

Peptide and protein drugs are in general poorly absorbed by mouth because of their high molecular weight, charge, and susceptibility to proteolytic enzymes. The main barriers to absorption of proteins are their size and charge (Table 12.6).

Large hydrophilic and charged molecules do not readily pass the cellular lipid bilayer membrane. Small peptides can be absorbed if they are relatively hydrophobic, or if specific transporters exist. Proteins can be transported by *transcytosis,* in which proteins enter cells at the basal surface via receptor-mediated endocytosis or fluid-phase pinocytosis into vesicles, are transported across the cell through the cytosol, and then released by

Table 12.6
Physical properties of some therapeutic proteins

Protein	Molecular wt (Da)	Isoelectric point
Somatostatin	1 600	10.4
Insulin	6 000	5.6
Human growth hormone	20 000	5.3
t-PA	60 000	9.1
Human serum albumin	66 000	5.3
IgG	150 000	Variable
Factor VIII	270 000	7.4
Typical small-molecule drug	< 500	Variable

Table 12.7
Exposure of protein/peptide drugs to protease activity by different routes of administration

Oral	Very high
Rectal	High
Buccal	Medium
Nasal	Medium
Vaginal	Medium
Transdermal	Low
Pulmonary	Low
Ocular	Low

with sonic energy (sonophoresis), electric current (iontophoresis) or electric field (electroporation). Table 12.7 compares different routes of non-parenteral dosing for the relative proteolytic activity to which a protein drug would be exposed.

Parenteral delivery

Oral or mucosal absorption of native, full-length proteins is inefficient even with enhancing strategies. Thus, many protein therapeutics are delivered parenterally by intravenous, intramuscular or subcutaneous injection. With intramuscular and subcutaneous administration sustained-release formulations can be used to increase the duration of action.

The blood–brain barrier is impermeable to most proteins and peptides, but possesses transporters that facilitate the entry of some, such as apolipoprotein E, transferrin and insulin. Linking active peptides to an antibody directed against the transferrin receptor has been shown in experimental animals to allow neurotrophic factors such as *nerve growth factor* (NGF) to enter the brain and produce neurotrophic effects when given systemically, and this strategy may prove applicable for human use.

Elimination of protein/peptide therapeutics

Most therapeutic proteins are inactivated by proteolysis, producing short peptides and amino acids which then enter dietary pathways. Unlike small-molecule drugs, metabolites of protein therapeutics are not considered to be a safety issue. The rate and extent of degradation of protein therapeutics before excretion depend on the route of administration. Breakdown occurs in both plasma and tissues. Attempts to minimize these losses include the use of glycosylated proteins, which more closely resemble the native protein, or chemical modification of the protein with polyethylene glycol (PEG) chains or other entities. PEGylation can increase the plasma half-life of a protein between three- and several hundredfold. Besides reducing proteolysis, PEGylation can shield antigenic sites, enhance protein solubility and stability, and prevent rapid uptake by organs. With small peptides, cyclization or the inclusion of D-amino acid residues, particularly at the N terminus, can be used to protect against exoproteolysis, though this approach is of course applicable only to synthetic peptides and not to biopharmaceuticals.

The kidney is an important organ for the catabolism and elimination of small proteins and peptides. Proteins of 5–6 kDa, such as insulin, are able freely to pass the glomerular filter of the kidney. Passage through the glomerulus decreases to about 30% for proteins of 30 kDa, and to less than 1% for 69 kDa proteins. Some proteins, such as calcitonin, glucagon, insulin, growth hormone, oxtocin, vasopressin and lysozyme, are reabsorbed by the proximal tubules via luminal endocytosis, and then are hydrolysed in lysosomes. Linear peptides less than 10 amino acids long are hydrolysed by proteases on the surface of brush border membranes of the proximal tubules.

Liver metabolism is highly dependent on specific amino acid sequences in proteins. Cyclic peptides, small (<1.4 kDa) and hydrophobic peptides are taken up by carrier-mediated transport and degraded. Large proteins use energy-dependent carrier-mediated transport, including receptor-mediated endocytosis and transcytotic pathways (polymeric IgA), and are targeted to lysosomes.

Summary

In the late 1970s recombinant DNA technology boosted biotechnology into a prominence it has not relinquished. Apart from fears about human genetic modification, the outlook has been positive for the production of new and better biopharmaceuticals. Whereas the traditional pharmaceutical companies were slow to embrace the new technology, a number of small biotech companies sprang up which have provided the innovative driving force for the protein and gene product industry. The genomic revolution is the latest manifestation of the technology, stimulating efforts to mine the information coming out of the various species genome projects for new products and therapies.

Recombinant DNA technology allows the production of individual proteins and peptides on a large scale regardless of their natural abundance. There are many advantages to recombinant production. Human sequence proteins reduce potential immunological problems and avoid potential infectious agents in materials isolated from natural sources. Proteins are expressed in a variety of cellular systems, determined by the properties of the molecule required. Bacterial systems are used wherever possible because of the high level of expression that can be obtained and the simplicity and availability of production. Bacteria, however, do not provide many of the post-translational modifications required for human protein stability and function, such as glycosylation, lipid modification, phosphorylation, sulfation and disulfide bond formation. Protein aggregation often occurs, and even though denaturation and refolding are successful for many proteins, some are problematic. In these cases eukaryotic systems, including various yeast species and cultured insect and mammalian cells, are used. Transgenic farm animals and plants are also coming into their own as protein 'factories'.

Antibodies in the form of animal sera were the first widely used protein therapeutics. Although immunization is still used as a prophylactic and as a therapeutic, recombinant DNA technology is used to produce both immunogen and antibodies. Hypersensitivity reactions are reduced by producing altered antibodies with the required epitope specificity. They are 'chimerized' (human constant domain) or 'humanized' (rodent complementarity-determining region (CDR), with human Fc portions for optimal interaction with the human complement system. Single-chain and multichain antibodies can be expressed intracellularly to attack previously sequestered antigens. These immunological agents are also used to target infectious organisms, deliver radioisotopes or cytotoxic agents to cancer cells, and to moderate tissue rejection in transplantation.

Proteins and enzymes have been engineered to hone their therapeutic usefulness. Protein structure can be stabilized or modified to slow degradation or increase uptake, and multiple functions can be built into the same molecule. Recombinant vaccine production of cloned protein domains uses these modifications to increase immunogenicity and avoid exposure to infectious agents. Delivery of synthetic vectors coding for antigenic epitopes into host tissues promotes endogenous antigen expression.

The biggest obstacle to the use of proteins and peptides as therapeutics is the delivery to the site of action of sufficient agent to create a biological effect. Formulating proteins and peptides to penetrate epithelial barriers in a biologically active form is difficult. Because of their size, charge and instability in the gastrointestinal tract, special delivery systems often must be used to achieve efficacious blood levels. Penetration through the blood–brain barrier can be even more challenging. Small-molecule drugs of <500 Da molecular weight have a much better record in this regard. Once in the blood, proteins are often rapidly eliminated by a variety of mechanisms, although there are modifications that can slow degradation.

Even though protein and peptide therapeutics faces significant pharmacokinetic and pharmacodynamic liabilities, much work is still being done on agents for which small molecules are not available to perform the same function.

Nucleic acids can be delivered into cells in a variety of ways. Complexation of the highly charged DNA with lipophilic cations, or derivitization of nucleic acid bases, sugars or the phosphodiester backbone can be efficient in cell culture, but less so in whole organisms. Ingenious schemes of antisense, RNAi, ribozyme, decoy sequences and RNA splicing inhibition are used to attain therapeutic effects. Viruses, Nature's DNA delivery machines, modified to eliminate their pathogenic capacity, are used in organisms to introduce the therapeutic gene into target cells. The inserted DNA directs the synthesis of a protein in the host cell, in the case of a growth factor deficiency in the brain providing a secreted product for the support of surrounding cells. Numerous gene therapy clinical trials are in progress, but the need to avoid side effects and host suppression of viral-based therapeutics has slowed progress.

References

Benhar I (2001) Biotechnological applications of phage and cell display. Biotechnology Advances 19: 1–33.

Biaggi E, Rousseau RF, Yvon E, Vigouroux S, Dotti G, Brenner MK (2002) Cancer vaccines: dream, reality, or nightmare? Clinical and Experimental Medicine 2: 109–118.

BSI Vaccine Immunology Group (2002) Vaccination against non infectious disease (BSI Vaccine Immunology Group/BSACI session). Immunology 107(Suppl 1): 67–70.

Buckel P (ed) (2001) Recombinant protein drugs. Basel: Birkhauser Verlag.

Capecchi B, Serruto D, Adu-Bobie J, Rappuoli R, Pizza M (2004) The genome revolution in vaccine research. Current Issues in Molecular Biology 6: 17–27.

Daniell H, Streatfield SJ, Wycoff K (2001) Medical molecular farming: production of antibodies, biopharmaceuticals and edible vaccines in plants. Trends in Plant Science 6: 219–226.

Denli AM, Hannon GJ (2003) RNAi: an ever growing puzzle. Trends in Biochemical Sciences 28: 196–201.

Dykxhoorn DM, Novina CD, Sharp PA (2003) Killing the messenger: short RNAs that silence gene expression. Nature Reviews Molecular Cell Biology 4: 457–467.

Frokjaer S, Hovgaard L (2000) Pharmaceutical formulation: development of peptides and proteins. Philadelphia, PA: Taylor & Francis.

Giddings G, Allison G, Brooks D, Carter A (2000) Transgenic plants as factories for biopharmaceuticals. Nature Biotechnology 18: 1151–1155.

Ho RJY, Gibaldi M (2003) Biotechnology and biopharmaceuticals. Transforming proteins and genes into drugs. Hoboken, NJ: Wiley-Liss.

Judge NA, Mason HS, O'Brien AD (2004) Plant cell-based intimin vaccine given orally to mice primed with intimin reduces time of Escherichia coli O157:H7 shedding in feces. Infection and Immunity 72: 168–175.

Kantak KM (2003) Anti-cocaine vaccines: antibody protection against relapse. Expert Opinion in Pharmacotherapy 4: 213–218.

Korban SS, Krasnyanski SF, Buetow DE (2002) Foods as production and delivery vehicles for human vaccines. Journal of the American College of Nutrition 21: 212S–217S.

Liu MA (2003) DNA vaccines: a review. Journal of Internal Medicine 253: 402–410.

Locher CP, Soong NW, Whalen RG, Punnonen J (2004) Development of novel vaccines using DNA shuffling and screening strategies. Current Opinion in Molecular Therapy 6: 34–39.

Manoj S, Babiuk LA, van Drunen Littel-van den Hurk S (2004) Approaches to enhance the efficacy of DNA vaccines. Critical Reviews in Clinical Laboratory Science 41: 1–39.

Powledge TM (2001) Tobacco pharming. A quest to turn the killer crop into a treatment for cancer. Scientific American 285: 25–26.

Rousseau RF, Hirschmann-Jax C, Takahashi S, Brenner MK (2001) Cancer vaccines. Hematology/Oncology Clinics of North America 15: 741–773.

Sofer G, Zabriskie DW (2000) Biopharmaceutical process validation. Vol. 25. New York: Marcel Dekker.

Streatfield SJ, Howard JA (2003) Plant production systems for vaccines. Expert Review on Vaccines 2: 763–775.

Tellier C (2002) Exploiting antibodies as catalysts: potential therapeutic applications. Transfusion Clinique et Biologique 9: 1–8.

van Berkel PH, Welling MM, Geerts M et al. (2002). Large scale production of recombinant human lactoferrin in the milk of transgenic cows. Nature Biotechnology 20: 484–487.

Walsh G (2003) Biopharmaceuticals, biochemistry, and biotechnology, 2nd edn. Chichester: John Wiley.

13 Patent issues in drug discovery

P Grubb

The nature of patent protection and the strategies that should be used to protect a compound in development are described in Chapter 19. However, some patent issues need to be considered at an earlier stage. Issues to be considered at the project planning stage are discussed briefly in Chapter 5. Here we consider issues that concern the selection of a compound as a development candidate. For a fuller account of pharmaceutical patents, see Grubb (2004).

The two questions that need to be answered before significant sums are invested in development activities are:

- What sort of protection can we get for this compound?
- What patent rights of others could prevent us from marketing this compound?

These are two completely different issues. As explained in Chapter 19, it is perfectly possible to have strong patent protection of one's own discoveries, yet still to be blocked by earlier dominating patent rights owned by someone else. The 'patent situation' for a compound should attempt to give the answers to both questions.

The state of the art

The answers to the two basic questions depend upon the *state of the art* – patent jargon for all material relating to the technical field that has been published at the relevant date. The state of the art (sometimes called the *prior art*) includes not only published scientific papers, but also, for example, what is in textbooks, manufacturers' brochures, newspaper articles, web pages on the Internet and oral presentations at conferences. It also includes patent documents, which may be granted patents or published applications.

Nothing can be patented that is already part of the state of the art, as a patentable invention must be *new* or *novel*. Also, a patentable invention must have an *inventive step*, that is, it must not be obvious, which means that anything very close to the state of the art may be very difficult to patent.

Patent documents as state of the art

A granted patent is not only a description, which, like any kind of prior publication, is part of the state of the art. It also contains *claims* defining a legal 'no-go area', so that anyone doing something that falls within the claims may be sued for infringement of the patent, and may be forced to stop these activities, as well as being liable for damages. Published patent applications also contain claims, but these are often much broader than the claims (if any) that will finally be granted.

Patent documents in the state of the art are therefore important in answering the second basic question, which concerns *freedom to operate*. Granted patents may be invalidated by a court, but as a rule they have a presumption of validity which is hard to challenge. Patent applications act as a warning flag for rights that may be granted in the future.

Evaluation by the scientist

The first person to evaluate the patent situation of a possible lead compound must be the research scientist responsible for the project. He or she should be aware of the work being published in the area, and should know who are the main players in the field, what journals and other information sources contain relevant information, and what competitor companies are likely to be filing relevant patent applications. To the extent that the chemical structure of the lead compound is a matter of choice, the research chemist should try to steer away from the known state of the art.

Where the research is in a field in which a number of competitors are active, it is clear that the closer you are to the competition, the closer you are to the prior art. And, as mentioned above, the closer you are to the prior art, the more difficult it is to obtain patent protection. Research managers are sometimes struck by what seems like a great idea – ask the patent department to check where there are gaps in the competitors' patent protection, and then try to work in these gaps. This is actually a very bad idea if the intention is to produce something innovative. Research must drive patenting, not the other way around, and the initial work should be done before the patent situation is checked.

Evaluation by the patent professional

A professional evaluation of the patent situation of a new chemical entity (NCE) needs to be made at about the same time that the filing of a patent application is being considered. The timing of this will depend upon the patent policy of the company or organization owning the invention, but will usually be at the time the compound is ready to enter the development process, i.e. at the time of transition of the compound to 'drug candidate' status.

The patent situation must be established on the basis of a search of the scientific and patent literature. Ideally, the search should be carried out by a professional patent searcher and evaluated by a patent attorney or patent agent. However, it is becoming more and more easy for a patent attorney or a scientist to carry out searches online, and while these are unlikely to be as complete as those done by a professional searcher, such a 'quick and dirty' search may be all that is required at this early stage. At some stage after a patent application has been filed, searches will be carried out in the major patent offices, and these can be used to supplement the search made at the time of filing.

More complete 'freedom to operate' searches must be made at later stages, for example to ensure that the proposed manufacturing process and the chosen pharmaceutical formulation are also free from third-party patent rights.

Sources of information

For patent literature there are now a number of databases available online which allow full-text searching by keywords. One, available on the website of the US Patent and Trademark Office (www.uspto.gov), contains fully searchable texts of all US patents since 1976, as well as image files of all US patents back to 1790. A similar database (Esp@cenet) available through the home page of the European Patent Office (www.european-patent-office.org) allows searching of European patent applications and PCT applications, although at the time of writing only recent applications are available in full-text form. For Japan, the database JAPIO (www.jpo.go.jp) gives English-language abstracts of all Japanese early-published applications from 1976 onwards. Use of these databases is free.

Other databases, maintained by commercial firms which charge user access fees, add value by high-quality abstracts and additional indexing possibilities, and downloading and printing information from these may be quicker and easier than it is from public domain Internet databases.

Chemical Abstracts (CA), published by the Ohio State University, abstracts both patents and scientific literature in the chemical field. The information retrieval system is based on a CA registry number allocated to every published chemical compound; once this has been identified, abstracts of all patents or literature articles mentioning the compound can be listed, and printed out if required.

Derwent Publications Ltd provides a wide range of abstracting and information retrieval systems for both scientific and patent literature. The latter includes the WPI (World Patent Index) database, covering all patents in the major countries issued since 1974. Searches can be made on the basis of keywords, or of partial structures of chemical compounds. Derwent also has a database covering all publications and patents in the field of biotechnology since 1982.

For the majority of these databases, specialized software is available from *Chemical Abstracts* to assist searching, ranging from STM-Express for experienced searchers, Scifinder for occasional users and STM-Easy for use with Internet access.

Results of the evaluation – NCEs

If the search shows that the compound lacks novelty, that is, has already been published, then the best course is to pick a different one for development. Even though it may be possible to obtain some form of secondary patent protection, for example the use of the compound as a medicament if it was previously known for a non-pharmaceutical use, most companies will not invest in the development of a compound unless it will be possible to patent the compound itself.

If the NCE appears to be novel but the search shows that very similar compounds are known, so that the compound may be judged to lack an inventive step, the best advice is to go ahead anyway. If the compound proves to have superior properties compared to the known product, these can be used to establish the inventive step. If it does not, it will drop out of development whatever the patent situation.

If the NCE, despite being apparently novel and inventive, appears to be covered by a third-party patent, the advice would be to go ahead only if the third-party patent appears to be invalid or will have expired before your product can reach the market, or if you are sure that you will be able to obtain a licence on acceptable terms.

Patenting of research tools

In addition to patent issues relating to the compound itself, research tools may also be covered by patents. By 'research tool' is meant anything that contributes to the discovery or development of a drug, without being part of the final product. Examples include genes, cell lines, reagents, markers, assays, screening methods, animal models etc.

A company whose business it is to sell drugs is not usually interested in patenting research tools, but it is the business of many biotech companies to develop and commercialize such tools, and these companies will naturally wish to obtain patent protection for them. For pharmaceutical companies, such research tool patents and applications raise issues of freedom to operate, particularly if they contain '*reach-through*' claims purporting to cover drugs found by using the patented tools.

Some scientists may believe that research activities, in contrast to the manufacture and sale of a product, cannot be patent infringement. This is not the case. If I have invented a process that is useful in research and have a valid patent for it, I can enforce that patent against anyone using the process without my permission. I can make money from my patent by granting licences for a flat fee, or a fee based on the extent to which the process is used; or by selling kits for carrying out the process or reagents for use in the process (for example the enzymes used in the polymerase chain reaction (PCR) process). What I am *not* entitled to do is to charge a royalty on the sale of drugs developed with the help of my process. I can patent an electric drill, but I should not expect to get a royalty on everything it bores a hole in.

Nevertheless, some patents have already been granted containing claims that would be infringed, for example, by the sale of a drug active in a patented assay, and although it is hoped that such claims would be held invalid if challenged in court, the risk that such claims might be enforceable cannot be dismissed.

Should research tool patents be the subject of a freedom to operate search at an early stage of product development? Probably not. There are simply too many of them, and if no research project could be started without clearance on the basis of such a search, nothing would ever get done. At least for a large company, it is an acceptable business risk to go ahead and assume that if problems arise they can be dealt with at a later stage.

Reference

Grubb P (2004) Patents for chemicals, pharmaceuticals and biotechnology: fundamentals of global law, practice and strategy, 4th edn. Oxford: Oxford University Press.

14 Organization and management of a large drug discovery department

P Herrling

Introduction

Historical perspective

Creative research and management are thought by some to be incompatible. It was at one time thought sufficient to hire excellent scientists, give them resources and a goal, and await a successful outcome. This view results partly from the origin of science, where individual scientists apparently generated most of the major advances in isolation. However, from the earliest times great thinkers built on knowledge generated by others before them: Thales' and Pythagoras' geometry builds on their learning experiences in Egypt (Nestle, 1922); Ibn Khaldun's alchemical treatises cite older authors such as Jabir ibn Hayyan (Rashid, 1996); Galileo's astronomical observations were influenced by his reading of Copernicus (Sobel, 1999), and he built his telescope after hearing of the technique to put two lenses together used by artisans in Holland (Bronowski and Mazlish, 1960). Merton (1961) discusses how this led eventually to the current practice of extensive – if sometimes very selective – citing in scientific papers and books. Nevertheless, the crucial contributions of individual creativity and intelligence in solving major scientific problems cannot be underestimated and must be taken into account in managing any scientific undertaking. Looking back to pre-19th century science, when few scientists were at work, the seminal contributions of a few creative giants, such as Galileo, Newton and Darwin, stand out clearly. Nevertheless, it can be argued that, had particular individuals not provided important new insights others would eventually have arrived at the same conclusion (Shepherd, 1991). Nowadays, with hundreds of thousands of professional scientists hard at work, the contribution of individuals is often less clear. There is evident redundancy in the sense that different research groups often publish the same discoveries simultaneously (Hu et al., 2003; Molinari et al., 2003; Oda et al., 2003; Verjovski-Almeida et al., 2003). Furthermore, the practice of interdisciplinary collaboration has greatly increased because many scientific problems are too broad to be solved within a single discipline or by only a few individuals. In particular, the discovery and development of new therapies is a complex problem that can only be successfully addressed by a large number of scientists and

199

specialists from many disciplines, who must work in closely integrated teams, often over many years.

In summary, the idea that it is sufficient to assemble excellent scientists and let them do 'excellent science', expecting innovative therapies to result, is clearly outdated. In view of the complexity and size of a modern drug discovery operation the process has to be carefully managed to be successful, and this chapter will outline a few organizational principles that have been found useful to improve both the quality of the new therapies and the productivity of discovery groups.

Assumptions

The research organization model will be discussed, taking into account some major basic assumptions:

- The model will focus on a scientific discovery organization that aims to deliver mostly highly innovative therapies with significant advantages over existing therapies, rather than so-called 'me-too' drugs. The aim is to deliver therapies which, at the time of their introduction, meet a significant medical need (i.e. covering conditions that are untreatable or only poorly treatable with existing medicines). This is in contrast to research organizations that focus on rapidly copying advances made by others, or mainly on prospecting outside through in-licensing activities.
- Such new therapies can only be discovered if the organization fosters cutting-edge science and technology and allows the best scientists to thrive.

- The organization takes into account that the discovery of new therapies necessitates working in multidisciplinary teams involving many scientific disciplines from the biological, physical, chemical and mathematical sciences (Figure 14.1).
- The organization must be built on a deep understanding of the underlying science (see below).
- Senior management must accept that, typically, research cycles last for 5–10 years (from the idea to clinical proof of concept), which means that the organization should not undergo frequent major reorganizations but rather steady evolutionary improvement.

Lessons from evolution: consequences for the drug discovery organization

In the 1970s and 1980s our knowledge of the biology of diseases was distinctly less than today, and industrial research groups were organized to address diseases according to medical classifications, the so-called *therapeutic areas*, such as cardiovascular diseases, psychiatry and neurology, dermatology, organ rejection, and metabolic and immunological diseases. This grouping created a natural bridge between the discovery scientists and the medical customers which helped to achieve the best use of newly discovered therapies.

Such therapeutic area-focused research groups, which are still the basic drug discovery units in many

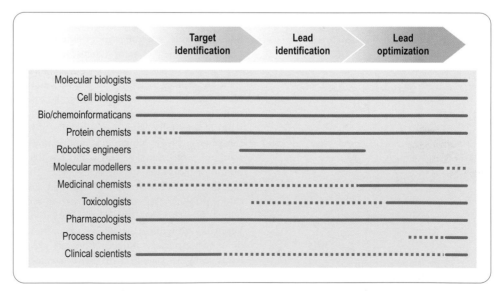

Fig. 14.1
The multidisciplinary nature of drug discovery. Some of the most important disciplines are mentioned and the time of their major involvement in the drug discovery process. Solid bars, major involvement; dotted bars, minor involvement.

pharmaceutical companies, are multidisciplinary, consisting of all chemical and biological disciplines required for the task of discovering new therapies. Their sizes range from a few dozen scientists to several hundreds in large companies. Often they have been established in small peripheral institutes on the principle that organization into small focused groups with clear tasks and ownership, where everybody knows each other, fosters creativity and minimizes of bureaucracy, providing an environment that was perceived to be the main advantage of small startup biotech companies.

Very often management also encouraged strong competition between the different therapeutic areas as a way of improving motivation and sense of ownership.

Multiple uses of therapeutic targets

The major advances in biomedical science over the last 30 years are beginning to challenge the appropriateness of this kind of organization. Isolated, competing research groups within one pharmaceutical company nowadays appear, in the author's view, much less efficient than a research organization that better reflects the 'new biology'.

Recent biological science shows that evolution does not often waste a good discovery. In the 1950s and 1960s pharmacological receptors were theoretical concepts derived from the study of agonists and antagonists and only a few were described, for example two types of noradrenergic and cholinergic receptor. Some were hotly disputed, such as the existence of a specific receptor for glutamate (Watkins and Evans, 1981). Nevertheless, simple mathematical models allowed pharmacologists to study their properties despite the fact that until then nobody had actually 'seen' a receptor. The biochemical isolation of receptors in the 1970s and 1980s, their characterization as proteins, and their cloning, brought them into the domain of protein sciences (Tanford and Reynolds, 2001) and genomics. It became increasingly apparent that receptors, as well as enzymes, ion channels and intracellular signalling molecules, actually occur in large 'families', i.e. groups of proteins with varying homologies derived from common ancestors. Different members of these families fulfil very diverse functions in different biological contexts, and this is often the reason for drug side effects. Because of the structural homology of the targets a single compound can interact with more than one of the targets, which can be either beneficial or deleterious in relation to its medical application. The structural relationships that define the molecular families to which drug targets belong show no respect for therapeutic area boundaries. Major families such as G-protein-coupled receptors, cation channels and kinase enzymes, for example, are involved in the pathophysiology of disorders in every therapeutic

area, from epilepsy to heart failure. A few concrete examples are:

- *Acetylcholinesterase (AChE) in muscle and brain.* AChE, the membrane-bound enzyme that cleaves the neurotransmitter acetylcholine occurs both in muscle and brain in slightly different forms. Irreversible and non-specific inhibitors of the enzyme (e.g. parathion) are used as insecticides; neostigmine (reversible) is used in myasthenia gravis; and newer brain-specific agents are used beneficially to treat Alzheimer's disease (Enz et al., 1993).
- *5HT4 receptors in brain and gut.* The serotonin 5HT4 receptor occurs in the hippocampus and is thought to be involved with memory. There have been many (so far unsuccessful) attempts to develop modulators aimed at improving cognition and memory (Bockaert et al., 1992). However, emerging from the same research programme, a partial agonist at the 5HT4 receptor (*tegaserod*) was found to affect gastric motility and is now available to treat patients with irritable bowel syndrome (IBS; Novick et al., 2002). Had the information on this agent remained exclusively within the nervous system therapeutic area, tegaserod would not now be available to IBS patients.
- *Tyrosine kinase inhibitors.* Chronic myelogenic leukaemia is a cancer of white blood cells resulting from a somatic translocation in white blood cells between chromosomes 9 and 22. This translocation caused a fusion of two normally independent tyrosine kinases, bcr and abl. The bcr-abl fusion protein kinase is the cause of the pathological cell division in this cancer. A specific antagonist was therefore developed (STI 571, Glivec, imatinib) by Novartis (Capdeville et al., 2002; see Chapter 4). Indeed, the new small molecular weight tyrosine kinase inhibitor turned out to be a breakthrough in cancer therapy because of its specificity to the biological mechanism of this cancer, being highly effective and having fewer side effects than the previous less specific treatments (Drucker, 2002). However, Glivec was not absolutely specific for the bcr-abl tyrosine kinase but also displayed affinity for c-kit, another kinase molecule found to be involved in a different cancer, gastrointestinal stromal tumour (GIST). Because of this additional property Glivec has proved to be highly effective in treating GIST, a condition for which no treatment was previously available (Van Oosterom et al., 2001). Other tyrosine kinase inhibitors are in development for the treatment of a much wider range of disorders, including immunological and neurological conditions, and Cohen (2002) speculates that tyrosine kinase represent 'the major drug targets of the 21st century'.

Examples such as these have major implications for the organization of large pharmaceutical discovery departments because quite often one therapeutic area's discard proves to be another's 'Holy Grail', or a particular therapeutic molecule (such as Viagra, see Chapter 4) proves to have beneficial effects in different areas from the one originally intended. The increasing number of such examples shows that different members (e.g. therapeutic area groups) of a large organization need to emphasize knowledge sharing rather than competition. It is also important to construct incentive systems that encourage such sharing.

Technologies

An additional strong argument for sharing rather than competing results from the trend in biology to complement the work of small individual laboratories with 'big science' technologies, where parts of the drug discovery process are automated, robotized and miniaturized in a high-throughput mode (see Chapter 8). What is needed is not a complete change from one to the other, but a constructive combination of both. Some problems are best solved by small teams; others are inaccessible without large high-throughput operations, because of the complexity of biology and the sheer amount of data that must be processed to achieve an understanding.

An illustrative example was the race for the sequencing of the human genome, which very clearly brought to the fore the clash between the two scientific cultures (Cooke-Deegan, 1994; Sulston and Ferry, 2002). Although many of the key discoveries needed for the Human Genome Project came from small teams or individuals, it took Venter at Celera to set up a factory floor full of sequencers and computers to achieve the draft of the *Drosophila*, mouse and human genomes via the 'shotgun' approach. Some fundamental discoveries about biology would not have been possible without the direct comparison of these genomes (Mural et al., 2002).

It can also be predicted that unravelling the large number of cellular signalling pathways will depend in future on large consortia of collaborating laboratories (Fisher, 2002).

It is undoubtedly much more efficient for large research organizations to set up the necessary high-throughput and other expensive technologies in such a way as to make them available to all research groups in the same company, albeit addressing very different problems. Often it is helpful if such technologies can be developed and tested with outside partners and internalized if successful, otherwise simply abandoned.

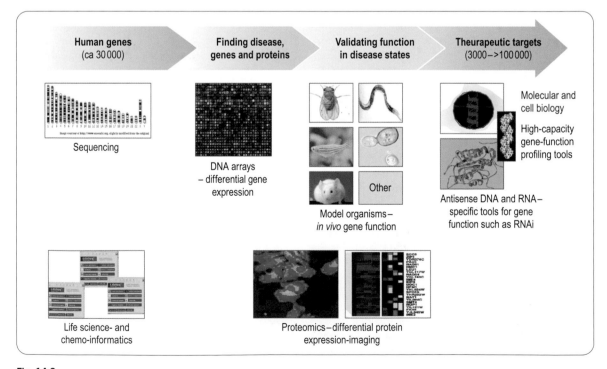

Fig. 14.2
Some technologies needed for functional genomics. A functional genomics platform can be established as a centre of excellence to apply and further develop these technologies before disseminating both technologies and results to therapeutic areas.

Advantages and disadvantages of size

A few years ago some thought that the research organizations of large pharmaceutical companies were going the way of dinosaurs, becoming extinct because of their large size and complexity, whereas the future lay with small biotech research groups able to maintain a flexible and fast culture of creativity and innovation. Indeed, some very important breakthroughs in technologies and therapeutics resulted from the biotech companies. However, the advent of 'big science' into biomedical research and drug discovery, with approaches such as high-throughput functional genomics (Figure 14.2), high-throughput screening (Chapter 8), combinatorial chemistry (Chapter 9) etc., necessitated a redesign of the drug discovery process in the direction of more industrialized processes. Only large pharmaceutical industry organizations can afford to do his and integrate the dozens of technologies and disciplines required.

For both of these reasons – access to and leveraging of expensive technologies as well as biological synergies across therapeutic areas – large research organization have an advantage over small ones, despite the increased effort required for communication and the disadvantages of bureaucracy and complexity in large organizations. Small biotech companies can typically only afford to cover a few technologies and therapeutic areas, forgoing the advantage afforded by multiple uses of the high investment in technologies, as well as the opportunity to leverage the scientific results in many disease areas as described. However, for a company to profit from the advantages of size it must avoid as far as possible the attendant disadvantages, namely, excessive complexity, communication difficulties, 'bureaucracy', managerial remoteness and slowness of decision making. The remainder of this chapter will describe some of the measures that have proved useful to maintain the advantages of small research groups while at the same time reaping the advantages of a large research organization.

Defining the research portfolio

A large pharmaceutical company will typically be active in most areas of medicine relevant to society, and will need this diversity to be able to generate the number of projects reaching the markets that are needed to sustain the growth rate expected by the company's investors.

Most large companies – those employing 3000–6000 discovery scientists – will work in most of the following broad therapeutic areas:

- *Psychiatric and neurological disorders*, including stroke, epilepsy, pain and neurodegenerative disorders;
- *Cancer;*
- *Cardiovascular disorders*, including hypertension, atherosclerosis, heart failure, dysrhythmias and peripheral vascular diseases;
- *Immunological disorders*, including allergies, transplant rejection, autoimmune diseases (e.g. rheumatoid arthritis, multiple sclerosis etc);
- *Infectious diseases*, including bacterial and viral infections such as hepatitis, AIDS and influenza;
- *Gastrointestinal disorders*, including inflammatory bowel diseases, peptic ulcers and irritable bowel syndrome;
- *Metabolic and endocrinological disorders,* including diabetes, obesity, disorders of the thyroid, parathyroid and pituitary, adrenal function and menopausal symptoms;
- *Respiratory disorders*, including asthma and chronic obstructive pulmonary diseases;
- *Musculoskeletal disorders*, including osteoarthritis, osteoporosis, Paget's disease and muscular dystrophies;
- *Skin diseases;*
- *Disorders of reproduction, fertility and sexual function.*

These are defined medical areas, but because of the underlying biology they will have a multitude of common biological mechanisms and related targets.

These general areas of activity will usually be decided by management to fit with the company's long-term commercial strategy, but the actual research strategy and target selection aimed at the solution of specific medical problems must always be generated by the scientists themselves, as they are the ones living at the relevant edge of scientific biomedical knowledge.

Competitive advantage

A key consideration in choosing a specific research strategy is that the resulting therapy must have a major competitive advantage over existing therapies when it enters clinical use, which is likely to be more than 10 years in the future. Such advantages can range over a wide spectrum, for example:

- The treatment of untreatable or poorly-treated medical conditions e.g. many cancers, neurodegenerative conditions such as Alzheimer's disease; Huntington's disease;
- Orally active drugs for conditions previously needing treatment by injections e.g. insulin or iron chelators for iron overload diseases;

● Drugs with improved efficacy, fewer side effects or reduced toxicity, e.g. antipsychotic drugs, antiepileptic drugs, antidysrhythmic drugs..

Whereas in the past many pharmaceutical companies were commercially successful exploiting so-called 'fast followers' and 'me-too' compounds of an established class with minor or no clinical advantages whose success depended mainly on the power of their marketing organizations, this is becoming increasingly difficult because of the resistance of payers and regulatory authorities to increasing healthcare costs unaccompanied by significant therapeutic improvements.

Currently, distinct superiority over existing therapy is increasingly required as a condition for regulatory approval. This is part of the reason why pipelines in the industry are deemed insufficient to sustain required growth. One other reason may be that the 'easy' targets have been addressed, and the recent explosion in biological knowledge and new technologies is only just beginning to translate into more and better drugs.

An important consequence of this trend is that research organizations that specialize in so-called 'fast followers' and 'me-too' drugs will find it increasingly difficult to survive, whereas companies with research organizations designed for innovation and major medical advantages will prevail.

Choice of drug target

Key elements of the research strategy for innovation are the choice and quality of the therapeutic target (see Chapter 6). Whereas until recently only a few hundred targets, mostly receptors or enzymes, were sufficiently defined to warrant intensive discovery work, the Human Genome Project has shown that the approximately 25 000 genes can code for more than 100 000 proteins, taking into account alternative splicing and post-translational modifications. There is an ongoing debate about how many of these will be 'druggable', i.e. amenable to pharmacological manipulation. The pessimists predict only a few thousand, but this is based on current chemical and pharmacological knowledge, and so it can be safely predicted that this is too few.

Ideally, the target will be one involved at the earliest stages of disease, in particular for long-lasting degenerative diseases, where the damage to the body takes years to become apparent, as is the case in Alzheimer's or Parkinson's diseases. Most of today's therapies are only applied when the symptoms become apparent, at a time when significant irreversible damage has already occurred.

The aim is to develop strategies that affect very early stages, so as to prevent or reverse deterioration of the organs involved. A therapy addressing such a target would be called 'disease-modifying' or 'causal'. This will necessitate treating patients who are symptom-free despite being judged to be at high risk, placing high demands on the safety and freedom from side effects of the drugs involved. The principle of using drugs prophylactically is already quite widely applied, for example in the use of statins to prevent atherosclerosis, antiepileptic drugs to prevent the development of epilepsy after head injury, or aspirin tablets to reduce the risk of deep vein thrombosis in long-haul airline passengers. There are many other examples, the key requirement being the presence of an identifiable risk factor or the availability of a predictive diagnostic test that justifies the administration of drugs to ostensibly healthy individuals. There are many conditions, such as Alzheimer's disease, where a preventive or disease-modifying therapy is greatly needed, though the prospect is some way off, although recent vaccination approaches in man have shown great promise (Hock et al., 2003) and the non-invasive imaging of plaque load approaches clinical testing.

Patenting

The discussion so far has emphasized the importance of selecting the right target and being ahead of the competition. This is where groups specializing in functional genomics and biological pathway analysis play a key role.

Recently, some companies, mainly startup biotech companies, have started to patent such targets, making them available on payment of a substantial licence fee to pharmaceutical companies wishing to use them in drug discovery programmes. This (see Chapter 13) has resulted in a change of patenting policy in many large pharmaceutical companies. Whereas previously such companies patented only the products they intended to sell, and the processes to make them, increasingly they now patent genes, targets, transgenic animal models and other scientific tools discovered in their laboratories. They do this not because they intend to sell them, but rather to protect themselves from having to pay licence fees for their use, and occasionally as objects of barter if they need access to proprietary tools belonging to another company. This is called *defensive patenting*, because the intention is not to prevent others from using the tools and targets but rather to protect the company's own freedom to use the tools.

Generally, it is advantageous and efficient for a pharmaceutical company that develops, for example, a new transgenic disease model to distribute the new strain widely, usually at no cost and without restriction on publication, to academic laboratories, so that it will be investigated and characterized extensively. The better a transgenic model or other research tool is characterized, the better the results obtained with it can be interpreted. An additional benefit is that this behaviour creates goodwill with academic scientists and good scientific networking.

Publishing

Companies need to balance the need for secrecy about some aspects of their research, which they do not wish to disclose to their competitors, against the advantages that come from publishing, and one of the more difficult tasks of a research manager is to judge where this balance should lie. An analysis of the publishing behaviour and citation frequency of several large pharmaceutical companies (Figure 14.3) reveals surprising differences. Some companies encourage their scientists to publish extensively, and they are then well cited, although the total citations do not correlate closely with the number of publications. Others of a similar size have a much more restrictive policy. It is the author's firm opinion that the former, more liberal publishing policy, provided it safeguards the company's intellectual property rights, has many advantages:

● Good scientists are highly motivated by having their work appear in the scientific literature, and are attracted to companies with a liberal policy.
● The scientific community accords status to scientists on the basis of their publications and presentations at scientific meetings. Acceptance by the scientific community is of great advantage to scientists in establishing good communications and fruitful collaborations.
● The company gains the benefit of independent peer review of its research, and its scientific reputation is enhanced by high-quality publications.

From the perspective of a company's in-house research community, the benefits of publication in general far outweigh the risks of divulging information to competitors. Nevertheless, the company must protect its intellectual property (see Chapter 19), as the strength of its patents is a major factor in determining the profitability of its products. Invariably, therefore, material intended for publication is scrutinized by the company's patent department before being released. The chemical structures of development compounds, or structures related to them, will naturally not be published until patent protection has been secured, and even then the company may not wish to disclose information that could be helpful to a competitor. This restriction means that compound-related information – a key part of the company's research output – will generally not be

published until the project is either advanced in development (i.e. several years after the research was done) or will be restricted to compounds that are no longer of interest as development candidates. Because of this, pharmaceutical companies inevitably gain a reputation for withholding publication of their most interesting data, and for a lack of openness in communicating with other scientists. The cultural barrier that this creates between academia and the pharmaceutical industry will probably always exist, but is likely to diminish as collaborations increase and as research managers move towards a more open publication policy.

External collaborations and partnerships

Similar arguments pertain to the desirability of external scientific collaborations. External collaborations are crucial even to the largest research organizations, as many essential discoveries and technologies come from outside, and it is important to access these whenever necessary. An organization that has learned to work efficiently with outside partners has a great advantage (Herrling, 1998). Establishing good relationships between the research scientists of the participating groups is critical for success, and a clear agreement on the goals of the project, and the division of responsibilities between the two groups, is also essential.

There are two basic types of external collaboration, each having different aims:

● *Academic collaborations*, funded by the pharmaceutical company, are ideally suited to access emerging basic knowledge in areas relevant to the company's goals. They also serve to foster the mutual understanding of industry and academic researchers. They may be set up as short-term collaborations in the context of a specific project, in which case clear-cut scientific objectives and milestones are agreed. Alternatively, a broadly based 'umbrella' collaboration agreement may be set up on a long-term basis, which gives the company privileged access to the data and expertise of the academic partner and provides a framework within which collaborations on specific projects can be established. Examples of such long-term agreements are Novartis' collaborations with the Dana Faber Cancer Institute in Boston, and with the Scripps Research Institute in La Jolla, and many other companies establish similar relationships with academic centers of excellence. Under such arrangements academic scientists can be very useful members of industrial management teams, and industry-based scientists may serve on the boards

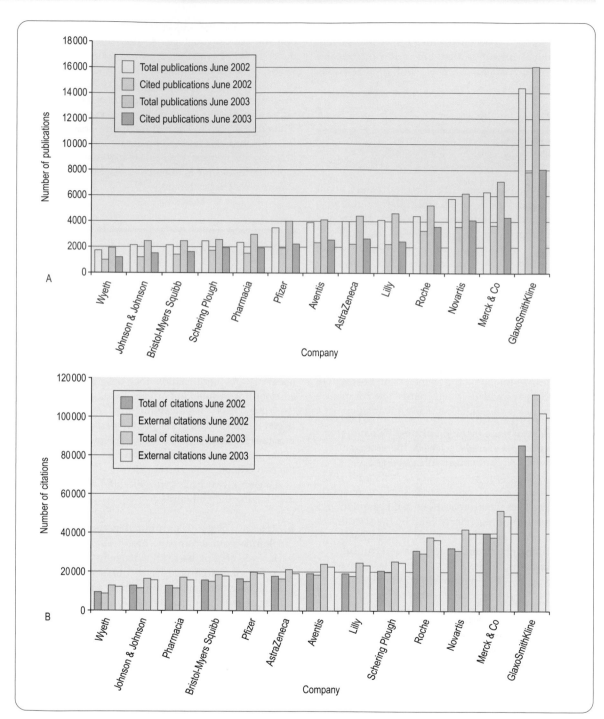

Fig. 14.3
Number of papers published by major pharmaceutical companies since 1997 and number of papers cited.
Source: M. Deuqud, Novartis Institutes for Biomedical Research.

of academic institutions. In such cases the exchange of sabbatical scholars or post-doctoral fellows is a very efficient tool for mutual knowledge transfer.

• *Partnerships with biotechnology companies* provide a useful way of exploring new technologies (e.g. the collaboration between Novartis and Celera on shotgun sequencing) or specific drug targets (e.g. the kinase collaboration between Vertex and Novartis). Under these arrangements each partner commits resources to the project, and both share in the rewards of success. For example, if the project is successful in producing a development compound, the biotechnology company may receive substantial milestone payments as the product reaches successive stages of development, and a royalty share on the sales of a marketed compound. Contract negotiations in these cases are often protracted and complex, and many different financial models have been devised to meet particular needs.

For any kind of formal collaboration a solid legal framework is essential, and a large pharmaceutical company will entrust the task of contract negotiation to its business development department. But just as importantly, the scientists and managers on each side must respect and trust each other and be able to communicate openly. Suspicions on either side that relevant information is being withheld, or that data are of poor quality, have a corrosive effect. There is no formula for avoiding this danger, apart from ensuring in advance that the scientists on both sides are actually enthusiastic about collaborating, and allowing them to communicate freely.

Contract research is different from collaborative research, in that the company simply commissions an external group, either a commercial contract research organization (CRO) or an academic group, to carry out research studies on a fee-for-service basis. In the field of drug discovery, compounds may be sent out for routine pharmacological profiling on a defined battery of standard assays, or for early-stage pharmacokinetic or toxicological investigation. If data are needed with a specialized animal model developed by an academic group, the group may be commissioned to investigate the effect of one or more compounds. Work of this kind is carried out on a simple fee-for-service basis, the data generated being the property of the company that pays for the work to be done.

A number of rules – learned the 'hard', i.e. the expensive, way – have to be followed to make external collaborations (as distinct from contract research agreements) successful and efficient:

- The goals of the partner need to be aligned with the company's goals with respect to the topic of the collaboration, and this can be achieved by appropriate structuring of the contracts (see below). Identity of goals is by no means automatic even in the case of commercial partners, because of the financial situation of many biotech partners and their dependence on making deals with big pharmaceutical companies. This carries the danger that once a deal is signed and the upfront monies paid, the temptation will be great to divert resources and management attention to establishing new projects aimed at securing future collaborations, paying less attention to addressing the goals of the first partner.
- External collaborations involving innovative science (as distinct from fee-for-service contracts for routine studies) must never follow the 'pay and forget' principle that is appropriate for contract research. This is a recipe for disaster, for several reasons.

Usually the project does not progress according to the original plan, since new discoveries are made and technologies change. Unless it remains actively engaged the customer company cannot influence the new directions. Additionally, it would forgo the opportunity to learn from the partner, and would have great difficulty integrating the results into its own operation. To avoid this it is helpful to set up an appropriately dimensioned *joint* research team composed of partner and customer scientists, and to have the research decisions entrusted to a joint steering committee, based on frequent project reviews, typically twice per year.

- Some of the greatest blunders of management with respect to external collaborations, with the concomitant waste of millions of dollars, have occurred when senior managers have taken the initiative in setting up external collaborations without sufficiently involving their own scientists. Even in cases where the need for external collaboration is justified from a scientific point of view, this top-down approach inevitably leaves the in-house scientific team feeling demotivated and under pressure to save resources that have been allocated to the external partner, and they may resent the fact that they will be called on subsequently to integrate the new technology and data into their project. To avoid this trap it is essential that 'ownership' of the project is conferred as far as possible on in-house scientists, who need to be closely involved at the planning stage and in the management of the project, even when the strategic decision for partnering is made at a higher management level. It is also important to encourage the in-house project team to bring forward proposals for external collaborations, recognizing that research scientists are best able to pick up emerging trends and opportunities in their field, and to judge when an external collaboration could help in meeting their project goals. A willingness to act on such 'bottom-up' proposals is extremely important, even though it sometimes requires senior managers to hold their egos in check.
- It must be recognized that academic scientists need to publish their work, and often rely on funding from public sources that support their laboratories and expect publication of the results. The commercial partner needs to retain control of publication, however, and it is essential that the limits of this control are clearly understood and agreed.

Certain aspects of the design and structure of the contract are crucial to help alleviate the problems outlined above:

- Upfront payments should be kept to a minimum. There must be clearly defined and frequently assessed milestones that must be reached before payment is triggered.

- The contract must ensure that technology, data and knowledge are transferred from the partner to the customer, a condition that precludes partnerships with collaborators who are not prepared to share such knowledge. Without this, the major advantage of a partnership – learning – is seriously impaired. At the same time the contract must stipulate which party 'owns' the data generated, as well as any restrictions on the use to which it may be put, including the right to publish or pass the data on to a third party.

Possible termination points must be built in at frequent intervals, for example yearly, with suitable 'wind-down' periods if the project is ended prematurely. The 'back-loading' of payments and the provision of termination points also maintain the customer's flexibility in case the scientific hypothesis behind the collaboration collapses, or the project is overtaken by competitors, avoiding long-term commitment of resources in a project that has become hopeless.

Contract research agreements are generally straightforward, as the deliverables and the timing of payments are simple, and the data will belong to the customer.

If the above points are duly taken into consideration, external collaborations can be a major competitive tool to make a pharmaceutical company more successful, to revitalize internal energies, and to continuously improve internal skills. However, there is a limit to the number and size of external collaborations a research department can take on, as each will require the allocation of significant internal resources if it is to succeed. Currently, it is generally thought that about 30% of the total discovery budget of a pharmaceutical company should ideally be allocated to external scientific collaborations. An important measure of success must be the answer to the following question: Which compounds or technologies in the pharmaceutical company's portfolio would not be available, or would have been significantly delayed or made more costly without the collaborations? This question can, of course, only be answered retrospectively, and judging the merits of collaboration proposals and negotiating appropriate contract terms is one of the more difficult tasks that research managers face.

Productivity measures in drug discovery research

The ultimate measure of productivity of a pharmaceutical research and development organization is the number of medically and commercially successful new therapies it delivers in relation to the investment made. However, in view of the long time that elapses between the research investment and its final output, and also the fact that the final outcome depends as much on the

quality and management of the development programme as on that of the discovery teams, intermediary or 'surrogate' measures are needed to assess how well the discovery groups are performing.

Drug discovery phases and attrition rates

Based on a company's long-term business strategy, the number and value of new therapies needed to sustain the required growth of the pharmaceutical company can be determined. From this productivity endpoint, taking

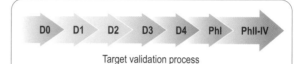

Target validation process

Definitions:

Phase D0 – Basic Research: Basic conceptual and exploratory research with the intent of identifying a therapeutic target.

Phase D1 – Screen (or Assay) Development: Target identified for initial screening. Applied research focused on assay development (e.g., receptor or enzyme assays, gene reporter assays, cell or tissue assays and whole animal models) for screening and evaluating compounds. The tests developed include those of high and low throughput, both in vitro and in vivo.

Phase D2 – Screening: Initial screening to discover chemical template for optimization (lead). Testing of compounds, either in vitro or in vivo, to determine their target effect (e.g., molecular interaction or biological effects) for the purpose of identifying a chemical template for optimization. Activities associated with screen development would be excluded.

Phase D3 – Lead Optimization: Medicinal chemistry optimization and biological testing of the compound intended for dosing in first GLP toxicology studies. The outcome should be the best structure in terms of potency and selectivity for the target selected, as well as indication for acceptable ADME properties.

Phase D4 – Completion of studies to allow first application in man. All studies from first GLP toxicology study to first dose in man. Includes extensive in vivo studies, pharmacokinetic and pharmacodynamic studies, stability and solubility studies, determination of surrogate markers for human studies.

Fig. 14.4
The phases of the drug discovery processes as generally defined by most large pharmaceutical research organizations. D0 is equivalent to 'target identification' elsewhere in this book; D1 and D2 are equivalent to 'lead identification', and D3 and D4 to 'lead optimization'. Each of these phases will be accompanied by a number of criteria specific to different companies, which will determine when the next phase can be undertaken. The actual molecular entities also go through criteria-determined phase transitions, e.g. lead (L, at early D3); early development candidate (EDC, occurs at the end of D3), and full development candidate (FDC, usually after proof of concept/mechanism in man, end of PhI).

Table 14.1
Calculation of numbers of new projects entering each phase required to generate three launches of new compounds per year

Phase	Success rate to next phase (%)	Number of new entries per year
D1	60	76
D2	60	46
D3	75	28
D4	80	21
Phase I POC	20	17
Phase III	90	3.3
Launch		3

These are very rough estimates by the author for purely illustrative purposes. Different numbers can be found in the literature (Center for Medicines Research; see Chapter 22) due to different phase transition criteria or very different success rates in different companies etc. It can be seen what major consequences changes in success rate can have, i.e. if the PhI to PhIII success rate is only 10% this would require 92 new targets screened in D2 and 56 new D3 phases per year, resulting in a significant readjustment of the drug discovery process.

into account the historical attrition rates at each stage of the research process, the number of projects required in each phase can be calculated. The discovery and development phases defined within the Novartis research organization are summarized in Figure 14.4, and Table 14.1 sets out fictitious attrition rates for projects at the various stages, suggesting that more than 70 new projects need to be initiated each year in order to generate three successful new launches, which is approximately the output that a major company requires to remain viable.

These figures also show how important it is to reduce the attrition rates by improving the predictive power of the data obtained at earlier stages for the ultimate outcome. Small improvements in the attrition rate will result in major increases in efficacy for the entire drug discovery organization.

An example of a productivity formula for drug discovery

In order to obtain an early warning of problems anywhere in the early pipeline we have developed a formula to estimate the contribution of discovery into the pipeline for any given resource investment, i.e. a 'productivity index'. A generic example of such a formula for calculating the *productivity index* P is given in Box 14.1.

The numerical value of P can be used to compare different research groups, but needs to be taken in conjunction with additional factors, such as the results of panel reviews and the state of development of the research group at the time of review. It is the task of research management to make these judgements. Evaluation by formula can be only one factor in the overall judgement.

> **Box 14.1 Calculating the productivity index**
>
> $$P = \frac{\sum_j (D3_j \times W_{D3j}) + 2\sum_j (EDC_j \times W_{EDCj}/T_{D3j}) + 4\sum_k (FDC_k \times W_{FDCk}/T_{EDCk})}{\text{Total resources allocated}}$$
>
> where:
> Σ = total number for the year analysed
> $j/i/k$ = running index on completed D3/EDC/FDC phases (see Figure 14.4 for definitions) achieved during the period, e.g. 1 year
> W = weight or 'value' of each project (determination method, see text) attributed by a panel of internal and/or external experts
> T = duration of D3/EDC phases preceding the phase transition, relative to the planned duration. For a T corresponding to the plan duration of a project, T = 1, for projects faster than the plan duration T <1, and for projects delayed beyond the planned duration T >1. The value of a candidate compound decreases with increased durations of the preceding D3/EDC/FDC phases because an early time to market is of high value. The decision as to how to weigh the time advantage/penalty will be handled differently by different companies.
> **Allocated resources** include all resources used to achieve the respective phase transitions, full internal costs and costs allocated externally
> **The factors 2 and 4 applied to EDC and FDC** indicate an estimation that an EDC is 'worth' twice as much as a D3, an FDC four times as much as a D3.
> P = a value that includes both numerical and 'value' estimates of the state of a pipeline, and can be attributed either to the whole discovery organization or to parts of it

Another very important aspect is the estimation of W, which represents the *value* of the various projects in the pipeline, and the following section will illustrate a few methods for making such estimates.

Portfolio management

The research portfolio of a large pharmaceutical company can cover more than 100 projects (D2/D3) and must be regularly evaluated because of the pace of scientific progress and the rapidly changing competitive situation. An additional argument relates to the fact that scientists and managers generally have a strong tendency to spread their resources too thinly and embark on too many projects, despite the fact that drug discovery needs multidisciplinary teams of a critical mass (sometimes up to 30–70 scientists per project) to move the projects forward beyond the exploratory phase. The review process must identify which projects have completed the exploratory phase and now need to be organized into larger teams, and also those that have fallen too far behind the competition or have reached a scientific dead end and must be terminated. The following system was developed by Novartis and used for many years.

Typically a yearly review cycle is chosen. There needs to be a balance between the timeliness of the review and the considerable preparatory work required from both the scientists reviewed and the review panel. The review panel might include:

- Basic scientists (internal and external) at the forefront of the basic sciences of the areas under review;
- Drug discovery scientists, both biologists and chemists;
- Clinicians knowledgeable about the details of the medical situation and the needs of patients, and having a good grasp of the current scientific knowledge about the disease area under review;
- Representatives of the development functions, in particular drug safety, chemical research and development, galenics, clinical pharmacology etc.
- Marketing experts with an atypically long time perspective (~10 years).

Each research project is presented by the teams in a structured format to allow comparisons across the entire portfolio. The presentation includes:

- A description of the scientific therapeutic hypothesis and its novelty or uniqueness, as well as the medical need;
- The state of validation of the concept or target;
- The estimated number and type of patients that could benefit from the approach;
- An evaluation of the competitive position in terms of benefit to patients and society, with a clear strategy as to how to maintain or improve it up to and beyond the launch date;

- A description of achievements during the period under review, in relation to goals for that period and measurable goals for next period;
- A summary of key achievements of the project team since its inception;
- Future plans and expectations for the project;
- Key issues to be discussed with the panel;
- A list of patents and publications by the team for the reporting period.

Following presentation and discussion of the project with the team, the review panel makes an assessment against a list of criteria reflecting the potential value of the project and performance measures representing operational factors, including for example:

- Measures of potential value of projects:
  - Novelty of scientific concept
  - Medical need/disease relevance
  - Estimation of feasibility
  - Relevance and level of validation of target
  - Potential competitive advantage at the time of introduction
  - Synergy potential (potential value to other teams and therapeutic areas)
  - Market potential.
- Performance measures of projects:
  - Quality of the team
  - Achievements respective to milestones
  - Quality of interactions with other parts of the organizations, in particular development functions
  - Quality and efficiency of external collaborations
  - Quality of the chemical leads
  - Competitive position of the project team, both direct and indirect
  - Required resources to next go/no-go decision point
  - Achieved synergies, i.e. have concepts, compounds, technologies from this team been used by other programmes? Have collaborations been established?

Finally, the review panel is asked to make recommendations to the team and management, including controversial issues.

The interpretation of these criteria needs to be well understood by panel and project teams and is often controversial, reflecting the respective experience of the panel members and scientists under review. A useful procedure is for the teams to make a self-evaluation which is then challenged, commented upon and refined by the review panel. The panel's comments and conclusions are communicated immediately to the teams in a feedback session attended by members of the panel, during which the project team is encouraged to respond to the comments and suggestions made. Carrying out the review in this open way helps to avoid misunderstandings, and greatly facilitates acceptance of the review panel's conclusions, even when difficult and unpopular decisions flow from the review. The contrasting system of reviews carried out behind closed doors with little or no participation of the project team members, though it may involve less time and effort, has little to commend it and can actually be damaging, as it tends to generate mistrust between scientists and managers. With this open system the mutual exchange of arguments is the main value of the exercise, helping the management to make prioritization decisions within the portfolio and giving the scientists the benefit of experienced input from the review panel.

Assessing the 'value' of a project

For comparison of projects across the portfolio it can be useful to assign a qualitative value (e.g. 'high', 'medium', 'low') to each of the parameters described above as a basis for evaluating the overall 'value' of each project. One model that has proved useful for estimating the overall value of a programme is shown in Figure 14.5. 'Potential value of projects' measures (see above) are represented on the vertical axis and 'performance of project' measures on the horizontal axis, and the size of the symbol represents the resources allocated. The result of both axes is an indication of the actual value of a

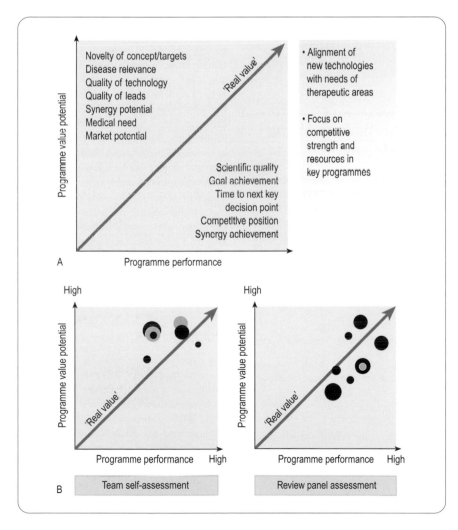

Fig. 14.5
(A) **Parameters to estimate the value of discovery programmes (see text).** (B) Actual examples from a portfolio review. Left side: self-evaluation of research teams. Right side: distribution of same teams after challenge by review panel. The size of the blobs indicates the relative resources allocated to programmes.

research programme. A programme appearing near the top but close to the *y*-axis is one based on an excellent idea but having little chance of success. A programme appearing in the opposite quadrant is performing well, but working on the wrong topic. The research manager's task is to place all programmes in the upper right quadrant while keeping the blobs as small as possible. A typical distribution of the projects within a therapeutic area, as assessed by the project team and by the review panel, is shown in Figure 14.5B. The entire drug discovery programme can be similarly depicted by symbols representing different therapeutic areas. An analysis of this kind, although the evaluation procedure can be criticized as simplistic, qualitative and subjective, provides a very useful overview of the strengths and weaknesses of the research programme, and has proved helpful in guiding decisions about redirecting drug discovery programmes and the reallocation of resources.

Building blocks of a drug discovery organization

Therapeutic areas, biological and technological platforms

Academic organizations traditionally group their sciences into broadly based departments such as chemistry, zoology, molecular biology, anatomy, physiology etc., each of which aims to achieve excellence in research and teaching. This type of organization, however, makes interdisciplinary collaboration more difficult.

As emphasized throughout this book, drug discovery research requires a finely tuned interdisciplinary collaboration, so the traditional discipline oriented academic model[1] is inappropriate.

Drug discovery research can be organized on the basis of various different principles, the main ones being:

- By medical specialty – the *therapeutic area* or *disease area* structure;
- By biological mechanism – the *biological platform* structure;
- By technological specialty – the *central support group* structure or technology platform;
- By project phase – the *drug discovery/translational research* structure.

---

[1]It should be pointed out, however, that traditional departmental structure in academia is rapidly changing towards more flexible groupings to facilitate interdisciplinary collaboration.

In practice, most companies adopt a hybrid system involving elements of all these. The terminology varies, and research managers love to juggle with it and shift the furniture, but the basic principles remain.

Therapeutic area research groups

A therapeutic area research group in a large company typically numbers about 200–400 scientists, sufficient to achieve competitive critical mass and to include most of the disciplines required, including synthetic and computational chemistry, molecular and cell biology, bioinformatics, pharmacology etc., as described in other chapters.

Medical professionals are organized into specialties, such as cardiology, rheumatology, endocrinology, neurology etc., so it is useful to organize drug discovery research on the same basis. The grouping of research know-how into particular disease areas facilitates communication of the research team with in-house and external medical experts, as well as the marketing organization and regulatory authorities. In many companies these groups form the major part of the drug discovery organization, and are responsible, with the help of central support groups, for taking the project all the way from target identification to identification of a drug candidate suitable for development (as described in previous chapters). They therefore include the necessary disease models and pharmacokinetic capabilities to take the project this far. However, some companies have taken the step of separating the task into (a) the early stages of *target identification* and *lead finding*, involving mainly biological platform groups for target identification, and central functions groups for screening and lead identification, and (b) the later stages of *lead optimization* and *compound profiling*, which are treated as translational research and performed by therapeutic area groups (see below).

Biological platforms

The exponential increase in biological knowledge has revealed that many therapeutic targets occur in large families, as described earlier (see also Chapter 6), such as kinases (Manning et al., 2002), proteases (Puente et al., 2003), G-protein-coupled receptors (Fantom Consortium and the RIKEN Genome Exploration Group, 2002) and ion channel proteins. There is a strong case for assembling groups of specialists (platforms) focusing on an entire target family on the assumption that the knowledge and methodology elaborated on one target will be applicable to others in the same family. A similar case can be made for some important biological mechanisms, such as angiogenesis, signal transduction pathways, autoimmunity, inflammation, cell cycle control etc., that are involved in many disease states.

Because such platform groups will yield results of use to more than one therapeutic area, good communication, and alignment of goals and incentives with those of the therapeutic area groups, is very important.

Platform groups will typically hand over ideas and lead compounds directed at new, experimentally validated therapeutic targets to the therapeutic area groups at the point where disease specific knowledge is required, as well as lead optimization to generate drug candidates whose properties are appropriate for the particular disease condition. A special form of a biological platform is the 'functional genomics' group, whose task is to identify and functionally characterize new disease relevant targets from the genome (Kramer and Cohen, 2004; see Chapter 6). This group needs expertise in all the relevant technologies (see Figure 14.2) for this task, and also has an important role in developing tools and methods that can be used throughout the discovery organization.

The function and organization of platform groups can be defined in various ways. They can be organized as service units, commissioned by therapeutic area groups to carry out particular studies needing special expertise or technology. For example, a diabetes research group might wish to know how experimental diabetes affects gene expression in particular tissues. Gene expression profiling (see Chapter 7) is best done by experts, and so such a project would be suitable for a functional genomics platform group. Alternatively, platform groups may be used to carry out exploratory research to elucidate mechanisms and potential drug targets in areas such as tissue regeneration, neurodegeneration or obesity, where new drug targets need to be found and there is a good possibility that modern biological approaches can reveal them. The 'deliverable' in this case might be a new target to be taken up by the appropriate therapeutic area group. In another model the platform group may take the project further, developing a suitable screening assay and identifying lead compounds suitable for optimization by therapeutic area groups. To do this, the platform group will need to include experts in assay development, as well as a substantial contingent of medicinal chemists. A logical extension of this may be to link the various platform groups representing different fundamental biological mechanisms together as a 'drug discovery centre', whose role is to deliver lead compounds to one or more therapeutic area groups, which pursue 'translational research', i.e. optimizing lead compounds to produce drug candidates for particular disease indications.

These multidisciplinary groups – therapeutic areas and platforms – are stable organizational units, the members of which are assigned as participants in one or more specific multidisciplinary research programme teams with a defined goal, such as drug discovery or technology development. The research programme teams can be flexibly created or disbanded, expanded or reduced, depending on the success of the scientific hypothesis and the performance of the teams. Each team is headed by an experienced team leader, who should have significant decision power over the resources allocated to their team.

It is recognized that the need for hands-on synthetic chemistry tends to fluctuate widely and unpredictably as a project proceeds, depending on the number of good chemical leads that have been identified and the need for optimization. It can therefore be useful to create, in addition to the chemists allocated to multidisciplinary therapeutic areas and platforms, a specific group of chemists that can be easily and flexibly deployed as 'flying squads' when a project needs additional chemistry capacity. This helps to avoid the upheaval of transferring scientists from their 'home' therapeutic area or platform

Central support groups

There are a number of activities where the economy of scale does not allow a deployment into all therapeutic areas or platform groups. Most frequent examples are:

- A high-throughput screening unit that is highly robotized, miniaturized, and operates as a quasi-industrialized process and includes the compound warehouse facility (see Chapter 8);
- The 'Kilolab', a chemistry laboratory that is equipped to synthesize compounds and intermediates, on a gram–kilogram scale. This is often needed for combinatorial chemistry operations, as well as for production of compounds needed for detailed pharmacological investigations. Medium-scale synthesis of this sort is not normally possible in a typical medicinal chemistry research laboratory;
- The animal facility, including laboratories equipped for in vivo experiments;
- Technologies needing large and expensive equipment which needs to be run and maintained by dedicated personnel. These include large MRI scanners, large-scale (up to 10 000 L) fermenters, high-field NMR (800 MHz to 1 GHz) and X-ray crystallography. Technologies such as these, which are, when first introduced, large, expensive and technically demanding on the user, tend with time to become cheaper, smaller and easier to use. As this happens (for example with mass spectrometry), they need to be transferred from central functions to end-user laboratories, allowing central functions to move into new, emerging technologies.

Management issues

An essential requirement for the successful operation of such a complex organization of interdependent scientific units, as described above, is that the goals of each need to be clearly defined and their incentives aligned with the common goal of drug discovery, which no group can achieve on its own. The provision of incentives is discussed in the next section.

Within the research organization each group needs to be *reactive* to the changing needs of current drug discovery projects, and at the same time *proactive* in anticipating how developments in its own scientific and technological field can best be utilized. If a group becomes too starry-eyed about future developments it risks being branded as an empire builder, neglectful of its day-to-day service role; nevertheless, it will quickly become out of date if it focuses only on its current tasks and neglects to keep up with new ideas and methods. Keeping a balance between short- and long-term needs is a constant theme in research management. Good goal-setting and alignment of goals and incentives between therapeutic areas, platforms and central groups is necessary to ensure that they adjust their skills and deliverables to the needs of the entire discovery operation.

Figure 14.6 summarizes the organization and relationships of the various types of research groups discussed above, with the caveat that many variants are to be found in different companies.

Incentives, culture and human resource aspects

Incentives

Scientists have special requirements with respect to incentives and environment, because of their characteristic scientific culture and unique way of applying science to discover new therapies. In particular, monetary and management-related rewards, although important, are for many scientists – or other professionals for that matter – not sufficient on their own to sustain motivation and focus. What is needed in addition is a challenging task and the resources to see it through. Lack of sufficient challenge generally detracts from motivation, and if their job is too easy scientists may lose the edge and urgency to discover new medicines. Drug discovery research is often tedious and frustrating: a year-long effort will often fail through no foreseeable fault of the scientists, because of an unexpected side effect, lack of predicted efficacy in the clinical environment or, as

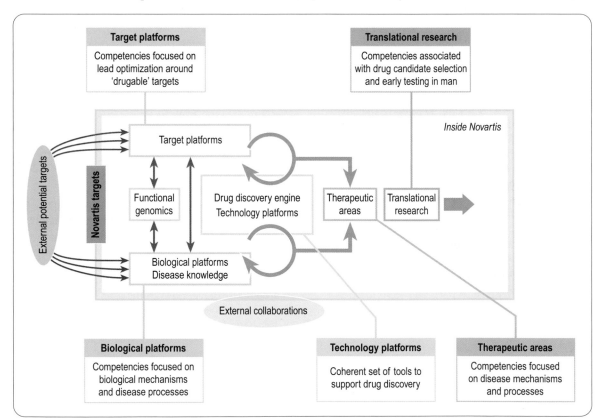

Fig. 14.6
Elements of a drug discovery organization. The yellow area denotes the internal organization. The ellipses indicate that external partnerships contribute throughout the process, from targets to technologies up to specific compound candidates. The arrows denote the iterative interactions between all elements of the process.

happens too often, strategic reorientation of the company.

It is important for bench scientists engaged in biomedical research to understand the clinical reality of the patients they intend to help. It can be a powerful experience for a scientist to see, for example, schizophrenic patients in a psychiatric ward and to learn from them and their doctors about their problems. It is often possible, with the help of cooperative clinicians, to provide basic scientists with the useful experience of seeing medicine at first hand.

It is also important during the selection process for new scientists to choose only those with a genuine interest in applying their science to solving medical problems, and to discourage those who seek only a secure base from which to pursue independent research. It is important for scientists coming from academia to realize that translating laboratory science into a new therapy that saves lives is every bit as demanding – albeit requiring a quite different mindset – as translating it into a significant scientific paper. Scientists in industry perforce work collaboratively in multidisciplinary groups, and need to have the communication skills, patience and adaptability to do this successfully; there are few niches where loners, however brilliant and creative, can fit comfortably, and recruiting policy has to take account of this.

Within a research organization the best incentive is to leave scientists as much room for scientific initiative as the drug discovery process allows. Typically, there is very little time for a scientist fully engaged in drug discovery to pursue independent research, but a period of sabbatical leave can provide a good opportunity to refresh scientific skills and interests in a new environment.

Providing support for postdoctoral fellows to work with scientists who have the ability and experience to direct them effectively enables speculative exploratory projects to be undertaken. Besides taking advantage of the creative ideas and new skills that postdoctoral fellows on short-term contracts bring into the research organization, such provision is much valued by the staff scientists involved. A large research organization, such as Novartis, would normally support more than 100 postdoctoral positions.

Another strong motivator is peer recognition, which can be encouraged, as discussed above, by a liberal publishing policy and by encouraging industry-based scientists to participate in external activities, such as the organization of scientific meetings, serving on editorial boards, teaching and other academic activities. A high-level company prize for the best scientific achievements can, if fairly and openly judged, be a valuable way to create role models to be followed by others.

In view of the particular importance of collaborative research and teamwork in drug discovery, special incentives need to be directed to this aspect. Sharing across organizational units must also be strongly fostered to increase the chances of success of the entire discovery operation. One way to achieve this is to ensure that members of one organizational unit are rewarded not only for the success of their own unit, but also if they contribute to the success of others. Indicators include the number of joint projects different units have, and even more importantly the number of projects in the pipeline that begin in one therapeutic area and find additional applications in others. Organizational units excelling at such sharing can be given significantly more resources.

Culture and scientific environment

Project decisions

In the drug discovery environment it is essential that active research scientists, as well as experienced managers, contribute to decision making. Decision making always needs to be as transparent and open as possible, to minimize rumour-mongering and distrust. Furthermore, scientists will be better prepared to accept difficult decisions that affect them (for example ending programmes or whole therapeutic areas) if they understand the objective arguments behind the decisions, which managers must be prepared to defend openly. An important example is phase transition decisions, where a senior management meeting decides on advancing, delaying or abandoning a compound as a development candidate. It must be borne in mind that successful drug discovery projects are difficult to achieve and quite rare in the productive life of an individual scientist. Drug discovery scientists need to be strongly committed to 'their' projects, and it is essential that they can participate in the decision making. A recommended procedure is to involve the entire scientific team in management meetings when decisions are made on their projects, so that they can witness the decision process, contribute their own detailed knowledge and participate in the arguments.

For phase transition decisions, the team prepares in advance the necessary documentation addressing all the key points relating to the project (based on guidelines or checklists applicable to the different phase transition decisions). At the meeting, an experienced member of the management team, who is not directly involved with the project, reviews the document and identifies the key issues that need to be resolved. This provides for a very structured discussion as to whether the proposed project should be promoted, amended or stopped. Experience shows that this refereeing process works well in achieving high-quality discussions and phase transition decisions. A similar process can be applied to decisions concerning major external collaborative projects proposed by managers or scientists.

Research conferences

A useful device for fostering collaboration is a regular global drug discovery conference, in the form of a scientific meeting at an attractive location where every scientist in the company participates in presentations, talks, workshops or posters. Such meetings are powerful in fostering collaborations between diverse and geographically distant groups, as well as a common culture of excellence.

Documentation

Scientific data represent the intellectual property of a research-based pharmaceutical company. Formal documentation and archiving is essential, not only for patenting reasons, but also to allow the information to be accessed and used throughout the organization, rather than being confined to the scientist who obtained the data. The principle of corporate, rather than individual, ownership of data is fundamental, and distinguishes industry from academia.

Documentation is time-consuming and takes time away from experimental research. However, science that is not formally reported, including details of the exact methods employed to obtain the results, is of little value. Because of the long duration of projects and the possibility that the responsible scientists may have left the company by the time the project comes under regulatory review, inadequate documentation can be a major liability for the company. Scientific documentation can be regarded as a form of internal publication, and in many cases approximates to the format of a scientific paper. Detailed methods reports are particularly important as a link to numerical databases (e.g. screening databases containing potency estimates for many compounds, where it is essential to define exactly the assay procedure for each data point; see Chapter 8). To achieve this kind of functionality, the document archive needs to be built as a relational database, searchable by subject, author, date, compounds studied, project etc., together with appropriate procedures for submitting, approving, amending and updating reports. In this context the reporting of negative, as well as positive, results is important.

The document database needs to be available to all scientists and managers in the organization, independent of their geographic site and of time of data entry. Its value becomes obvious when data summaries need to be produced as a basis for management decisions or submissions to regulatory authorities. Equally important in a global organization is its value for communication. Any scientists can quickly check on previous works on a particular subject or compound, and thus avoid repetitions, or identify experts in other locations who can offer useful advice. There are today many software solutions for maintaining searchable document archives and linking them to other bioinformatics resources, such as laboratory management systems and compound databases (see Chapter 7). For success, however, research managers must enforce strong discipline to ensure that all relevant data are entered into the databases in a timely and qualitative fashion. Ways to do this include the linkage of complete documentation to phase transitions or personal incentives and job descriptions.

Summary

A discovery organization will include most of the elements shown in Figure 14.6. A successful large modern industrial organization must take the following key factors into consideration:

- The environment must allow top-level scientists to work creatively.
- The scientists selected must have the motivation to address major medical problems. This is overwhelmingly the major motivational drive for pharmaceutical scientists, the others being merely supportive.
- Drug discovery scientists must be skilled in working as members of an interdisciplinary team and must be willing to share their expertise with scientists in other disciplines.
- Incentive systems must encourage collaboration and excellence.
- Communication systems and quality-controlled databases must be in place to allow easy global access to research data.
- The organization must reflect and evolve with advances in science and technology. The consequence is a research organization that itself is constantly changing, and its members must accept this and thrive in the changing environment and not be confused or distracted by it. Science is about bringing about change.
- Management decisions must be fully discussed with and explained to the scientists affected by them.
- The company should foster a culture that encourages sharing within the organization and (so far as the limits of intellectual property rights allow) also with external scientists and organizations.
- Research centres must be established in or near the main centres of biomedical research excellence, and close collaboration with academic research centres encouraged.
- Drug discovery is one of the most complex human endeavours, and therefore the organization will always be complex. The often-heard call for

'simplicity' is a recipe for failure, as the organization will not reflect the needs of the discovery activity. Here the saying: 'Make things as simple as possible, but not more' must be the guiding principle.

Acknowledgments

This chapter is based on a talk given at Harvard Business School in 2001 by invitation of Srikant Datar, and includes his input. Daniel Vasella and Joerg Reinhardt also contributed significantly during many debates about the management of drug discovery research, but the views presented are entirely those of the author.

References

Bockaert J, Fozard JR, Dumuis A, Clarke DE (1992) The 5-HT$_4$ receptor: a place in the sun. Trends in Pharmacological Sciences 131: 141–145.

Bronowski J, Mazlish B (1960) The western intellectual tradition. London: Hutchinson.

Capdeville R, Buchdunger E, Zimmermann J, Matter A (2002) Glivec (STI 571, imatinib), a rationally developed targeted anticancer drug. Nature Reviews Drug Discovery 1: 495–502.

Cohen P (2002) Protein kinases – the major drug targets of the 21st century? Nature Reviews Drug Discovery 1: 309–316.

Cooke-Deegan R (1994) The gene wars. New York: WW Norton.

Drucker BJ (2002) STI 571 (Gleevec™) as a paradigm for cancer therapy. Trends in Molecular Medicine 8: 14–18.

Enz A, Amstutz R, Boddeke H, Gmelin G, Malanowski J (1993) Brain selective inhibition of acetylcholinesterase: a novel approach to the therapy for Alzheimer's disease. Progress in Brain Research 98: 431–438.

Fantom Consortium and the RIKEN Genome Exploration Research Group Phase I and II Team (2002) Analysis of the mouse transcriptome based on functional annotation of 60770 full length cDNAs. Nature 420: 563–573.

Fisher K (2002) 'Glue grant' boosts cell signaling consortium. Science 289: 1854.

Herrling PL (1998) Maximizing pharmaceutical research by collaboration. Nature 292(Suppl April): 32–35.

Hock C, Konietzko U, Streffer JR et al. (2003) Antibodies against β-amyloid slow cognitive decline in Alzheimer's disease. Neuron 38: 547–554.

Hu W, Yan Q, Shen DK et al. (2003) Evolutionary and biomedical implications of a *Schistosoma japonicum* complementary DNA resource. Nature Genetics 35: 139–147.

Kramer R, Cohen D (2004) Functional genomics to new drug targets. Nature Reviews Drug Discovery 3: 965–972.

Manning G, Whyte DB, Martinez R, Hunter T, Sudarsanam S (2002) The protein kinase complement of the human genome. Science 298: 1912–1934.

Merton RK (1961) On the shoulders of giants. New York: Free Press.

Molinari M, Calanca V, Galli C, Lucca P, Paganetti P (2003) Role of EDEM in the release of misfolded glycoproteins from the calnexin cycle. Science 299: 1397–1400.

Mural RJ, Adams MD, Myers EW et al. (2002) A comparison of whole-genome shotgun-derived mouse chromosome 16 and the human genome. Science 296: 1661–1671.

Nestle W (1922) Die Vorsokratiker. Jena: Diederichs.

Novick J, Miner P, Krause R et al. (2002) A randomized, double blind, placebo-controlled trial of tegaserod in female patients suffering from irritable bowel syndrome with constipation. Alimentary Pharmacology and Therapeutics 16: 1877–1888.

Oda Y, Hosokawa N, Wada I, Nagata K (2003) EDEM as an acceptor of terminally misfolded glycoproteins released from calnexin. Science 299: 1394–1397.

Puente X, Sanchez LM, Overall CM, Lopez-Otin C (2003) Human and mouse proteases: a comparative genomic approach. Nature Review Genetics 4: 544–558.

Rashid R (ed) (1996) Encyclopedia of the history of Arabic science. Vol 3. London: Routledge, 879–885.

Shepherd GM (1991) Foundations of the neuron doctrine. Oxford: Oxford University Press.

Sobel D (1999) Galileo's daughter. London: Fourth Estate.

Sulston J, Ferry G (2002) The common thread. Washington DC: Joseph Henry Press.

Tanford C, Reynolds J (2001) Nature's robots. Oxford: Oxford University Press.

Van Oosterom AT, Judson I, Verweij J et al. (2001) Safety and efficacy of imatinib (STI 571) in metastatic gastrointestinal stromal tumors: a phase I study. Lancet 358: 1421–1423.

Verjovski-Almeida S, DeMarco R, Martins EA et al. (2003) Transcriptome analysis of the acoelomate human parasite *Schistosoma mansoni*. Nature Genetics 35: 148–157.

Watkins JC, Evans RH (1981) Excitatory amino acid transmitters. Annual Review of Pharmacology and Toxicology 21: 165–204.

DRUG DEVELOPMENT

15 Drug development: introduction

H P Rang

Introduction

Drug development comprises all the activities involved in transforming a compound from drug candidate (the end-product of the discovery phase) to a product approved for marketing by the appropriate regulatory authorities. Efficiency in drug development is critical for commercial success, for two main reasons:

- Development accounts for about two-thirds of the total R&D costs. Because the number of development projects is much smaller than the number of discovery projects, the cost per project is very much greater in the development phase, and increases sharply as the project moves into the later phases of clinical development. Keeping these costs under control is a major concern for management. Failure of a compound late in development represents a lot of money wasted.
- Speed in development is an important factor in determining sales revenue, as time spent in development detracts from the period of patent protection once the drug goes to market. As soon as the patent expires, generic competition sharply reduces sales revenue.

Despite a high level of awareness in the pharmaceutical industry of the need to reduce the money and time spent on development, both have actually increased significantly over the last two decades (see Chapter 22). This is mainly due to external factors, particularly the increased stringency applied by regulatory authorities in assessing the safety and efficacy of new compounds (see Chapter 20). The development burden is therefore tending to increase, thereby increasing the need for companies to improve their performance in this area in order to remain profitable and competitive.

The nature of drug development

Drug discovery, as described in Section 2, is invariably an exploration of the unknown, and successful projects may end up with compounds quite different from what had originally been sought: there is a large component of 'unplannability'. In contrast, drug development has a very clear-cut goal: to produce the drug in a marketable form, and to gain regulatory permission to market it for use in the target indication(s) as quickly as possible. The work required to do this falls into three main parts, respectively *technical, investigative* and *managerial*:

- Technical development – solving technical problems relating to the synthesis and formulation of the drug substance, aimed mainly at ensuring the *quality* of the end-product;
  - Main functions involved: chemical development, pharmaceutical development.
- Investigative studies – establishing the *safety* and *efficacy* of the product, including assessment of whether it is pharmacokinetically suitable for clinical use in man;
  - Main functions involved: safety pharmacology, toxicology, clinical development.
- Managerial functions:
  - Coordination – managing quality control, logistics, communication and decision making in a large multidisciplinary project to ensure high-quality data and to avoid unnecessary delays;
    - Main function involved: project management.
  - Documentation and liaison with regulatory authorities – collating and presenting data of the type, quality and format needed to secure regulatory approval;
    - Main function involved: regulatory affairs.

An important distinction between the technical and investigative aspects of development is that, in tackling technical problems, it is assumed that a solution does exist, and so the team's task is to find and optimize it as quickly as possible, whereas in assessing safety and efficacy it cannot be assumed that the compound reaches the required standards – rather, the object is to discover this as quickly and cheaply as possible. In other words, technical development is essentially an exercise in problem solving, whereas clinical and toxicological development is a continuing investigation of the properties of the compound. Although technical problems, such as an unacceptably complex and poor-yielding synthesis route, or difficulty in developing a satisfactory formulation, can result in abandonment of the project, this is relatively uncommon. Failure on account of the drug's biological properties, such as toxicity, poor efficacy or unsatisfactory pharmacokinetics, is, however, very common, and largely accounts for the fact that only 10–20% of compounds entering Phase I clinical trials are eventually marketed. An important aspect of the management of drug development projects, therefore, is to establish firm 'no-go' criteria, and to test the compound against them as early as possible.

Development proceeds along much more clearly defined lines than discovery, and is consequently more 'plannable', particularly the non-clinical studies, where standard experimental protocols exist for most of the work that needs to be carried out. This applies also in Phase I clinical studies. Delays can nevertheless occur if unexpected findings emerge, for example poor oral absorption in humans, or species-specific toxic effects, which require additional work to be carried out before clinical trials can proceed.

Beyond Phase I, the route to be followed is generally much less well charted, and success depends to a much greater extent on strategic decisions by the project team as to which clinical indications should be investigated (see Chapter 18). They will need to assess, for example, whether recruiting patients to the trial will be easy or difficult, what exclusion criteria should apply, what clinical outcome measures should be used, and how long the treatment and assessment periods will need to be. To achieve registration as quickly as possible, it may, for example, be expedient to select a relatively low-market, but quick-to-test, clinical indication for the initial trials, and to run these trials in parallel with more prolonged trials in the major indication. Careful attention needs to be given to the patient group selected for the trial, so as to maximize the chance of success in obtaining a clear-cut result. Experience shows that inconclusive clinical trials resulting from poor decisions of this sort are a common cause of failure or delay in drug development.

Components of drug development

Figure 15.1 summarizes the main activities involved in developing a typical synthetic compound. It shows the main tasks that have to be completed before the compound can be submitted for regulatory approval, but needs to be translated into an operational plan (Figure 15.2) that will allow the project to proceed as quickly and efficiently as possible. It is obvious that certain tasks have to be completed in a particular order. For example, a supply of pure compound, prepared in an acceptable formulation, has to be available before Phase I clinical studies can begin. Animal toxicity data must also be available before the compound can be given to humans. Deciding on the dosage schedule to be used in efficacy trials requires knowledge of the pharmacokinetics and metabolism of the compound in humans. Because the data generated will be included in the final registration proposal, it is essential that each part of the work should be formally reported and 'signed off' by the group responsible, and archived for future reference. A typical development project is likely to involve several hundred individuals, expert in different disciplines and working on different aspects of the project, and coordinating their work is a complex and demanding task. For this reason, most companies assign specialist project managers to this task. Their role is to design a project plan, based on input from the experts involved, to monitor progress and to adapt the plan accordingly. As well as being good organizers, project managers need to be excellent communicators, diplomatic, and with a good understanding of the scientific and technological aspects of the project. Figure 15.2 is a much-simplified outline of a project plan of the development of a typical orally active drug. Each 'task', represented by an arrow, starts and ends at a circular symbol (representing an 'event'), and decision points are marked by diamond symbols. This type of graphical format, which is widely used as a project management tool and implemented in many commercially available software packages, is known as a PERT (project evaluation and review technique) chart. By assigning times – shortest possible, maximum, and expected – to each task, the timing of the whole project can be assessed and the *critical path* – i.e. the sequence of tasks that need to be completed on time in order to avoid an overall delay – defined. In Figure 15.2 the process has been reduced to a bare minimum to allow representation on a single page; in practice, each of the 'tasks' shown (e.g. develop formulations, perform Phase I studies etc.) needs to be further subdivided into a series of subtasks and timings to enable the project to be planned and monitored at the operational level. The complete diagram for a typical drug development project will be of such size and complexity as to frighten all but the most hardened project management profes-

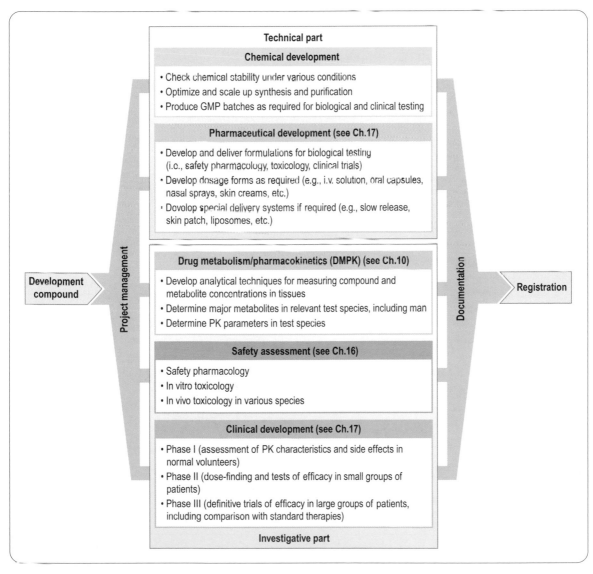

Fig. 15.1
The main technical and investigative components of a typical drug development project.

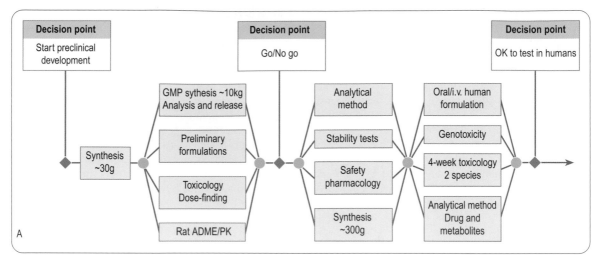

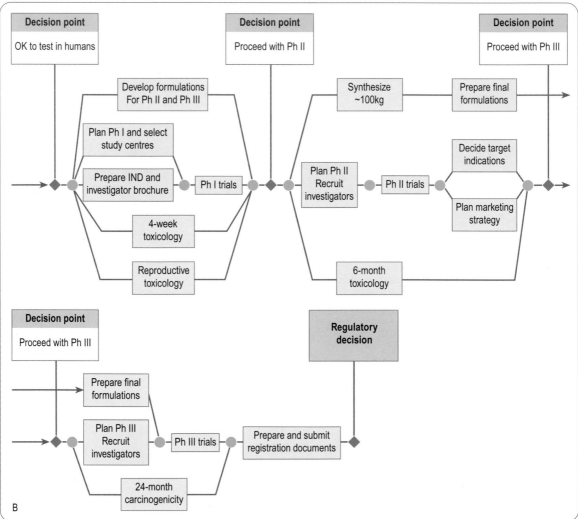

Fig. 15.2

Simplified flowchart showing the main activities involved in drug development. The nodes indicated by circles represent the start and finish points of each activity, and the diagram indicates which activities need to be completed before the next can begin. By assigning timescales to each activity, the planned overall development time can be determined and critical path activities identified. (A) Preclinical development. (B) Clinical development.

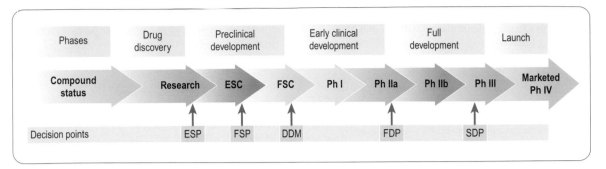

Fig 15.3
Strategic decision points in drug development. ESP, early selection point; FSP, final selection point; DDM, decision to develop in man; FDP, full development; SDP, submission decision point.

sionals. Software tools, fortunately, are available which allow the project to be viewed in different ways, such as Gantt charts, which are barcharts set against a calendar timescale, showing the expected start and completion dates for each task, many of which will be running simultaneously on any given date[1].

In this section of the book we outline the main technical and experimental parts of the work that goes into drug development, namely toxicology, pharmaceutical development and clinical studies. Chapter 19 discusses the principles underlying the patenting of drugs. Chapter 20 describes how regulatory bodies go about evaluating new compounds for registration, and Chapter 21 presents an introduction to the principles of pharmaceutical marketing. Chemical development, covering the specialized technical aspects of producing the drug substance economically and safely on a large scale, as well as the control measures needed to ensure consistent high quality of the final product, is beyond the scope of this book (see Repic, 1998, for a full account of this subject).

pharmacokinetic, toxicological or stability problems. Whereas in vitro tests of absorption and metabolism were traditionally performed on individual compounds during the development phase, they are now being incorporated into medium-throughput screens in the discovery phase (Chapter 10), as are in vitro toxicity tests. Formulation work also often begins during the discovery phase, particularly if the characteristics of the lead compounds suggest that specialized formulations are likely to be required for use in pharmacological profiling of compounds in vivo. Furthermore, the selection of one compound for development will often be deferred until data from Phase I trials have been obtained. Thus, the preliminary work needed before Phase I, and the Phase I trials themselves, will need to be performed on a group of candidate compounds. This is clearly more expensive than choosing the development compound before Phase I, but may be justified as a strategy for reducing the risk of failure.

The interface between discovery and development

For the purposes of this book, drug development is presented as an operation separate from discovery and following on from it, but the distinction is actually not clear-cut. Increasingly, as has been stressed in Chapters 9 and 10, activities previously undertaken during development are taking place earlier, as an integral part of the discovery process. The emphasis on the 'druggability' of leads (Chapter 9) reflects a concern for focusing on structures that are least likely to have unsatisfactory

Decision points

The decision to advance a drug candidate into early development is the first of several key strategic decision points in the history of the drug development project. The timing, nomenclature and decision-making process vary from company to company, and Figure 15.3 shows a typical scheme, developed by Novartis.

● The early selection point (ESP) is the decision to take the drug candidate molecule into early (preclinical) development. The proposal will normally be framed by the drug discovery team and evaluated by a research committee, which determines whether the criteria to justify further development have been met. After this checkpoint, responsibility normally passes to a multidisciplinary team with representatives from research, various development functions, patents, regulatory affairs and marketing, under the

---

[1] In Robert Burns' words 'The best-laid plans of mice and men gang aft agley' Drug development is no exception to this principle – managers prefer the euphemism 'slippage'.

direction of a professional project manager. In a large multinational company the team will have international representation, and the development plan will be organized to meet global development standards as far as possible.

- The decision to develop in man (DDM) controls entry of the compound into Phase I, based on the additional information obtained during the preclinical development phase (i.e. preliminary toxicology, safety pharmacology, pharmacokinetics etc.). An important task once this decision point is passed is normally the production of a sufficient quantity (usually 2–5 kg) of clinical-grade material. Passing this decision point takes the project into Phase I and Phase IIa clinical studies, described in more detail in Chapter 18, which are designed to reveal whether the drug has an acceptable pharmacokinetic and side-effect profile in normal volunteers (Phase I), and whether it shows evidence of clinical efficacy in patients (Phase IIa). For drugs acting by novel mechanisms, Phase IIa provides the all-important first 'proof of concept', on which the decision whether or not to proceed with the serious business of full development largely rests[2].
- The full development decision point (FDP) is reached after the Phase I and Phase IIa ('proof-of-concept') studies have been completed, this being the first point at which evidence of clinical efficacy in man is obtained. It is at this point that the project becomes seriously expensive in terms of money and manpower, and has to be evaluated strictly in competition with other projects. Evaluation of the likely commercial returns, as well as the chances of successful registration and the time and cost of the 'pivotal' Phase III studies, are therefore important considerations at this point.
- The submission decision point (SDP) is the final decision to apply for registration, based on a check that the amount and quality of the data submitted are sufficient to ensure a smooth passage through

the regulatory process. Hold-ups in registration can carry serious penalties in terms of the cost and time required to perform additional clinical studies, as well as loss of confidence among financial analysts, who will have been primed to expect a new product to bring in revenues according to the plan as originally envisaged.

A couple of aphorisms are often applied to drug development, namely:

- In research, surprise = discovery; in development, surprise = disaster.
- It is as valuable to stop a project as to carry one forward.

Like most aphorisms they contain a grain of truth, but only a small one. With regard to the first, equating surprise with disaster applies, if at all, only to the technical parts of development, not to the investigational parts, which are, as discussed above, a continuation of research into the properties of the drug. Surprises in this arena can be good or bad for the outcome of the project. Finding, to the company's surprise, that sildenafil (Viagra) improved the sex life of trial subjects, set the development project off in a completely new, and very successful, direction.

The value attached to stopping projects reflects the frustration – commonly felt in large research organizations – that projects that have little chance of ending in success tend to carry on, swallowing resources, through sheer inertia, sustained mainly by the reluctance of individuals to abandon work to which they may have devoted many years of effort. In practice, of course, the value of stopping a project depends only on the possibility of redeploying the resources to something more useful, i.e. on the 'opportunity cost'. If the resources used cannot be redeployed, or if no better project can be identified, there is no value in stopping the project. What is certain is that it is only by carrying projects forward that success can be achieved. Despite the aphorism, it is no surprise that managers who regularly lead projects into oblivion achieve much less favourable recognition than those who bring them to fruition!

---

[2]The division of Phase II clinical trials, which are exploratory tests involving relatively small numbers of patients (100–300), and lack the statistical power of the later 'pivotal' Phase III trials, into two stages (a and b) is a fairly recent idea, now widely adopted. Phase IIa is essentially a quick look to see whether the drug administered in a dose selected on the basis of pharmacokinetic, pharmacodynamic and toxicological data has any worthwhile therapeutic effect. Phase IIb, also on small numbers, is aimed at refining the dosage schedule to optimize the therapeutic benefit, and to determine the dosage to be tested in the large-scale, definitive Phase II trials. It marks the beginning of full development, following the key decision (FDP) whether to proceed or stop. For the discovery team, the outcome of Phase IIa largely determines whether they throw their hats in the air or retire to lick their wounds.

The need for improvement

As emphasized elsewhere in this book, innovative new drugs are not being registered as fast as the spectacular developments in biomedical science in the last decades of the 20th century had led the world to expect. The rate of new drug approvals in recent years has shown a disheartening decline and little sign of the anticipated surge (see Figures 1.3 and 22.1), despite a steadily rising R&D spend. This worrying problem has been analysed in a 2004 report by the FDA, which lays the blame firmly on the failure of the development process to keep up with advances in biomedicine. The report comments: '….the applied sciences needed for medical product development have not kept pace with the tremendous advances in the basic sciences.' The report points to a historical success rate (i.e. chance of reaching the market) of new compounds entering Phase I clinical trials of 14%, and comments that this figure did not improve between 1985 and 2000. Furthermore, a recent analysis cited in this report shows that the cost of development, per compound registered, almost doubled in 2000–2002 compared with 1995–2000, whereas the cost of discovery changed very little. In their view, too little effort is being made to develop an improved 'product development toolkit' that places more reliance on early laboratory data, and relies less on animal models and clinical testing in assessing safety and efficacy. The FDA and other regulatory bodies hold a large amount of data which could be used to analyse in a much more systematic way than has so far been done by the predictive value of particular laboratory tests in relation to clinical outcome. New screening technologies and computer modelling approaches need to be brought into the same frame. Currently, extrapolation from laboratory and animal data to the clinical situation relies largely on biological intuition – it is assumed, for example, that a compound that does not cause hepatotoxicity in animals is unlikely to do so in man – but there may well be cheaper and quicker tests that would be at least as predictive. There are many other examples, in the FDA's view, where new technologies offer the possibility of replacing or improving existing procedures, with substantial savings of money and time. The task is beyond the capabilities of any one pharmaceutical company, but needs collaboration and funding at the national or international level.

The remaining chapters in this section give a simple overview of the main activities involved in drug development. Griffin and O'Grady (2002) describe the drug development process in more detail.

References

FDA Report (2004) Innovation stagnation: challenge and opportunity on the critical path to new medical products. www.fda.gov/oc/initiatives/criticalpath/whitepaper.html

Griffin JP, O'Grady JO (2002) The textbook of pharmaceutical medicine, 4th edn. London: BMJ Books.

Repic O (1998) Principles of process research and chemical development in the pharmaceutical industry. New York: John Wiley.

16 Assessing drug safety

H P Rang

Introduction

Since the thalidomide disaster, ensuring that new medicines are safe when used therapeutically has been one of the main responsibilities of regulatory agencies. Of course, there is no such thing as 100% safety, much as the public would like reassurance of this. Any medical intervention – or for that matter, any human activity – carries risks as well as benefits, and the aim of drug safety assessment is to ensure, as far as possible, that the risks are commensurate with the benefits.

Safety is addressed at all stages in the life history of a drug, from the earliest stages of design, through preclinical investigations (discussed in this chapter) and preregistration clinical trials (Chapter 18), to the entire post-marketing history of the drug. The ultimate test comes only after the drug has been marketed and used in a clinical setting in many thousands of patients, during the period of Phase IV clinical trials (post-marketing surveillance). It is unfortunately not uncommon for drugs to be withdrawn for safety reasons after being in clinical use for some time (for example *practolol*, because of a rare but dangerous oculomucocutaneous reaction, *troglitazone* because of liver damage, *cerivastatin* because of skeletal muscle damage, *terfenadine* because of drug interactions, *rofecoxib* because of heart attacks), reflecting the fact that safety assessment is fallible. It always will be fallible, because there are no bounds to what may emerge as harmful effects. Can we be *sure* that drug X will not cause kidney damage in a particular inbred tribe in a remote part of the world? The answer is, of course, 'no', any more than we could have been sure that various antipsychotic drugs – now withdrawn – would not cause sudden cardiac deaths through a hitherto unsuspected mechanism, hERG channel block (see later). What is not hypothesized cannot be tested. For this reason, the problem of safety assessment is fundamentally different from that of efficacy assessment, where we can define exactly what we are looking for.

Here we focus on non-clinical safety assessment – often called preclinical, even though much of the work is done in parallel with clinical development. We describe the various types of in vitro and in vivo tests that are used to predict adverse and toxic effects in humans, and which form an important part of the data submitted to the regulatory authorites when approval is sought (a) for the new compound to be administered to humans for the first time (IND approval in the USA; see Chapter 20), and (b) for permission to market the drug (NDA approval in the USA, MAA approval in Europe; see Chapter 20).

The programme of preclinical safety assessment for a new synthetic compound can be divided into the following main chronological phases, linked to the clinical trials programme (Figure 16.1):

● *Exploratory toxicology*, aimed at giving a rough quantitative estimate of the toxicity of the compound when given acutely or repeatedly over a short period (normally 2 weeks), and providing an indication of the main organs and physiological systems involved. These studies provide information for the guidance of the project team in making further plans, but are not normally part of the regulatory package that has to be approved before the drug can be given to humans, so they do not need to be perfomed under good laboratory practice (GLP) conditions.

● *Regulatory toxicology*. These studies are performed to GLP standards and comprise (a) those that are required by regulatory authorities, or by ethics committees, before the compound can be given for the first time to humans; (b) studies required to support an application for marketing approval, which are normally performed in parallel with clinical trials. Full reports of all studies of this kind are included in documentation submitted to the regulatory authorities.

Regulatory toxicology studies in group (a) include 28-day repeated-dose toxicology studies in two species (including one non-rodent, usually dog), in vitro and in vivo genoxocity tests, safety pharmacology and reproductive toxicity assessment. In vitro genotoxicity tests, which are cheap and quick to perform, will often have been performed much earlier in the compound selection phase of the project, as may safety pharmacology studies.

The nature of the tests in group (b) depends greatly on the nature and intended use of the drug, but they will include chronic 3–12-month toxicological studies in two or more species, long-term (18–24 months) carcinogenicity tests and reproductive toxicology, and often interaction studies involving other drugs that are likely to be used for the same indications.

The basic procedures for safety assessment of a single new synthetic compound are fairly standard, although the regulatory authorities have avoided applying a defined checklist of tests and criteria required for regulatory approval. Instead they issue guidance notes (available on relevant websites – USA: www.fda.gov/cder/; EU: www.emea.eu.int; draft international guidelines: www.ich.org), but the onus is on the pharmaceutical company to anticipate and exclude any unwanted effects based on the specific chemistry, pharmacology and intended therapeutic use of the compound in question.

There are many types of new drug applications that do not fall into the standard category of synthetic small molecules, where the safety assessment standards are different. These include most biopharmaceuticals (see

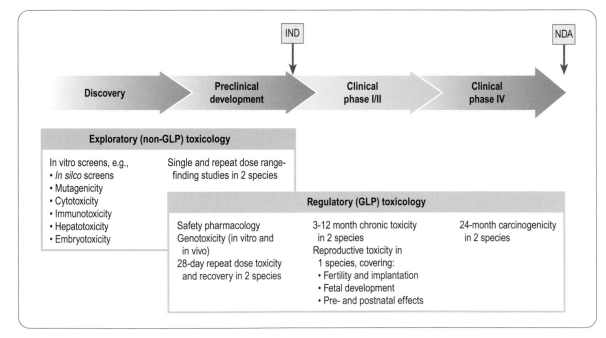

Fig. 16.1
Timing of the main safety assessment studies during drug discovery and development.

Chapter 12), as well as vaccines, cell and gene therapy products (see below). Drug combinations, and non-standard delivery systems and routes of administration, are also examples of special cases where safety assessment requirements differ from those used for conventional drugs. These special cases are not discussed in detail here; Gad (2002) gives a comprehensive account.

Types of adverse drug effect

Adverse reactions in man are of four general types:

- Exaggerated pharmacological effects – sometimes referred to as *hyperpharmacology* – which are dose related and in general predictable on the basis of the principal pharmacological effect of the drug. Examples include hypoglycaemia caused by antidiabetic drugs, hypokalaemia induced by diuretics, immunosuppression in response to steroids, etc.
- Pharmacological effects associated with targets other than the principal one – covered by the general term *side effects*. Examples include hypotension produced by various antipsychotic drugs which block adrenoceptors as well as dopamine receptors (their principal target), and cardiac arrythmias associated with hERG-channel inhibition (see below). Many drugs inhibit one or more forms of cytochrome P450, and hence affect the metabolism of other drugs. Provided the pharmacological profile of the compound is known in sufficient detail, effects of this kind are also predictable.
- Dose-related *toxic effects* that are unrelated to the intended pharmacological effects of the drug. Commonly such effects, which include toxic effects on liver, kidney, endocrine glands, immune cells and other systems, are produced not by the parent drug, but by chemically reactive metabolites. Examples include the gum hyperplasia produced by the antiepileptic drug phenytoin, hearing loss caused by aminoglycoside antibiotics, and peripheral neuropathy caused by thalidomide[1]. Genotoxicity and reproductive toxicity (see below) also fall into this category. Such adverse effects are not, in general, predictable from the pharmacological profile of the compound. It is well known that certain chemical structures are

associated with toxicity, and so these will generally be eliminated early in the lead identification stage. The main function of toxicological studies in drug development is to detect dose-related toxic effects of this unpredictable nature.

- Rare, and sometimes serious, adverse effects, known as *idiosyncratic reactions*, that occur in certain individuals and are not dose related. Many examples have come to light among drugs that have entered clinical use, e.g. aplastic anaemia produced by *chloramphenicol*, anaphylactic responses to *penicillin*, oculomucocutaneous syndrome with *practolol*, bone marrow depression with *clozapine*. Toxicological tests in animals rarely reveal such effects, and because they may occur in only one in several thousand humans they are likely to remain undetected in clinical trials, coming to light only after the drug has been registered and given to thousands of patients. (The reaction to clozapine is an exception. It affects about 1% of patients and was detected in early clinical trials. The bone marrow effect, though potentially life-threatening, is reversible, and clozapine was successfully registered, with a condition that patients receiving it must be regularly monitored.)

Safety pharmacology testing and *dose range-finding studies* are designed to detect pharmacological adverse effects; *chronic toxicology testing* is designed to detect dose-related toxic effects, as well as the long-term consequences of pharmacological side effects; idiosyncratic reactions may be revealed in Phase III clinical trials, but are likely to remain undetected until the compound enters clinical use.

Safety pharmacology

The pharmacological studies described in Chapter 11 are exploratory (i.e. surveying the effects of the compound with respect to selectivity against a wide range of possible targets) or hypothesis driven (checking whether the expected effects of the drug, based on its target selectivity, are actually produced). In contrast, safety pharmacology comprises a series of protocol-driven studies, aimed specifically at detecting possible undesirable or dangerous effects of exposure to the drug in therapeutic doses (see ICH Guideline S7A). The emphasis is on acute effects produced by single-dose administration, as distinct from toxicology studies, which focus mainly on the effects of chronic exposure. Safety pharmacology evaluation forms an important part of the dossier submitted to the regulatory authorities.

ICH Guideline S7A defines a *core battery* of safety pharmacology tests, and a series of *follow-up* and *supplementary tests* (Table 16.1). The core battery is normally

---

[1]This notorious drug is undergoing a therapeutic revival in the treatment of myeloma, a serious type of bone marrow cancer, progressive muscle weakness and sensory loss due to peripheral neuropathy being the most common and troublesome side effects.

Drug development

performed on all compounds intended for systemic use. Where they are not appropriate (e.g. for preparations given topically) their omission has to be justified on the basis of information about the extent of systemic exposure that may occur when the drug is given by the intended route. Follow-up studies are required if the core battery of tests reveals effects whose mechanism needs to be determined. Supplementary tests need to be performed if the known chemistry or pharmacology of the compound gives any reason to expect that it may produce side effects (e.g. a compound with a thiazide-like structure should be tested for possible inhibition of insulin secretion, this being a known side effect of thiazide diuretics; similarly, an opiate needs to be tested for dependence liability and effects on gastrointestinal motility). Where there is a likelihood of significant drug interactions, this may also need to be tested as part of the supplementary programme.

The core battery of tests listed in Table 16.1 focuses on acute effects on cardiovascular, respiratory and

Table 16.1
Safety pharmacology

Type	Physiological system	Tests

Core battery	Central nervous system	Observations on conscious animals
		    Motor activity
		    Behavioural changes
		    Coordination
		    Reflex responses
		    Body temperature

	Cardiovascular system	Measurements on anaesthetized animals
		    Blood pressure
		    Heart rate
		    ECG changes
		    Tests for delayed ventricular repolarization (see text)

	Respiratory system	Measurements on anaesthetized or conscious animals
		    Respiratory rate
		    Tidal volume
		    Arterial oxygen saturation

Follow-up tests (examples)	Central nervous system	Tests on learning and memory More complex test for changes in behaviour and motor function Tests for visual and auditory function
	Cardiovascular system	Cardiac output Ventricular contractility Vascular resistance Regional blood flow
	Respiratory system	Airways resistance and compliance Pulmonary arterial pressure Blood gases
Supplementary tests (examples)	Renal function	Urine volume, osmolality, pH Proteinuria Blood urea/creatinine Fluid/electrolyte balance Urine cytology
	Autonomic nervous system	Cardiovascular, gastrointestinal and respiratory system responses to agonists and stimulation of autonomic nerves
	Gastrointestinal system	Gastric secretion Gastric pH Intestinal motility Gastrointestinal transit time
	Other systems (e.g. endocrine, blood coagulation, skeletal muscle function etc.)	Tests designed to detect likely acute effects.

nervous systems, based on standard physiological measurements.

The follow-up and supplementary tests are less clearly defined, and the list given in Table 16.1 is neither prescriptive nor complete. It is the responsibility of the team to decide what tests are relevant and how the studies should be performed, and to justify these decisions in the submission to the regulatory authority.

Tests for QT interval prolongation

The ability of a number of therapeutically used drugs to cause a potentially fatal ventricular arrhythmia ('torsade de pointes') has recently been a cause of major concern to clinicians and regulatory authorities (see Committee for Proprietary Medicinal Products, 1997; Haverkamp et al., 2000). The arrhythmia is associated with prolongation of the ventricular action potential (delayed ventricular repolarization), reflected in ECG recordings as prolongation of the QT interval. Drugs known to possess this serious risk, many of which have been withdrawn, include several *tricyclic antidepressants*, some antipsychotic drugs (e.g. *thioridazine, droperidol*), antidysrhythmic drugs (e.g. *amiodarone, quinidine, disopyramide*), antihistamines (*terfenadine, astemizole*) and certain antimalarial drugs (e.g. *halofantrine*). The main mechanism responsible appears to be inhibition of the potassium channel, termed the hERG channel, which plays a major role in terminating the ventricular action potential (Netzer et al., 2001).

Screening tests have shown that QT interval prolongation is a common property of 'drug-like' small molecules, and the patterns of structure–activity relationships have revealed particular chemical classes associated with this effect. Ideally, these are taken into account and avoided at an early stage in drug design, but the need remains for functional testing of all candidate drug molecules as a prelude to tests in humans.

Proposed standard tests for QT interval prolongation have been formulated as ICH Guideline S7B. They comprise (a) testing for inhibition of hERG channel currents in cell lines engineered to express the hERG gene; (b) measurements of action potential duration in myocardial cells from different parts of the heart in different species; and (c) measurements of QT interval in ECG recordings in conscious animals. These studies are usually carried out on ferrets or guinea pigs, as well as larger mammalian species, such as dog, rabbit, pig or monkey, in which hERG-like channels control ventricular repolarization, rather than in rat and mouse. In vivo tests for proarrhythmic effects in various species are being developed (De Clerck et al., 2002), but have not yet been evaluated for regulatory purposes.

Because of the importance of drug-induced QT prolongation in man, and the fact that many diverse groups of drugs appear to have this property, there is a need for high-throughput screening for hERG channel inhibition to be incorporated early in a drug discovery project. The above methods are not suitable for high-throughput screening, but alternative methods, such as inhibition of binding of labelled *dofetilide* (a potent hERG-channel blocker), or fluorimetric membrane potential assays on cell lines expressing these channels, can be used in high-throughput formats. Such assays are now becoming widely used, though neither is reliably predictive of a lack of QT prolongation in functional tests.

Exploratory (dose range-finding) toxicology studies

The first stage of toxicological evaluation usually takes the form of a *dose range-finding study* in a rodent and/or a non-rodent species. The species commonly used in toxicology are mice, rats, guinea pigs, hamsters, rabbits, dogs, minipigs and non-human primates. Usually two species (rat and mouse) are tested initially, but others may be used if there are reasons for thinking that the drug may exert species-specific effects. A single dose is given to each test animal, preferably by the intended route of administration in the clinic, and in a formulation shown by previous pharmacokinetic studies to produce satisfactory absorption and duration of action. Generally, widely spaced doses (e.g. 10, 100, 1000 mg/kg) will be tested first, on groups of three to four rodents, and the animals will be observed over 14 days for obvious signs of toxicity. Alternatively, a *dose escalation* protocol may be used, in which each animal is treated with increasing doses of the drug at intervals (e.g. every 2 days) until signs of toxicity appear, or until a dose of 2000 mg/kg is reached. With either protocol, the animals are killed at the end of the experiment and autopsied to determine which target organs are grossly affected. The results of such dose range-finding studies provide a rough estimate of the *no toxic effect level* (NTEL, see Toxicity Measures, below) in the species tested, and the nature of the gross effects seen is often a useful pointer to the main target tissues and organs.

The dose range-finding study will normally be followed by a more detailed single-dose toxicological study in two or more species, the doses tested being chosen to span the estimated NTEL. Usually four or five doses will be tested, ranging from a dose in the expected therapeutic range to doses well above the estimated NTEL. A typical protocol for such an acute toxicity study is shown in Figure 16.2. The data collected consist of regular systematic assessment of the animals for a range of clinical signs on the basis of a standardized

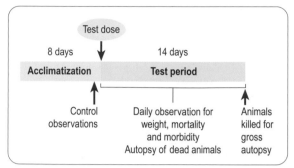

Test dose

8 days	14 days
Acclimatization	**Test period**

Control observations | Daily observation for weight, mortality and morbidity | Animals killed for gross autopsy
Autopsy of dead animals

Fig. 16.2
Typical protocal for single-dose toxicity study.

checklist, together with gross autopsy findings of animals dying during a 2-week observation period, or killed at the end. The main signs that are monitored are shown in Table 16.2.

Single-dose studies are followed by a multiple dose-ranging study in which the drug is given daily or twice daily, normally for 2 weeks, with the same observation and autopsy procedure as in the single-dose study, in order to give preliminary information about the toxicity after chronic treatment.

The results of these preliminary in vivo toxicity studies will help in the planning and design of the next

Table 16.2
Clinical observations in acute toxicity tests

System	Observation	Signs of toxicity
Nervous system	Behaviour	Sedation Restlessness Aggression
	Motor function	Twitch Tremor Ataxia Catatonia Convulsions Muscle rigidity or flaccidity
	Sensory function	Excessive or diminished response to stimuli
Respiratory	Respiration	Increased or decreased respiratory rate Intermittent respiration Dyspnoea
Cardiovascular	Cardiac palpation	Increase or decrease in rate or force
	?Electrocardiography	Disturbances of rhythm. Altered ECG pattern (e.g. QT prolongation)
Gastrointestinal	Faeces	Diarrhoea or constipation Abnormal form or colour Bleeding
	Abdomen	Spasm or tenderness
Genitourinary	Genitalia	Swelling, inflammation, discharge, bleeding
Skin and fur		Discoloration Lesions Piloerection
Mouth		Discharge Congestion Bleeding
Eye	Pupil size	Mydriasis or miosis
	Eyelids	Ptosis, exophthalmos
	Movements	Nystagmus
	Cornea	Opacity
General signs	Body weight	Weight loss
	Body temperature	Increase or decrease

steps of the development programme; they will also help to decide whether or not it is worthwhile to continue the research effort on a given chemical class.

As mentioned above, these toxicology studies are preliminary, and usually they are not sufficient for supporting the first human evaluation of the medicine. Very often, they are not conducted under good laboratory practice (GLP) conditions, nor are they conducted with test material which has been produced according to good manufacturing practice (GMP).

Subsequent work is guided by regulatory requirements elaborated by the International Conference of Harmonization or by national regulatory authorities. Their published guidelines specify/recommend the type of toxicological evaluation needed to support applications for carrying out studies in humans. These documents provide guidance for example on the duration of administration, on the design of the toxicological study, including the number of animals to be studied, and stipulate that the work must be carried out under GLP conditions and that the test material must be of GMP standard. The test substance for the toxicology evaluation has to be identical in terms of quality and characteristics to the substance given to humans.

Genotoxicity

Foreign substances can affect gene function in various ways, the two most important types of mechanism in relation to toxicology being:

- *Mutagenicity*, i.e. chemical alteration of DNA sufficient to cause abnormal gene expression in the affected cell and its offspring. Most commonly, the mutation arises as a result of covalent modification of individual bases (point mutations). The result may be the production of an abnormal protein if the mutation occurs in the coding region of the gene, or altered expression levels of a normal protein if the mutation affects control sequences. Such mutations occur continuously in everyday life, and are counteracted more or less effectively by a variety of DNA repair mechanisms. They are important particularly because certain mutations can interfere with mechanisms controlling cell division, and thereby lead to malignancy or, in the immature organism, to adverse effects on growth and development. In practice, most carcinogens are mutagens, though by no means all mutagens are carcinogens. Evidence of mutagenicity therefore sounds a warning of possible carcinogenicity, which must be tested by thorough in vivo tests.
- *Chromosomal damage*, for example chromosome breakage (clastogenesis), chromosome fusion,

translocation of stretches of DNA within or between chromosomes, replication or deletion of chromosomes etc. Such changes result from alterations in DNA, more extensive than point mutations and less well understood mechanistically; they have a similar propensity to cause cancerous changes and to affect growth and development.

The most important end results of genotoxicity – carcinogenesis and impairment of fetal development (teratogenicity) – can only be detected by long-term animal studies. There is therefore every reason to pre-screen compounds by in vitro methods, and such studies are routinely carried out before human studies begin. Because in many cases the genotoxicity is due to reactive metabolites rather than to the parent molecule, the in vitro tests generally include assays carried out in the presence of liver microsomes or other liver-derived preparations, so that metabolites are generated. Often, liver microsomes from rats treated with inducing agents (e.g. a mixture of chlorinated biphenyls known as Arochlor 1254) are used, in order to enhance drug metabolizing activity.

Selection and interpretation of tests

Many in vitro and in vivo test systems for mutagenicity have been described, based on bacteria, yeast, insect and mammalian cells (see Gad, 2002 for details). The ICH Guidelines S2A and S2B, stipulate a preliminary battery of three tests:

- *Ames test: a test of mutagenicity in bacteria*. The basis of the assay is that mutagenic substances increase the rate at which a histidine-dependent strain of *Salmonella typhimurium* reverts to a wild type that can grow in the absence of histidine. An increase in the number of colonies surviving in the absence of histidine therefore denotes significant mutagenic activity. Several histidine-dependent strains of the organism which differ in their susceptibility to particular types of mutagen are normally tested in parallel. Positive controls with known mutagens that act directly or only after metabolic activation are routinely included when such tests are performed.
- *An in vitro test for chromosomal abnormalities in mammalian cells or an in vitro mouse lymphoma tk cell assay*. To test chromosomal damage Chinese hamster ovary (CHO) cells are grown in culture in the presence of the test substance, with or without liver microsomes. Cell division is arrested in metaphase, and chromosomes are observed

microscopically to detect structural aberrations, such as gaps, duplications, fusions or alterations in chromosome number. The mouse lymphoma cell test for mutagenicity involves a heterozygous (*tk* +/−) cell line that can be killed by the cytotoxic agent BrDU. Mutation to the *tk* −/− form causes the cells to become resistant to BrDU, and so counts of surviving cells in cutures treated with the test compound provide an index of mutagenicity. The mouse lymphoma cell mutation assay is more sensitive than the chromosomal assay, but can give positive results with non-carcinogenic substances. These tests are not possible with compounds that are inherently toxic to mammalian cells.

- *An in vivo test for chromosomal damage in rodent haemopoietic cells.* The mouse micronucleus test is commonly used. Animals are treated with the test compound for 2 days, after which immature erythrocytes in bone marrow are examined for micronuclei, representing fragments of damaged chromosomes.

If these three tests prove negative, no further tests of genotoxicity are generally needed before the compound can be tested in humans. If one or more is positive, further in vitro and in vivo genotoxicity testing will usually be carried out to assess more accurately the magnitude of the risk. In a few cases, where the medical need is great and the life expectancy of the patient population is very limited, development of compounds that are clearly genotoxic – and, by inference, possibly carcinogenic – may still be justified, but in most cases genotoxic compounds will be abandoned without further ado.

Whereas early toxicological evaluation emcompasses acute and subacute types of study, the full safety assessement is based on subchronic and chronic studies. The focus is more on the harmful effects of long-term exposure to 'low' doses of the agent. The chronic toxic effects can be very different from the acute toxic effects, and could accumulate over time. Three main categories of toxicological study are required according to the regulatory guidelines, namely chronic toxicity, special tests and toxicokinetic analysis.

Chronic toxicology studies

The object of these studies is to look for toxicities that appear after repetitive dosing of the compound, when a steady state is achieved, i.e. when the rate of drug administration equals the rate of elimination. In long-term toxicity studies three or more dose levels are tested, in addition to a vehicle control. The doses will include one that is clearly toxic, one in the thera-peutic range, and at least one in between. Ideally, the in-between doses will exceed the expected clinical dose by a factor of 10 for rodents and 5 for non-rodents, yet lack overt toxicity, this being the 'window' normally required by regulatory authorities. At least one recovery group is usually included, i.e. animals treated with the drug at a toxic level and then allowed to recover for 2–4 weeks so that the reversibility of the changes observed can be assessed. The aim of these studies is to determine (a) the cumulative biological effects produced by the compound, and (b) at what exposure level (see below) they appear. The initial repeated-dose studies, by revealing the overall pattern of toxic effects produced, also give pointers to particular aspects (e.g. liver toxicity, bone marrow depression) that may need to be addressed later in more detailed toxicological investigations.

The standard procedures discussed here are appropriate for the majority of conventional synthetic compounds intended for systemic use. Where drugs are intended only for topical use (skin creams, eye drops, aerosols etc.) the test procedures are modified accordingly. Special considerations apply also to biopharmacaceutical preparations, and these are discussed briefly below.

Experimental design

Chronic toxicity testing must be performed under GLP conditions, with the formulation and route of administration to be used in humans. Tests are normally carried out on one rodent (usually rat) and one non-rodent species (usually dog), but additional species (such as monkey or pig) may be tested if there are special reasons for suspecting that their responses may predict effects in man more accurately than those of dogs. Pharmaco-kinetic measurements are included, so that extrapolation to humans can be done on the basis of the concentration of the drug in blood and tissues, allowing for differences in pharmacokinetics between laboratory animals and humans. Separate male and female test groups are used. The recommended number of animals per test group (see Gad, 2002) is shown in Table 16.3. There are strong reasons for minimizing the number of animals used in such studies, and the figures given take this into account, representing the minimum shown by experience to be needed for statistically reliable conclusions to be drawn. An average study will require 200 or more rats and about 60 dogs, dosed with compound and observed regularly, including blood and urine sampling, for several months before being killed and autopsied, with tissue samples being collected for histological examination. It is a massive and costly experiment requiring large amounts of compound prepared to GMP standards, the conduct and results of which will receive detailed scrutiny by regulatory authorities, and so careful planning and scrupulous execution are essential.

Table 16.3
Recommended numbers of animals for chronic toxicity studies (Gad, 2002)

Study duration	Rats (per sex)	Dogs (per sex)	Primates (per sex)
4 weeks	5–10	3–4	3
3 months	20	6	5
6 months	30	8	5
12 months	50	10	10
2-year (carcinogenicity)	50–80		

Regulatory authorities stipulate the duration of repeat-dose toxicity testing required before the start of clinical testing, the ICH recommendations being summarized in Table 20.1. These requirements can be relaxed for drugs aimed at life-threatening diseases, the spur for this change in attitude coming from the urgent need for anti-HIV drugs during the 1980s. In such special cases chronic toxicity testing is still required, but approval for clinical trials – and indeed for marketing – may be granted before they have been completed.

Evaluation of toxic effects

During the course of the experiment all animals are inspected regularly for mortality and gross morbidity, severely affected animals being killed, and all dead animals subjected to autopsy. Specific signs (e.g. diarrhoea, salivation, respiratory changes etc.) are assessed against a detailed checklist, and specific examinations (e.g. blood pressure, heart rate and ECG, ocular changes, neurological and behavioural changes etc.) are also conducted regularly. Food intake and body weight changes are monitored, and blood and urine samples collected at intervals for biochemical and haematological analysis.

At the end of the experiment all animals are killed and examined by autopsy for gross changes, samples of all major tissues being prepared for histological examination. Tissues from the high-dose group are examined histologically, and any tissues showing pathological changes are also examined in the low-dose groups to enable a dose threshold to be estimated. The reversibility of the adverse effects can be evaluated in these studies by studying animals retained after the end of the dosing period.

As part of the general toxicology screening described above, specific evaluation of possible *immunotoxicity* is required by the regulatory authorities, the main concern being immunosuppression. If effects on blood, spleen or thymus cells are observed in the 1-month repeated-dose

studies, additional tests are required to evaluate the strength of cellular and humoral responses in immunized animals. A battery of suitable tests is included in the FDA Guidance note (2002).

The large body of data collected during a typical toxicology study should allow conclusions to be drawn about the main physiological systems and target organs that underlie the toxicity of the compound, and also about the dose levels at which critical effects are produced. In practice, the analysis and interpretation are not always straightforward, for a variety of reasons, including:

● Incorrect choice of doses;
● Variability within the groups of animals;
● Spontaneous occurrence of 'toxic' effects in control or vehicle-treated animals;
● Missing data, owing to operator error, equipment failure, unexpected death of animals etc.;
● Problems of statistical analysis (qualitative data, multiple comparisons etc.).

Overall, it is estimated that correctly performed chronic toxicity tests in animals successfully predict 70% of toxic reactions in humans (Olson et al., 2000); skin reactions in humans are the least well predicted.

Biopharmaceuticals

Biopharmaceuticals now constitute more than 25% of new drugs being approved. For the most part they are proteins made by recombinant DNA technology, or monoclonal antibodies produced in cell culture. As a rule, proteins tend to be less toxic than synthetic compounds, mainly because they are normally metabolized to smaller peptides and amino acids, rather than to reactive compounds formed from many synthetic compounds, which are the cause of most types of drug toxicity, especially genotoxicity. Biopharmaceuticals are therefore generally less toxic than synthetic compounds. Their unwanted effects are associated mainly with 'hyperpharmacology' (see above), lack of pharmacological specificity, or immunogenicity. Many protein therapeutics are highly species specific. This applies to biological mediators, such as hormones, growth factors, cytokines etc., as well as to monoclonal antibodies. The presence of impurities in biopharmaceutical preparations has an important bearing on safety assessment, as unwanted proteins or other cell constituents are often present as contaminants, and may vary from batch to batch. Quality control presents more problems than with conventional chemical products, and is particularly critical for biopharmaceuticals.

The safety assessment of new biopharmaceuticals is discussed in ICH Guidance Note S6. The main aspects that differ from the guidelines relating to conventional drugs are: (1) careful attention to choice of appropriate species; (2) no need for routine genotoxicity and carcinogenicity testing (though carcinogenicity testing may be required in the case of mediators, such as growth factors, which may regulate cell proliferation); and (3) specific tests for immunogenicity, expressed as sensitization, or the development of neutralizing antibodies.

Newer types of biopharmaceuticals, such as DNA- and cell-based therapies (see Chapter 3), pose special questions in relation to safety assessment (see FDA Guidance Note, 1998). Particular concerns arise from the use of genetically engineered viral vectors in gene therapy, which can induce immune responses and in some cases retain potential infectivity. The possibility that genetically engineered foreign cells might undergo malignant transformation is a further worrisome risk. These specialized topics are not discussed further here.

Special tests

In addition to the the general toxicological risks addressed by the testing programme discussed above, the risks of carcinogenicity and effects on reproduction (particularly on fertility and on pre- and postnatal development) may be of particular concern, requiring special tests to be performed.

Carcinogenicity testing

Carcinogenicity testing is normally required before a compound can be marketed – though not before the start of clinical trials – if the drug is likely to be used in treatment continuously for 6 months or more, or intermittently for long periods. It is also required if there are special causes for concern, for example if:

- The compound belongs to a known class of carcinogens, or has chemical features associated with carcinogenicity; nowadays such compounds will normally have been eliminated at the lead identification stage (see Chapter 9);
- Chronic toxicity studies show evidence of precancerous changes;
- The compound or its metabolites are retained in tissues for long periods.

If a compound proves positive in tests of mutagenicity (see above), it must be *assumed* to be carcinogenic and its use restricted accordingly, so no purpose is served by in vivo carcinogenicity testing. Only in very exceptional cases will such a compound be chosen for development.

ICH Guidelines S1A, S1B and S1C on carcinogenicity testing stipulate one long-term test in a rodent species (usually rat), plus one other in vivo test, which may be either (a) a short-term test designed to show high sensitivity to carcinogens (e.g. transgenic mouse models) or to detect early events associated with tumour initiation or promotion; or (b) a long term carcinogenicity test in a second rodent species (normally mouse). If positive results emerge in either study, the onus is on the pharmaceutical company to provide evidence that carcinogenicity will not be a significant risk to humans in a therapeutic setting. Until recently, the normal requirement was for long-term studies in two rodent species, but advances in the understanding of tumour biology and the availability of new models that allow quicker evaluation have brought about a change in the attitude of regulatory authorities such that only one long-term study is required, together with data from a well-validated short-term study.

Long-term rat carcinogenicity studies normally last for 2 years and are run in parallel with Phase III clinical trials. (Oral contraceptives require a 3-year test for carcinogenicity in beagles.)

Three or four dose levels are tested, plus controls. Typically, the lowest dose tested is close to the maximum recommended human dose, and the highest is the maximum tolerated dose (MTD) in rats (i.e. the largest dose that causes no obvious side effects or toxicity in the chronic toxicity tests). Fifty to 80 animals of each sex are used in each experimental group (see Table 16.3), and so the complete study will require about 600–800 animals. Premature deaths are inevitable in such a large group and can easily ruin the study, so that housing the animals under standard disease-free conditions is essential. At the end of the experiment, samples of about 50 different tissues are prepared for histological examination, and rated for benign and malignant tumour formation by experienced pathologists. Carcinogenicity testing is therefore one of the most expensive and time-consuming components of the toxicological evaluation of a new compound.

Several transgenic mouse models have been developed which provide data more quickly (usually about 6 months) than the normal 2-year carcinogenicity study (Gad, 2002). These include animals in which human proto-oncogenes, such as hRas, are expressed, or the tumour suppressor gene P53 is inactivated. These mice show a very high incidence of spontaneous tumours after about 1 year, but at 6 months spontaneous tumours are rare. Known carcinogens cause tumours to develop in these animals within 6 months.

Advances in this area are occurring rapidly, and as they do so the methodology for carcinogenicity testing is expected to become more sophisticated and faster than the conventional long-term studies used hitherto.

Reproductive/developmental toxicology studies

Two incidents led to greatly increased concern about the effects of drugs on the fetus. The first was the thalidomide disaster of the 1960s. The second was the high incidence of cervical and vaginal cancers in young women whose mothers had been treated with diethylstilbestrol (DES) in early pregnancy with the aim of preventing early abortion. DES was used in this way between 1940 and 1970, and the cancer incidence was reported in 1971. These events led to the introduction of stringent tests for teratogenicity as a prerequisite for the approval of new drugs, and from this flowed concern for other aspects of reproductive toxicology which now must be fully evaluated before a drug is marketed. Current requirements are summarized in ICH Guideline S5A.

Drugs can affect reproductive performance in three main ways:

- Fertility (both sexes, fertilization and implantation), addressed by *Segment 1* studies;
- Embryonic and fetal development or teratology, addressed by *Segment 2* studies;
- Peri- and postnatal development, addressed by *Segment 3* studies.

It is usually acceptable for Phase I human studies on male volunteers to begin before any reproductive toxicology data are available, so long as the drug shows no evidence of testicular damage in 2- or 4-week repeated-dose studies. The requirement for reproductive toxicology data as a prelude to clinical trials differs from country to country, but as a general rule clinical trials involving women of childbearing age should be preceded by relevant reproductive toxicology testing. In all but exceptional cases, such as drugs intended for treating life-threatening diseases, or for use only in the elderly, registration will require comprehensive data from relevant toxicology studies so that the reproductive risk can be assessed.

Segment 1 tests of fertility and implantation involve treating both males (for 28 days) and females (for 14 days) with the drug prior to mating, then measuring sperm count and sperm viability, numbers of implantation sites and live and dead embryos on day 6 of gestation. For drugs that either by design or by accident reduce fertility, tests for reversibility on stopping treatment are necessary.

Segment 2 tests of effects on embryonic and fetal development are usually carried out on two or three species (rat, mouse, rabbit), the drug being given to the female during the initial gestation period (day 6 to day 16 after mating in the rat). Animals are killed just before parturition, and the embryos are counted and assessed for structural abnormalities. In vitro tests involving embryos maintained in culture are also possible. The main stages of early embryogenesis can be observed in this way, and the effects of drugs added to the medium can be monitored. Such in vitro tests are routinely performed in some laboratories, but are currently not recognized by regulatory authorities as a reliable measure of possible teratogenicity.

Segment 3 tests on pre- and perinatal development entail dosing female rats with the drug throughout gestation and lactation. The offspring are observed for motility, reflex responses etc. both during and after the weaning period, and at intervals some are killed for observations of structural abnormalities. Some are normally allowed to mature and are mated, to check for possible second-generation effects. Mature offspring are also tested for effects on learning and memory.

Reproductive and developmental toxicology is a complex field in which standards in relation to pharmaceuticals have not yet been clearly defined. The experimental studies are demanding, and the results may be complicated by species differences, individual variability and 'spontaneous' events in control animals.

It is obvious that any drug given in sufficient doses to cause overt maternal toxicity is very likely to impair fetal development. Non-specific effects, most commonly a reduction in birthweight, are commonly found in animal studies, but provided the margin of safety is sufficient – say 10-fold – between the expected therapeutic dose and that affecting the fetus, this will not be a bar to developing the compound. The main aim of reproductive toxicology is to assess the risk of specific effects occurring within the therapeutic dose range in humans. Many familiar drugs and chemicals are teratogenic in certain species at high doses. They include *penicillin, sulfonamides, tolbutamide, diphenylhydantoin, valproate, imipramine, acetazolamide, ACE inhibitors* and *angiotensin antagonists*, as well as many *anticancer drugs* and also *caffeine, cannabis* and *ethanol*. Many of these are known or suspected teratogens in humans, and their use in pregnancy is to be avoided.

A classification of drugs based on their safety during pregnancy has been developed by the FDA (A, B, C, D or X). Category A is for drugs considered safe in human pregnancy, that is, adequate and well-controlled studies in pregnant women have failed to demonstrate a risk to the fetus in any trimester of pregnancy. Few drugs belong to this category. Category X is reserved for drugs (e.g. *isotretinoin, warfarin*) that have been proved to cause fetal abnormalities in man, and are therefore contraindicated in pregnancy. Category B covers drugs with no evidence of risk in humans; category C covers drugs in which a risk cannot be ruled out; and category D covers drugs with positive evidence of risk.

Other studies

The focus of this chapter is on the core battery of tests routinely used in assessing drug safety at the preclinical level.

In practice, depending on the results obtained from these tests, and on the particular therapeutic application and route of administration intended for the drug, it is nearly always necessary to go further with experimental toxicology studies in specific areas. It must be remembered that the regulatory authorities put the onus firmly on the pharmaceutical company to present a dossier of data that covers all likely concerns about safety. Thus, where toxic effects are observed in animals, evidence must be presented to show either that these are seen only at exposure levels well outside the therapeutic range, or that they involve mechanisms that will not apply in humans. If the compound is observed to cause changes in circulating immune cells, or in lymphoid tissues, further tests for immunosuppression will be needed, as well as studies to determine the mechanism. Potential toxicological problems, not necessarily revealed in basic toxicology testing, must also be anticipated. Thus, if the compound is potentially immunogenic (i.e. it is a peptide or protein, or belongs to a known class of haptens), tests for sensitization will be required. For drugs that are intended for topical administration, local tissue reactions, including allergic sensitization, need to be investigated. For some classes of drugs skin photosensitization will need to be tested.

Interaction toxicology studies may be needed if the patients targeted for the treatment are likely to be taking another medicine whose efficacy or toxicity might be affected by the new therapeutic agent.

In summary, it is essential to plan the toxicology testing programme for each development compound on a case-by-case basis. Although the regulatory authorities stipulate the core battery of tests that need to be performed on every compound, it is up to the development team to anticipate other safety issues that are likely to be of concern, and to address them appropriately with experimental studies. In planning the safety assessment programme for a new drug, companies are strongly advised to consult the regulatory authorities, who are very open to discussion at the planning stage and can advise on a case-by-case basis.

Toxicokinetics

Toxicokinetics is defined in ICH Guideline S3A as 'the generation of pharmacokinetic data, either as an integral component in the conduct of non-clinical toxicity studies, or in specially designed supportive studies, in order to assess systemic exposure'. In essence, this means pharmacokinetics applied to toxicological studies, and the methodology and principles are no different from those of conventional absorption, distribution, metabolism and excretion (ADME) studies. But whereas ADME studies address mainly drug and metabolite *concentrations* in dif-

ferent body compartments as a function of dose and time, toxicokinetics focuses on *exposure*. Although exposure is not precisely defined, the underlying idea is that toxic effects often appear to be a function of both local concentration and time, a low concentration persisting for a long time being as likely to evoke a reaction as a higher but more transient concentration. Depending on the context, exposure can be represented as peak plasma or tissue concentration, or more often as average concentrations over a fixed period. As with conventional pharmacokinetic measurement, attention must be paid to plasma and tissue binding of the drug and its metabolites, as bound material, which may comprise 98% or more of the measured concentration, will generally be pharmacologically and toxicologically inert. The principles of toxicokinetics as applied to preclinical studies are discussed in detail by Baldrick (2003).

Despite the difficulties of measuring and interpreting exposure, toxicokinetic measurements are an essential part of all in vivo toxicological studies. Interspecies comparisons, and extrapolation of animal data to humans, are best done on the basis of measured plasma and tissue concentrations, rather than administered dose, and regulatory authorities require this information to be provided.

As mentioned earlier, the choice of dose for toxicity tests is important, and dose-limiting toxicity should ideally be reached in toxicology studies. This is the reason why the doses administered in these studies are always high, unless a maximum limit based on technical feasibility has been reached.

Toxicity measures

Lethal dose (expressed as LD_{50}, the estimated dose required to kill 50% of a group of experimental animals) has been largely abandoned as a useful measure of toxicity, and no longer needs to be measured for new compounds. Measures commonly used are:

- *No toxic effect level* (NTEL), which is the largest dose in the most sensitive species in a toxicology study of a given duration which produced no observed toxic effect;
- *No observed adverse effect level* (NOAEL), which is the largest dose causing neither observed tissue toxicity nor undesirable physiological effects, such as sedation, seizures or weight loss;
- *Maximum tolerated dose* (MTD), which usually applies to long-term studies and represents the largest dose tested that caused no obvious signs of ill-health;
- *No observed effect level* (NOEL), which represents the threshold for producing any observed pharmacological or toxic effect.

The estimated NTEL in the most sensitive species is normally used to determine the starting dose used in the first human trials. The safety factor applied may vary from 100 to 1000, depending on the information available, the type and severity of toxicities observed in animals, and whether these anticipated toxicities can be monitored by non-invasive techniques in man.

Variability in responses

The response to a given dose of a drug is likely to vary when it is given to different individuals, or even to the same individual on different occasions. Factors such as age, sex, disease state, degree of nutrition/malnutrition, co-administration of other drugs and genetic variations may influence drug response and toxicity. As elderly people have reduced renal and hepatic function they may metabolize and excrete drugs more slowly, and therefore may require lower doses of medication than younger people. In addition, because of multiple illnesses elderly people often may be less able than younger adults to tolerate minor side effects. Likewise, children cannot be regarded as undersized adults, and drug dosages relative to body weight may be quite different. Drug distribution is also different between premature infants and children. The dosages of drugs for children are usually calculated on the basis of weight (mg/kg) or on the basis of body surface area (mg/m^2). These important aspects of drug safety cannot be reliably assessed from preclinical data, but the major variability factors need to be identified and addressed as part of the clinical trials programme.

Conclusions and future trends

No drug is completely non-toxic or safe[2]. Adverse effects can range from minor reactions, such as dizziness or skin reactions, to serious and even fatal effects such as anaphylactic reactions. The aims of preclinical toxicology are (a) to reduce to a minimum the risk to the healthy volunteers and the patients to whom the drug will be given in clinical trials; and (b) to ensure that the risk in patients treated with the drug once it is on the market is commensurate with the benefits. The latter is also a major concern during clinical development, and beyond in Phase IV.

It is important to understand the margin of safety that exists between the dose needed for the desired effect and the dose that produces unwanted and possibly dangerous side effects. But the extrapolation from animal toxicology to safety in man is difficult because of the differences between species in terms of physiology, pathology and drug metabolism.

Data from preclinical toxicity studies may be sufficiently discouraging that the project is stopped at that stage. If the project goes ahead, the preclinical toxicology data provide a basis for determining starting doses and dosing regimens for the initial clinical trials, and for identifying likely target organs and surrogate markers of potential toxicity in humans. Two particular trends in preclinical toxicology are noteworthy:

- Regulatory requirements tend to become increasingly stringent, and toxicology testing more complex, as new mechanisms of potential toxicity emerge. This has has been one cause, over the years, of the steady increase in the cost and duration of drug development (see Chapter 22). Only in the last 5–10 years have serious efforts been made to counter this trend, driven by the realization that innovation and therapeutic advances are being seriously slowed down, to the detriment, rather than the benefit, of human healthcare. The urgent need for effective drugs against AIDS was the main impetus for this change.

- In an effort to reduce the time and cost of testing, and to eliminate development compounds as early as possible, early screening methods are being increasingly developed and applied during the drug discovery phase of the project, with the aim of reducing the probability of later failure. One such approach is the use of cDNA microarray methods (see Chapter 7) to monitor changes in gene expression resulting from the application of the test compound to tissues or cells in culture. Over- or underexpression of certain genes is frequently associated with the occurrence of specific toxic effects, such as liver damage (Nuwaysir et al., 1999; Pennie, 2000), so that detecting such a change produced by a novel compound makes it likely that the compound will prove toxic, thereby ruling it out as a potential development candidate. Such high-throughput genomics-based approaches enable large databases of gene expression information to be built up, covering a diverse range of chemical structures. The expectation is that the structure–activity patterns thus revealed will enable the prediction in silico of the likely toxicity of a wide range of hypothetical compounds, enabling exclusion criteria to be applied very early in the

[2]Nor, of course, are any other everyday technologies, such as ladders, kitchen knives, pots of paint or trains. None the less, public opinion seems particularly sensitive to iatrogenic medical risks and is inclined to demand what is impossible, namely 'proof that this drug/vaccine/procedure is 100% safe'.

discovery process. This field of endeavour, dubbed 'toxicogenomics', is expected by many to revolutionize pharmaceutical toxicology (Castle et al., 2002).

At present, extensive toxicity testing in vivo is required by regulatory authorities, and data from in vitro studies carry little weight. There is no likelihood that this will change in the near future (Snodin, 2002). What is clearly changing is the increasing use of in vitro toxicology screens early in the course of a drug discovery programme to reduce the risk of toxicological failures later (see Chapter 10). The main impact of new technologies will therefore be – if the prophets are correct – to reduce the attrition rate in development, not necessarily to make drug development faster or cheaper.

References

Baldrick P (2003) Toxicokinetics in preclinical evaluation. Drug Discovery Today 8: 127–133.

Castle AL, Carver MP, Mendrick DL (2002) Toxicogenomics: a new revolution in drug safety. Drug Discovery Today 7: 728–736.

Committee for Proprietary Medicinal Products (1997) Points to consider for the assessment of the potential QT prolongation by non-cardiovascular medicinal products. Publication CPMP 986/96. London: Human Medicines Evaluation Unit.

De Clerk, F, Van de Water A, D'Aubiol J et al. (2002) In vivo measurement of QT prolongation, dispersion and arrhythmogenesis: application to the preclinical cardiovascular safety pharmacology of a new chemical entity. Fundamental and Clinical Pharmacology 16: 125–140.

FDA Guidance Note 1998 Cell therapy and gene therapy products. http://www.fda.gov/cber/gdlns/somgene.pdf

FDA Guidance note (2002) Immunotoxicology evaluation of investigational new drugs. www.fda.gov/guidance/index.htm

Gad SC (2002) Drug safety evaluation. New York: Wiley Interscience.

Haverkamp W, Breitlandt G, Comm AJ et al. (2000) The potential for QT prolongation and proarrhythmias by non-anti-arrhythmic drugs: clinical and regulatory implications. European Heart Journal 21: 1232–1237.

ICH Guideline S1A: Guideline on the need for carcinogenicity studies of pharmaceuticals. www.ich.org

ICH Guideline S1B: Testing for carcinogenicity of pharmaceuticals. www.ich.org

ICH Guideline S1C: Dose selection for carcinogenicity studies of pharmaceuticals and S1C(R): Addendum: addition of a limit dose and related notes. www.ich.org

ICH Guideline S2A: Genotoxicity: guidance on specific aspects of regulatory tests for pharmaceuticals. www.ich.org

ICH Guideline S2B: Genotoxicity: a standard battery for genotoxicity testing for pharmaceuticals. www.ich.org

ICH Guideline S3A: Note for guidance on toxicokinetics: the assessment of systemic exposure in toxicity studies. www.ich.org

ICH Guideline S5A: Detection of toxicity to reproduction for medicinal products. www.ich.org

ICH Guideline S6: Preclinical safety evaluation of biotechnology-derived pharmaceuticals. www.ich.org

ICH Guideline S7A: Safety pharmacology studies for human pharmaceuticals. www.ich.org

ICH Guideline S7B: Safety pharmacology studies for assessing the potential for delayed ventricular repolarization (QT interval prolongation) by human pharmaceuticals. www.ich.org

Netzer R, Ebneth E, Bischoff U, Pongs O (2001) Screening lead compounds for QT interval prolongation. Drug Discovery Today 6: 78–84.

Nuwaysir EF, Bittner M, Trent J, Barrett JC, Afshari CA (1999) Microassays and toxicology; the advent of toxicogenomics. Molecular Carcinogenesis 24: 152–159.

Olson H, Betton G, Robinson D et al. (2000) Concordance of the toxicity of pharmaceuticals in humans and animals. Regulatory Toxicology and Pharmacology 32: 56–67.

Pennie WD (2000) Use of cDNA microassays to probe and understand the toxicological consequences of altered gene expression. Toxicology Letters 112: 473–477.

Snodin DJ (2002) An EU perspective on the use of in vitro methods in regulatory pharmaceutical toxicology. Toxicology Letters 127: 161–168.

17 Pharmaceutical development

H P Rang

Introduction

Pure compounds are never used clinically as white powders straight from the bottle. Invariably they must be *formulated*, i.e. combined with other substances, made into tablets, capsules, injection solutions etc., in order to produce dosage forms that can be used clinically.

Pharmaceutical development comprises the range of tasks required to develop such physical dosage forms for a compound identified as a drug candidate, to enable the drug to work reliably when it is put on the market. To scientists involved in drug discovery it often comes as a surprise to discover how complex, time-consuming and expensive it can be to design a formulation for their beloved compound, whose biological properties they have been studying for years, so as to turn it into a product that can be sold and used. 'We know it works', they may grumble, 'just put it into pills and let's get on with testing it in the clinic.'

Increasingly, some initial issues in pharmaceutical development are being addressed as part of the process of lead optimization, before development proper begins. Just as with preliminary pharmacokinetic and toxicological evaluations, described in Chapter 10, it is recognized that the physicochemical properties of potential drug candidates play an important part in determining whether formulation is likely to be straightforward or troublesome, and so these properties will generally be evaluated during the discovery phase, before the drug candidate is selected – work often termed *preformulation* studies.

This chapter describes briefly the main considerations that need to be taken into account during pharmaceutical development, and some of the experimental approaches used. The main emphasis is on conventional drug delivery, particularly the use of oral formulations. The special types of formulation needed for topical application of drugs, for example skin creams, eye drops, suppositories etc., and the special problems associated with the administration of biopharmaceuticals, are not discussed here; detailed information on these topics can be found in textbooks (Ansel et al., 1999: Hillery et al., 2001; Allen, 2002; Aulton, 2002; Banker and Rhodes 2002).

Much effort is currently going into the development of more sophisticated drug delivery systems, particularly those designed to target drugs more precisely to relevant cells and tissues, and so-called 'intelligent' systems designed to adjust dosage according to clinical response.

243

Although there is abundant recent literature about the clever technologies being applied in this area, few clinically proven therapeutic products have so far been developed. The development of such systems requires substantial investment in research at the preclinical level, as well as evidence from clinical trials that the new formulation represents a significant improvement. Manufacturing costs are invariably much greater than those of conventional formulations. These factors mean that such products will be considerably more expensive, and healthcare providers may balk at this unless the advantages are substantial. Currently, most of this very specialized and high-risk development work is being undertaken by biotechnology companies, rather than by large pharmaceutical companies. We discuss briefly some of the principles of drug targeting and controlled release; the above-cited textbooks, and review articles (Pillai and Panchagnula, 2001; Garnett, 2001; Kumar and Kumar, 2001; Gregoriadis, 2003) should be consulted for more detailed information.

Routes of administration and dosage forms

The preferred dosage form for therapeutic agents is almost always an oral tablet or capsule, either taken as needed to control symptoms, or taken regularly once or twice a day. However, there are many alternatives, and Table 17.1 lists some of the main ones. An important consideration is whether it is desirable to achieve *systemic exposure* (i.e. distribution of the drug to all organs via the bloodstream) or *selective local exposure* (e.g. to the lungs, skin or rectum) by applying the drug topically. In most cases systemic exposure will be required, and an oral capsule or tablet will be the desired final dosage form. Even so, an intravenous formulation will normally be required for use in safety pharmacology, toxicology and pharmacokinetic studies in man.

Preformulation studies

As a preliminary to developing dosagse forms, various physical and chemical properties of the drug substance need to be investigated. These investigations are termed *preformulation studies*. Most synthetic drugs are either weak bases (~75%) or weak acids (~20%), and will generally need to be formulated as salts. Salts of a range of acceptable conjugate acids or bases therefore need to be prepared and tested. Intravenous formulations of relatively insoluble compounds may need to include non-aqueous solvents or emulsifying agents, and the

Table 17.1
The main routes of administration and dosage forms

Exposure required	Routes of administration	Dosage forms	
Systemic	Oral	Tablet, capsule, solution, suspension, emulsion	Liquid forms are particularly suitable for children, and for patients unable to swallow tablets. Unsuitable for foul-tasting medicines
	Parenteral		
	Injection (intravenous, subcutaneous, intramuscular) Needle-free injection)	Solution, emulsion, suspension, implant)	Examples: cytotoxic drugs liable to damage GI tract, drugs needed for unconscious patients, drugs unstable in GI tract (e.g. peptide hormones)
	Percutaneous	Skin patches	
	Inhalation	Gas, vapour	Applicable mainly to anaesthetic agents
	Intranasal	Aerosol	Used for some hormone preparations that are not absorbed orally, e.g. vasopressin analogues, gonadotrophin-releasing hormone
Topical	Skin	Ointment, cream, gel, aerosol	
	Respiratory tract	Aerosol, inhaled powder	
	Rectum, vagina	Suppository	
	Eye	Solution, ointment	

compatibility of the test substance with these additives, as well as with the commonly used excipients that are included in tablets or capsules, will need to be assessed.

The main components of preformulation studies are:

- Development of a suitable spectroscopic assay method for determining concentration and purity;
- Determination of solubility and dissolution rates of parent compound and salts in water and other solvents;
- Chemical stability of parent compound and salts in solution and solid state;
- Determination of pK_a and pH dependence of solubility and chemical stability;
- Determination of lipophilicity (i.e. oil:water partition coefficient, expressed as K_d);
- Determination of particle morphology, melting point and suitability for milling;

Theoretical treatments of these molecular properties, and laboratory methods for measuring them, which are beyond the scope of this book, are described in textbooks such as Allen (2002), Aulton (2002) and Burger and Abraham (2003). Here we consider some issues that commonly arise in drug development.

Solubility and dissolution rate

The question of solubility, already emphasized in Chapters 9 and 10, is particularly important in relation to pharmaceutical formulation. It is measured by standard laboratory procedures and involves determining the concentration of the compound in solution after equilibration – usually after several hours of stirring – with the pure solid. In general, compounds whose aqueous solubility exceeds 10 mg/mL present no problems of formulation. Compounds with lower solubility are likely to require conversion to salts, or the addition of non-aqueous solvents, in order to achieve satisfactory oral absorption. Because the extreme pH values needed to induce ionization of very weak acids or bases are likely to cause tissue damage, the inclusion of a miscible solvent of relatively low polarity, such as 20% propylene glycol or some other biocompatible solubilizing agent (see below), will often be required for preparing injectable formulations. Complications may arise with oral formulations if the solubility is highly dependent on pH, because of the large pH difference between the stomach and the small intestine. Gastric pH can range from near neutrality in the absence of any food stimulus to acid secretion, to pH 1–2, whereas the intestinal pH is around 8. Basic substances that dissolve readily in the stomach can therefore precipitate in the intestine and fail to be absorbed. Compounds that can exist in more than one crystal form can also show complex behaviours. The different lattice energies of molecules in the

different crystal forms mean that the intrinsic solubility of the compound is also different. This means that if different crystal forms coexist in the solid material that is in contact with the solution, the solid will gradually be converted to the lowest-energy, least soluble form, and the dissolved compound will spontaneously precipitate on storage. The different crystal forms may correspond to different hydration states of the compound, so that a solution prepared from the unhydrated solid may gradually precipitate as hydrated crystals. Selecting the best salt form to avoid complications of this sort is an important aspect of preformulation studies.

Compounds that have low intrinsic solubility in aqueous media can often be brought into solution by the addition of a water-miscible *solubilizing agent*, such as polysorbates, ethanol or polyethylene glycol (PEG). Preformulation studies may therefore include the investigation of various solubilizing agents, such as methylcellulose or cyclodextrin, which are known to be relatively free of adverse effects in man.

As well as intrinsic solubility, *dissolution rate* is important in determining the rate of absorption of an oral drug. The process of dissolution involves two steps: (a) the transfer of molecules from the solid to the immediately adjacent layer of fluid, known as the *boundary layer*; and (b) escape from the boundary layer into the main reservoir of fluid, which is known as the *bulk phase* and is assumed to be well stirred so that its concentration is uniform. Step (a) is invariably much faster than step (b), so the boundary layer quickly reaches saturation. The overall rate of dissolution is limited by step (b), and depends on the intrinsic solubility of the compound, the diffusion coefficient of the solute, the surface area of the boundary layer, and the geometry of the path leading from boundary layer to the bulk phase.

In practice, dissolution rates depend mainly on:

- Intrinsic solubility (since this determines the boundary layer concentration);
- Molecular weight (which determines diffusion coefficient);
- Particle size and dispersion of the solute (which determine the surface area of the boundary layer and the length of the diffusion path).

In pharmaceutical development, dissolution rates are often manipulated intentionally by including different polymers, such as methylcellulose into tablets or capsules, to produce 'slow-release' formulations of drugs such as *diclofenac*, allowing once-daily dosage despite the drug's short plasma half-life.

Stability

For routine use, a drug product is expected to have a shelf-life, representing less than 5% decomposition and no significant physical change under normal storage conditions, of at least 3 years.

During the preformulation studies stability tests are often carried out for 1–4 weeks. The chemical stability of the solid is measured at temperatures ranging from 4 to 75°C, and moisture uptake at different relative humidities is also assessed.

Measurements of stability in solution at pH values ranging from 1 to 11, at room temperature and at 37°C will be performed, including formulations with solubilizing agents where appropriate. Sensitivity to UV and visible light, and to exposure to oxygen, is also measured.

The rate of degradation in short-term studies under these harsh conditions is used to give a preliminary estimate of the likely rate of degradation under normal storage conditions. Sensitivity to low pH means that degradation is likely to occur in the stomach, requiring measures to prevent release of the compound until it reaches the intestine.

These preformulation stability tests serve mainly to warn that further development of the compound may be difficult or even impossible. Definitive tests of the long-term (3 years or more) stability of the formulated preparation will be required for regulatory purposes.

Particle size and morphology

Ideally, for incorporation into a tablet or capsule the drug substance needs to exist in small, uniformly sized particles, forming a smoothly flowing powder which can be uniformly blended with the excipient material. Rarely, the compound will emerge from the chemistry laboratory as non-hygroscopic crystals, and the melting point will be sufficiently high that it can be reduced to a uniform fine powder by mechanical milling. More often it will take the form of an amorphous, somewhat waxy solid, and additional work will be needed later in development to produce it in a form suitable for incorporation into tablets or capsules.

Preformulation studies are designed to reveal how far the available material falls short of this ideal. Various laboratory methods are available for analysing particle size and morphology, but in the preformulation stage simple microscopic observation is the usual method. Particles larger than a few micrometres, particularly if the particle size is very variable, are difficult to handle and mix uniformly. Hygroscopic materials and polymorphic crystal forms are a disadvantage, as already mentioned. These issues are unlikely to matter greatly in the early stages of development, as Phase I studies can usually be carried out with liquid formulations if necessary, but can be a major hurdle later, so the main aim of the preformulation studies is to give a warning of likely problems to come.

Formulation

Routine formulation of an oral drug into tablet or capsule form, where there are no special requirements for modified release, still involves a good deal of engineering. The drug substance must be dried and converted to a powder form that can be precisely dispensed. The conditions required for different compounds will vary, and have to be selected by trial and error. For various reasons, other substances have to be included in the tablet or capsule. Slippery, non-adherent materials, such as magnesium stearate, may be needed to ensure that the powdered form runs smoothly. Inert diluents, such as lactose or starch, are added to produce tablets of a manageable size (generally 50–500 mg). Other substances, such as cellulose, may be needed to assist compaction into a solid tablet that will not crumble, and to ensure that the tablet disintegrates rapidly in the gastrointestinal tract. The tablet may need to be coated with cellulose or sugar to disguise its taste. The modest white pill that goes into the bathroom cabinet is actually the product of a lot of development and testing.

A two-piece gelatin capsule is often more convenient than a tablet formulation to contain the drug-containing powder. Such capsules can also be used to contain drugs in semisolid or liquid form. Capsule formulations are often used for initial clinical trials, as they are generally simpler to develop than compressed tablets, but are less suitable for controlled-release formulations (see below).

As already mentioned, the 'ideal' drug substance, intended for use as a once-daily oral preparation, has the following characteristics:

● Water solubility
● Chemical stability (including stability at low pH)
● Permeability across the gastrointestinal epithelium
● Good access to site of action (e.g. blood–brain barrier penetration, if intended to work in the brain)
● Resistance to first-pass metabolism
● Plasma half-life of several hours
● Sufficient therapeutic window that peak–trough oscillations are immaterial.

If these conditions are met the formulation of oral or injectable preparations presents no special problems, but, needless to say, they rarely are, and it falls to the pharmaceutical development group to develop formulations that successfully overcome the shortcomings of the compound.

In reality, formulation development has to take into account not only the properties of the drug substance, but also the desired delivery system and the form of the final product. In developing a new nitrate preparation for treating angina, for example, the preferred delivery system might be a skin patch to be packaged in a foil sachet, or a nasal spray to be packaged as a push-button aerosol can. Although a simple oral preparation may be feasible, the company's marketing objective might be to develop a different dosage form, and the development plan would have to be directed towards this more demanding task.

Drug delivery systems

In recent years, drug delivery systems have become progressively more sophisticated, for three main reasons. First, biopharmaceuticals represent an increasing proportion of new drugs. They are very unlikely to conform to the 'ideal' profile summarized above, and so ingenuity in formulation is often needed to turn them into viable products. Second, there is increasing emphasis on selective targeting of drugs to sites of disease via the use of specialized delivery systems. This is particularly relevant for anticancer drugs. Third, controllable delivery systems are being developed for a variety of different

applications. The use of electrophoresis to provide a steady flux of drug through the skin (see below) is experimental and appears promising. A further step is to incorporate sensors (e.g. for blood glucose concentration) into devices that control the delivery of insulin, in order to provide feedback control of blood glucose. An important component of many of the newer drug formulations and delivery systems which is currently receiving much attention is the use of polymer technology, and in the next section we discuss some of the properties and applications of polymers in pharmaceutical development.

Polymers and surfactants

Combining the drug substance with different polymers and surfactants permits it to adopt states that are intermediate between the pure solid and a free aqueous solution. Polymers in colloidal, gel or solid form can be used to entrap drug molecules, and have many applications in formulation (Kumar and Kumar, 2001; Torchilin, 2001; Dimitriu, 2002).

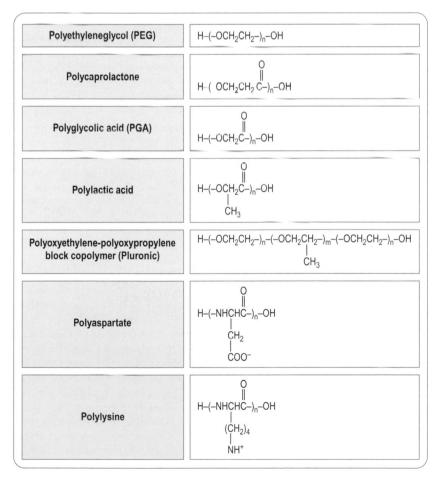

Fig. 17.1
Amphiphilic polymer.

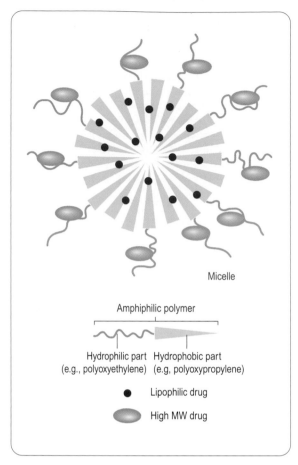

Fig. 17.2
Structures of some common pharmaceutical polymers.

- Polymers and surfactants in liquid form give rise to micelles or emulsions, which can greatly enhance the solubility of drug molecules while at the same time protecting them from chemical attack, and sometimes improving permeation through tissue barriers, such as the gastrointestinal epithelium and the blood–brain barrier.
- Polymers that form soft hydrated gels are used mainly in topical dermatological preparations.
- Solid gel formulations can be used as implantable depot preparations which can be inserted under the skin to give sustained release of the drug (see below). Skin patches can be made from sheet of such a flexible polymer, loaded with the drug substance.

The range of polymers available for drug formulation is vast. A few important examples are shown in Figure 17.1. By combining hydrophilic and hydrophobic domains in a single polymer, as in 'Pluronic', micelle formation is encouraged (see below). The inclusion of acidic or basic side chains, as in polyaspartate or polylysine, enables the polymer to bind oppositely charged drug molecules, thereby increasing their effective solubility.

Micelles

Micelles (Figure 17.2) consist of aggregates of a few hundred *amphiphilic* molecules that contain distinct hydrophilic and hydrophobic regions. In an aqueous medium, the molecules cluster with the hydrophilic regions facing the surrounding water and the hydrophobic regions forming an inner core. Micelles typically have diameters of 10–80 nm, small enough not to sediment under gravity, and to pass through most filters. Micelle-forming substances have limited aqueous solubility, and when the free aqueous concentration reaches a certain point – the *critical micelle concentration* – typically in the millimolar range, micelles begin to form; further addition of the substance increases their abundance. With some compounds, as the density of micelles increases a gel is formed, consisting of a loosely packed array of micelles interspersed with water molecules. Lipophilic drug molecules often dissolve readily in the inner core, allowing concentrations to be achieved that greatly exceed the aqueous solubility limit of the drug. Amphiphilic substances also tend to associate with micelles, as do high molecular weight substances such as peptides and proteins, which have affinity for surfaces, on account of the large surface area which micelles present.

Micelle formation is a natural property of bile acids, which are secreted into the duodenum under physiological conditions and which play an important role in fat absorption by the intestine. Micellar drug formulations are thus an extension of a normal physiological process. Micellar absorption by the gastrointestinal tract is directed mainly to the lymphatic system rather than the vascular system. Thus, unlike substances absorbed directly from aqueous solution, micelle-associated compounds tend to bypass the hepatic portal circulation, and thereby escape first-pass metabolism.

Micelle formation is a general property of amphiphilic molecules, and many chemical forms have been developed for pharmaceutical use (Pillai and Panchagnula, 2001; Torchilin, 2001). Some examples are shown in Figure 17.2, and additional information on the many types of polymers used in pharmaceutical formulation is given by Kumar and Kumar (2001), as well as in many textbooks (e.g. Ansel et al., 1999; Aulton, 2002, Dimitriu 2002). A particularly versatile group is that of *copolymers*, containing more than one type of polymer unit, one of which, typically, is hydrophilic (e.g. polyethylene glycol), whereas the other is hydrophobic (e.g. polypropylene glycol). Alternating blocks of these two units form a copolymer (known commercially as Pluronic, see Figure 17.2) which is commonly used in drug formulations. Copolymers of this sort at low concentrations form a liquid micellar suspension, but at higher concentrations the micelles may aggregate in an ordered array to form a water-containing gel. Such gel formulations are commonly used to prepare controlled-release preparations (see below). The polymer components may include anionic or cationic groups, which have the effect of altering their affinity for charged drug molecules, and also of altering their pharmacokinetic behaviour.

Micelles and other drug vehicles, such as cyclodextrins and liposomes (see below), have a considerable – and generally beneficial – effect on the pharmacokinetic properties of the drug. Often, but not invariably, absorption from gastrointestinal tract is improved, though the reasons for this are not well understood. Preferential uptake into lymphatics, as mentioned above, reduces the extent of first-pass metabolism. Circulating micelles protect the drug from metabolic degradation, so the plasma half-life is generally prolonged. Micelles are too large to cross 'tight' capillary endothelium, so transfer across the blood–brain barrier is not increased. They are able to cross the fenestrated capillaries that occur in most tissues, but the rate of permeation is less than that of the uncomplexed drug. Malignant tumours and inflamed tissues generally have rather leaky capillaries with large fenestrations, so that transfer of micellar drug complexes into such tissues is more rapid than into normal tissues. This mechanism results in a degree of selectivity in the distribution of the drug to diseased tissues, a phenomenon known as *passive targeting* (see below).

Solid polymers

Cross-linked polymers, such as polyacrylamide (Figure 17.1), will often form soft hydrated gels when placed in aqueous media, and these are able to accommodate and release drug molecules, the rate of release depending on the degree of hydration, the diffusion characteristics of the gel and the length of the diffusion path. Such solid polymers can exist in many forms, including slabs and cylinders suitable for subcutaneous depot or transdermal administration (see below), or as *microspheres* sufficiently small to be introduced directly into the circulation, whose properties are similar to those of the colloidal forms discussed above. A microsphere formulation was used to improve the poor oral bioavailability of the immunosuppressant drug *ciclosporin*.

Liposomes

Liposomes were first discovered in 1965 and proposed as drug carriers soon afterwards (see Gregoriadis, 2003 for a recent short review). They are microscopic vesicles formed when an aqueous suspension of phospholipid is exposed to ultrasonic agitation. Depending on the conditions, large multilayered vesicles 1–5 μm in diameter, or small single-layered vesicles 0.02–0.1 μm in diameter, may be formed. The vesicles are bounded by a phos-

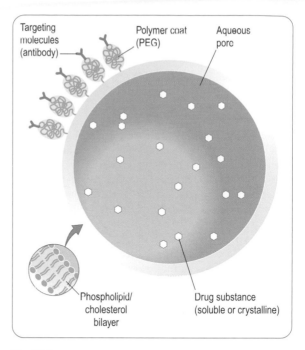

Fig. 17.3
Structure of drug delivery liposome.

pholipid bilayer, which is impermeable to non-lipophilic compounds. They can act as drug carriers in various ways (Figure 17.3).

- Non-lipophilic drugs are carried in solution in the aqueous core, by adding them to the aqueous medium in which the liposomes are produced. Techniques for introducing drug molecules into preformed liposomes have also been described.
- Lipophilic drugs occupy the phospholipid membrane phase.
- Some peptides and proteins, as well as amphiphilic drugs, can be sequestered at the lipid–water interface

These drug-containing vesicles are easy and cheap to manufacture, and in most cases are stable as aqueous suspensions. Simple phospholipid-based liposomes are unsatisfactory as drug carriers for several reasons: they are relatively permeable to drug molecules and tend to disintegrate in the circulation, and so fail to retain the drug satisfactorily; and their circulating half-life is short, because they are rapidly taken up by tissue macrophages, mainly in liver and spleen, so these tissues receive most of the drug as a brief bolus. The biological characteristics of liposomes can, however, be improved by chemical modifications of various kinds:

- The inclusion of cholesterol, and other alterations of the phospholipid composition, improves the stability of liposomes and renders them less permeable to drug molecules.

- Attaching other substances to their surface. Such substances include polyethylene glycol (PEG; see Figure 17.3), charged compounds, or antibodies directed at antigens expressed by tissues in which the drug is intended to act.

Altering the size, lipid composition and charge on the vesicle surface affects the rate at which circulating liposomes are taken up by tissue macrophages. Liposomes are not generally suitable for oral administration, as they are destroyed by enzymes and bile acids in the small intestine. Nor do they cross the blood–brain barrier, so they cannot be used to improve the access of drugs to the brain. Despite an extensive literature acclaiming liposomes as the answer to almost every imaginable formulation problem, the application of liposome technology in commercial products is so far limited to a very few examples, in the field of anticancer and antifungal drugs. Recent reviews providing information on trends and expectations in this field include Harrington et al. (2002), Barratt (2003) and Sapra and Allen (2003).

The main purpose of using liposomes is to improve the pharmacokinetic behaviour of drugs. Drugs contained in liposomes are inaccessible to metabolizing enzymes and transport systems, and their effective biological half-life is determined by the rate of clearance of the liposomes. The effect is therefore to produce a circulating reservoir of sequestered drug, which is able to exert an effect only when the liposome is disrupted. Liposomes are too large to escape from capillaries in most tissues, so their distribution volume is much smaller than that of the free drug. Circulating liposomes are taken up mainly by tissue macrophages, the principal sites of uptake being the liver and spleen. These cells are specialized to ingest phospholipid-containing cellular debris, which becomes coated with plasma-derived proteins known as *opsins*, to render the particles susceptible to ingestion macrophages. Liposomes are taken up in the same way, and the released drug may act locally in the liver or spleen, or escape into the circulation to act elsewhere. In tissues that are the seat of tumours or inflammatory changes, the capillary fenestrations that control permeability are enlarged and the tissues become more readily accessible to liposomes, allowing a degree of selective targeting of drugs to these tissues. This is termed *passive targeting*, as no mechanism of active recognition of the liposomes by malignant tissues is involved. Cytotoxic drugs such as *doxorubicin* are available as injectable liposomal preparations for treating solid tumours. Because of passive targeting these preparations act more selectively and therefore produce fewer side effects than conventional formulations. The antifungal drug *actinomycin* is also available as a liposomal formulation for use against systemic fungal infections, where it is desirable to target tissue macrophages in which the microorganism lodges.

Liposome technology has received much attention in the design of drug delivery systems (Garnett, 2001; Harrington et al., 2002; Sapra and Allen, 2003), though the developments remain mostly at the experimental stage. One successful approach has been to attach polyethylene glycol residues by conjugation to the surface of the liposomes, which has the effect of preventing opsonization and thus making them invisible to macrophages and greatly increasing their circulating half-life and the availability of the contained drug to relevant target tissues. Such so-called *stealth liposomes* have proved useful as delivery vehicles for cytotoxic drugs such as *daunorubicin* and *doxurubicin,* and others in clinical trials. They are also used as transdermal delivery vehicles (see below). Another much-studied approach has been to attach recognition molecules – mainly antibodies – to the surface of drug-containing liposomes so that the liposomes bind to tumour-specific antigens and release their load of cytotoxic drug in the close vicinity of tumour cells. A wide variety of such modified liposome formulations has been tested, and several have been shown to improve the efficacy of cytotoxic drugs in experimental animal tumour models. However, results with the few that have undergone clinical trials have generally so far proved disappointing. There is nevertheless considerable confidence that such approaches will soon prove their value in the clinic.

Cyclodextrins

Cyclodextrins are water-soluble compounds consisting of six to eight glucose molecules arranged in a cyclical conformation, forming a hollow cylinder with a hydrophilic exterior and a relatively hydrophobic cavity, able to accommodate drug molecules of low water solubility. Like the polymers and surfactants already described, cyclodextrins are used as solubilizing agents and, by mechanisms not fully understood, are able to enhance absorption from the gastrointestinal tract and other epithelial surfaces, such as the nasal cavity. Cyclodextrins are less toxic to epithelial cells than most of the commonly used surfactants, such as detergents, phospholipids etc.

Modified-release drug formulations

One of the most common requirements in drug formulation is to increase the duration of action of a drug by causing it to be absorbed gradually. Ideally, the rate of absorption should reach a steady level that is maintained for hours or days, depending on the application, until the reservoir is used up. This is known as *sustained release*. It is widely used to produce once-daily oral preparations, or long-lasting depot injections (e.g. contraceptives, hormone replacements, antipsychotic drugs) where the drug effect is required to last for weeks or months.

Other types of modified release include *delayed release*, used mainly for oral drugs that are unstable at the low pH of the stomach, and *controlled release*, produced by specialized devices that allow the rate of release to be adjusted according to need. Some of the approaches used to develop controlled-release formulations are discussed briefly below.

There are many different ways of producing sustained-release oral preparations, some of which are shown in Figure 17.4. They rely mainly on the use of impermeable coatings that are slowly eroded as the pill passes through the gut, or water-absorbing polymer gels which slowly become hydrated. Injectable implants operate in the same way over a longer period, and have the advantage that they can be removed if necessary. Depot injections of drugs dissolved in oil can also be used to provide long-lasting sustained release, but these generally produce a less constant rate of administration and cannot be removed.

Osmotic minipumps, which absorb water at a constant rate through a semipermeable membrane, and displace the drug solution from a separate compartment through a tiny laser-drilled hole, provide another means of producing sustained release which can be used orally or as an implant. These devices are not yet in routine use, though implanted minipumps are widely used for drug administration in animal studies..

Controlled release represents a stage beyond sustained release and involves coupling a sensing mechanism, responding to changes in temperature or pH, for example, to the drug release mechanism. Examples of the many kinds of device that could meet this need include

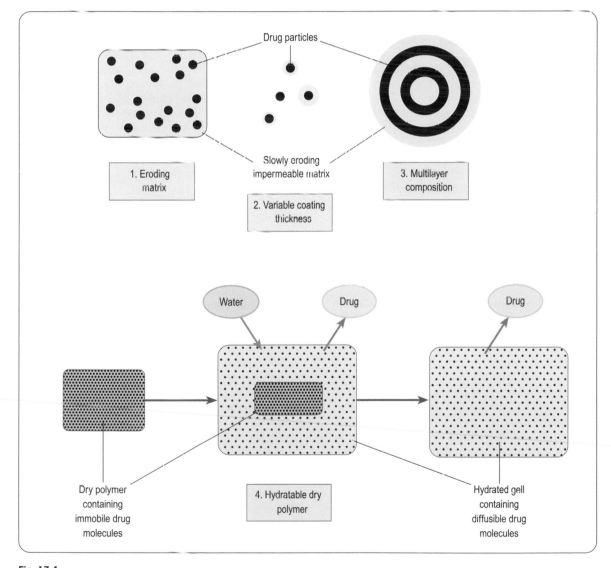

Fig. 17.4
Types of sustained-release preparation.

temperature-sensitive liposomes, which disintegrate when the temperature is increased to, say, 40°C, and temperature-sensitive polymers which aggregate into a gel when the temperature is increased. The idea is that local heating of a tumour will cause the drug to be released at that site. pH-sensitive systems are also in development which can be used to delay the release of acid-sensitive drugs (particularly peptides) until they have passed beyond the stomach. Drug delivery can also, in principle, be targeted to regions of low pH, such as inflamed or hypoxic tissues, by the use of pH-sensitive polymers. A particularly ingenious approach is to incorporate insulin into pH-sensitive gels loaded with glucose oxidase (known to specialists in this field as *GOD-gels*). If the ambient glucose concentration increases, enzymic oxidation causes a fall in pH and the release of insulin. For more details of 'responsive' polymers and their application in controlled drug delivery, see Kumar and Kumar (2001), Soppimath et al. (2002) and Gupta et al. (2002).

Drug delivery to the central nervous system

Brain capillaries, unlike those in most parts of the body, are non-fenestrated, so that drug molecules must traverse the endothelial cells, rather than passing between them, to move from circulating blood to the extracellular space of the brain (see Chapter 10). Three main routes of access are important (Scherrmann, 2002):

- Lipophilic compounds of low molecular weight cross the membrane of endothelial cells very easily, and comprise the great majority of CNS-acting drugs. Peptides, proteins, non-lipophilic or ionized drugs are for the most part unable to cross the endothelial cell membrane.
- The endothelial cells also possess various active transport mechanisms that can allow certain non-lipophilic compounds to enter the brain. Examples include *levodopa*, used for treating Parkinson's disease, *baclofen*, a GABA analogue used to treat spasticity, and the cytotoxic drug *melphalan*, all of which are transported across the blood–brain barrier by the amino acid transporter. Attempts have been made to couple other drugs with amino acids or sugars which are transported in the same way. Despite being successful in animal models, however, such compounds have not been developed for clinical use. Active transport out of the brain also occurs with many compounds, including drugs such as *penicillins*, which are able to enter passively.
- Molecules can be carried as endocytotic vesicles across the endothelial cells. This type of transcytosis occurs with molecules that are bound to receptors or other proteins on the endothelial cell surface. An approach that has been tested extensively, though not yet applied for clinical use, is to couple active peptides and proteins to the monoclonal antibody OX26, which recognizes the endothelial transferrin receptor. Binding to this receptor stimulates transcytosis, carrying the antibody and its cargo across the blood–brain barrier. Transcytosis can also be stimulated by the non-specific binding of small cationic peptides to the acidic glycoprotein components of the endothelial cell surface. Conjugates of various cytotoxic and antimicrobial drugs to such peptides show improved brain penetration in animal models, and may prove to be applicable clinically.

Recent approaches for improving drug delivery to the brain are described in more detail by Scherrmann (2002) and Misra et al. (2003).

Enabling impermeant drugs to reach the brain represents a major challenge for formulation chemists, and there are actually very few examples where it has been overcome. Most often, the drug molecule has to be redesigned to increase its lipophilicity. Formation of a lipid-soluble prodrug is one strategy, but is rarely effective in this context because conversion to the active, non-lipophilic compound is likely to take place in the circulation before the drug reaches the brain.

Other routes of administration

The main routes of administration for drugs acting systemically, apart from oral and injectable formulations, are *transdermal* and *intranasal. Rectal, vaginal* and *pulmonary* routes are also used in some cases, though these are used mainly for drugs that act locally.

Transdermal administration of drugs formulated as small adhesive skin patches has considerable market appeal, even though such preparations are much more expensive than routine formulations. To be administered in this way, drugs must be highly potent, lipid soluble and of low molecular weight. Examples of commercially available patch formulations include *nitroglycerin, scopolamine, fentanyl, nicotine, testosterone, oestradiol* and *ketoprofen*, and the list will undoubtedly grow. The main limitation is the low permeability of the skin to most drugs and the small area covered, which mean that dosage is limited to a few milligrams per day, so only very potent drugs can be given systemically in this way. Variations in skin thickness affect the rate of penetration, and the occurrence of local skin reactions is also a problem with some drugs. Various penetration enhancers, mainly surfactant compounds of the sort discussed above, are used to improve transdermal absorption. The transfer rate can be greatly enhanced by applying a small and painless electric current (about 0.5 mA/cm²), and this is effective in achieving transfer of peptides (e.g. *calcitonin*) and even *insulin* through the skin. It also offers promise as a route of administration of oligonucleotides in gene therapy applications (see Chapter 12). These procedures are being used experimentally in the clinic, but are not yet available as commercial products for routine clinical use. Ultrasonic irradiation is also under investigation as a means of facilitating transdermal delivery. These procedures would also allow the administration to be controlled according to need.

Intranasal drug administration (Illium, 2002, 2003) is another route that has been used successfully for a few drugs – and is, of course, a procedure familiar to cocaine users. The nasal epithelium is much more permeable than skin and allows the transfer of peptide drugs as well as low molecular weight substances, and commercially available preparations have been developed for peptide hormones, such as *vasopressin analogues*, *calcitonin*, *buserelin* and others, as well as for conventional drugs such as *triptans*, *opiates* etc. The main disadvantages are that substances are quickly cleared from the nasal epithelium by ciliary action, as well as being metabolized, and the epithelial permeability is not sufficient to allow most proteins to be given in this way. Ciliary clearance can be reduced by the use of gel formulations, and surfactant permeability enhancers can be used to improve the penetration of larger molecules. The possibility of administering insulin, growth factors or vaccines by this route is the subject of active research efforts. Some studies have suggested (see Illium, 2003) that substances absorbed through the nasal epithelium reach the brain more rapidly than if they are given intravenously, possibly bypassing the blood–brain barrier by reaching the olfactory bulb directly.

Even in cases where no problems are encountered, formulation studies require considerable time and resources. The end result has to be a product that can be manufactured on a large scale and meet strict quality control standards, and can be stored in thousands of homes under varying conditions of temperature and humidity without significant deterioration.

Very often pharmaceutical development is called on to improve the characteristics of the drug substance, for example by improving its solubility, disguising its taste, increasing its plasma half-life or reducing unwanted effects, and work of this kind increases the time and costs of the process. Increasing use is being made of colloidal systems, such as micelles, polymers and liposomes, as vehicles for drug molecules. Such formulations have a considerable effect on the drug's pharmacokinetic properties, and can also be used to achieve a degree of targeting of the drug to the tissues on which it is required to act. Drug targeting based on these principles is currently the subject of much experimental work. The principles have only proved applicable so far to a few anticancer and antifungal drugs, but many more applications are expected in the foreseeable future.

Overall, work on more sophisticated formulations and delivery systems for currently used drugs is thought likely to contribute as much to improved therapeutics as the discovery of new drugs, and is seen by the pharmaceutical industry as an important parallel approach to drug discovery, particularly at times – like the present – when drug discovery runs into a phase of disappointing productivity.

Summary

Pharmaceutical development comprises all the activities needed to turn a therapeutic drug substance into a marketable product that will perform reliably when used in real life. Preformulation studies consist of a series of chemical investigations on the drug substance which indicate the kinds of formulation that are likely to be satisfactory. In some cases problems (for example poor chemical stability) will emerge at this stage, requiring modification of the drug molecule before development can proceed – in other words, back to the drawing board.

The process of formulation will depend greatly on the intended route of administration of the drug. In most cases, where the intention is to produce a tablet or capsule for oral use, an intravenous formulation will also be developed for use in clinical trials, and the oral form used in initial efficacy trials (clinical Phase II) may not be the same as the intended market form.

References

Allen LV (2002) The art, science and technology of pharmaceutical compounding, 2nd edn. Washington DC: American Pharmaceutical Association.

Ansel HC, Allen LV, Popovich NG (1999) Pharmaceutical dosage forms and drug delivery systems, 7th edn. Baltimore: Lippincott Williams & Wilkins.

Aulton ME (ed) (2002) Pharmaceutics. The science of dosage form design, 2nd edn. Edinburgh: Churchill Livingstone.

Banker GS, Rhodes CT (eds) (2002) Modern pharmaceutics. New York: Marcel Dekker.

Barratt G (2003) Colloidal drug carriers: achievements and perspectives. Cellular and Molecular Life Sciences 60: 21–37.

Burger A, Abraham D (eds) (2003) Burger's medicinal chemistry and drug discovery. New York: John Wiley and Sons.

Dimitriu S (ed) (2002) Polymeric biomaterials. New York: Marcel Dekker.

Garnett M C (2001) Targeted drug conjugates: principles and progress. Advanced Drug Delivery Reviews 53: 171–216.

Gregoriadis G (2003) Liposomes in drug and vaccine delivery. Drug Delivery Systems and Sciences 2: 91–97.

Griffin JP, O'Grady JO (2002) The textbook of pharmaceutical medicine, 4th edn. London: BMJ Books.

Gupta P, Vermani K, Garg S (2002) Hydrogels: from controlled release to pH-responsive drug delivery. Drug Discovery Today 7: 569–579.

Harrington KJ, Syrigos KN, Vile RG (2002) Liposomally targeted cytotoxic drugs for the treatment of cancer. Journal of Pharmaceutics and Pharmacology 54: 1573–1600.

Hillery AM, Lloyd AW, Swarbrick J (2001) Drug delivery and targeting. London: Taylor & Francis.

Illium L (2002) Nasal drug delivery: new developments and strategies. Drug Discovery Today 7: 1184–1189.

Illium L (2003) Nasal drug delivery – possibilities, problems and solutions. Journal of Controlled Release 87: 187–198.

Kumar RMNV, Kumar H (2001) Polymeric controlled drug-delivery systems: perspective issues and opportunities. Drug Development and Industrial Pharmacy 27: 1–30.

Misra A, Shahiwala A, Shah SP (2003) Drug delivery to the central nervous system: a review. Journal of Pharmaceutics and Pharmaceutical Science 5: 252–273.

Pillai O, Panchagnula R (2001) Polymers in drug delivery. Current Opinion in Chemical Biology 5: 447–451.

Sapra P, Allen TM (2003) Ligand-targeted liposomal anticancer drugs. Progress in Lipid Research 42: 439–462.

Scherrmann J-C (2002) Drug delivery to the brain via the blood–brain barrier. Vascular Pharmacology 38: 349–354.

Soppimath KS, Aminabhavi TM, Dave AM, Kumbar SG, Rudzinski WE (2002) Stimulus-responsive 'smart' hydrogels as novel drug delivery systems. Drug Development and Industrial Pharmacy 28: 957–974.

Torchilin V (2001) Structure and design of polymeric surfactant-based drug delivery. Journal of Controlled Release 73: 137–172.

Clinical development

C Easdale

C W Vose

Introduction

The clinical development of new drugs is both a science and an art, requiring technical expertise, sound judgement and commercial awareness. At its best, it brings new medicines quickly and safely to patients who need them and delivers a sound financial return on the investment needed to take them from discovery to the market. Estimates of this investment vary, but most sources agree that, including the cost of failures and the cost of capital, the total cost is currently around $800 000 000 per registered drug, spread over an average 12-year development cycle (http://csdd.tufts.edu/NewsEvents/RecentNews.asp?newsid=5) (Pharma 2005, 1998). Most (70–80%) of this cost is incurred during clinical development, the stage at which the drug is tested in man (http://www.jpma.or.jp/12english/publications/pub022e_time/). However, only one in five compounds entering this costly process will ever be approved for use (Kuhlmann, 1997).

When things go wrong, unsafe drugs can reach the market only to be withdrawn again when their toxicity becomes apparent or, alternatively, potentially helpful drugs fail to reach the market at all. Both scenarios derive from shortcomings in the clinical development programme.

Around 30% of all drugs that fail in clinical development do so because they fail to show efficacy (Peck, 1997), though whether this is because they are actually ineffective or because poorly designed trials have failed to allow their efficacy to be demonstrated may never be known. Another 25% of failures occur for safety reasons. Had unacceptable toxicity been identified earlier, development could have been halted and resources and money diverted to better candidates. The overall cost of drug development is therefore inflated by the inefficiency of the current process. As well as inflating the price of drugs on the market, this burdens the pharmaceutical industry – the major drug development sponsor – with the cost of wasted time, resources and opportunity, and reduces the return on its research and development investment.

Governments also have a stake in drug development, as it affects the health of their citizens and their healthcare budgets. Increasingly, therefore, their decisions on licensing new drugs are influenced by evidence not only of efficacy and safety, but also of cost-effectiveness. Most of the drugs on the market today only work in a proportion of patients for whom they are prescribed. Drugs for hypertension are a good example. Most authorities agree that, quite apart from improving quality of life and reducing mortality, effective antihypertensive treatment reduces the healthcare cost of treating the long-term effects of uncontrolled hypertension, such as angina, peripheral ischaemia, heart failure and strokes to an extent that far outweighs the cost of treatment. The problem is, however, that even though there are many different types of antihypertensive drug available, none is effective in all hyper-

Table 18.1
Phases of clinical development

Clinical phase	General aim	Subjects/design	Data collected	Approx number of subjects	Approx cost ($ 000)	Approx time required
Ia	Exploratory; safety, tolerability and PK to support patient studies	Healthy subjects Escalating single-dose, placebo-controlled, randomized, double-blind	Adverse events PK parameters PD measures (sometimes)	40–60	200–400	6 months
Ib	Exploratory; safety, tolerability and PK to support patient studies	Healthy subjects Escalating repeat-dose, placebo-controlled, randomized double-blind	Adverse events PK parameters PD measures (sometimes)	30–50	200–400	6 months
IIa	Exploratory; preliminary safety and efficacy to support go/no-go decision	Patients; intended clinical dose and regimen based on Ph I results. Usually placebo-controlled randomized double-blind, but sometimes open label	Adverse events PK parameters Preliminary evidence of efficacy. 'Proof of concept'	50–200	500–1000	9 months–2 years
IIb	Confirmatory; dose selection to support registration	Patients in one or more indications; Selected dose levels/ regimens compared to placebo and/or standard treatment, randomized double-blind	Statistically rigorous analysis of dose–response relationships Confirmation of clinical dose and regimen for optimum efficacy, safety and tolerability	200–500	2000–5000+	2–3 years
III	Confirmatory; efficacy and safety data to support registration; may include pharmacoeconomic evaluation	Patients in target indication(s) but including different groups (age, ethnicity etc.). Selected dose level compared with placebo and/or standard treatment(s) randomized double blind	Statistically rigorous measurements demonstrating safety and efficacy in comparison with placebo or existing therapies May include pharmacoeconomic analysis	500–1000+	2000–10 000+	2–5+ years
IV	Obligatory postmarketing surveillance to reveal unexpected adverse effects or toxicity	Treated patients	Adverse events	10 000+	10 000+	2–4+ years

tensive patients. It is common for several different drugs to be tried before discovering by trial and error which, or which combination, if any, works for a particular patient. This process can last for months or years before the right treatment is identified, and the cost of trying several unsuccessful drugs is a drain on healthcare resources.

The characterization of the human genome promises a new approach (Cadman and Connor, 2003). In future, it may be possible by genotyping to identify specific subgroups of patients who share a common genetic basis for their disease and treat them with drugs customized to their particular disease subtype. Such personalized medicine promises drugs that are effective in almost all members of a specifically screened and identified patient subgroup, wasting less money on trial-and-error prescribing. Similarly, this approach may identify subgroups of patients likely to suffer adverse effects from particular drugs. Since 1993, seven drugs that were approved and then later withdrawn may have contributed to over 1000 deaths in the United States (Lasser et al., 2002). Clearly, therefore, personalized medicine is desirable to patients and governments, which, through their drug regulatory authorities, may drive drug development in this direction in future. The implications for the pharmaceutical industry are profound. Currently, only one in eight marketed drugs makes an adequate return on investment (Price-Waterhouse Coopers, 1995). Nonetheless, the pharmaceutical industry remains profitable because successful blockbuster drugs make very large returns indeed, and the industry still relies on them for its profitability. However, if in future there is to be pressure towards personalized medicine, and drugs are increasingly licensed for use in tightly defined patient subtypes, the opportunities for blockbusters will diminish as potential markets become fragmented. It may therefore be necessary for the pharmaceutical industry to develop many more drugs, specifically targeted at identified patient subtypes, and to develop them faster, more accurately and much more cost-effectively. These changes are causing drug development sponsors to reconsider their strategies for all stages of development, including clinical development.

Clinical trials

Clinical trials involve the administration of new, potentially therapeutic substances to man under controlled conditions for the purpose of determining their bioavailability, efficacy, safety, tolerability and acceptability. The clinical development process is divided into four phases, summarized in Table 18.1:

- *Phase I*: first administration and safety evaluation in man, usually in healthy volunteers;
- *Phase II*: early exploratory and dose-finding studies in patients;

- *Phase III*: large-scale studies in patients;
- *Phase IV*: post-marketing safety monitoring of patients.

In most parts of the world, clinical trials are a legal requirement before a new drug can be sold[1] or any claims made for its therapeutic benefit or safety. All clinical trials, including Phase I studies, are subject to international, national, and sometimes also local regulation. International regulatory requirements for human administration of a new active substance (NAS) are set out in a series of guidelines published by the International Committee on Harmonization (ICH; see Chapter 20). This committee was formed to harmonize the regulation of clinical trials in the three major pharmaceutical development regions (European Union, USA and Japan), with the aim of avoiding duplication of clinical research programmes when applying for approval in all three ICH regions. National and local regulations still exist and may vary from country to country within these regions, but ICH guidelines still apply and usually have the force of law. Clinical development of new drugs for registration in any of these regions must comply, and be seen to comply, with ICH guidelines if the data are to be accepted for registration purposes in the ICH regions, irrespective of where in the world they were generated. This means it is not possible to sidestep the requirements of the ICH guidelines by developing drugs outside the ICH regions in a manner that would not comply with them. As the EU, USA and Japan represent the three biggest world markets for new drugs, there is little incentive for non-compliance.

All human studies are performed according to strict ethical requirements. The Declaration of Helsinki (2000) sets the rules for all clinical development. In one sentence, the message comes through: 'It is the duty of the physician in medical research to protect the life, health, privacy, and dignity of the human subject'.

ICH requirements for all clinical trials include the following elements of good clinical practice (CPMP/ICH/286/95, released November 2000. http://www.emea.eu.int/index/indexh1/htm):

- The risks and potential benefits must be assessed before trials are initiated, and the benefits must outweigh the risks.
- The interests of the individual study subjects must take precedence over those of science or society.

---

[1]This does not apply currently to a wide variety of 'alternative' medicines, including plant extracts which may contain pharmacologically active substances. Anyone can market such a product without having to subject it to clinical trials. There are moves to tighten the regulation of herbal medicines, which may or may not be efficacious but can and do produce adverse effects. It is a sensitive area, however, and governments are proceeding very cautiously.

- All trial subjects must freely give their informed consent prior to participation.
- Trials must be scientifically sound and clearly described in a trial protocol.
- The trial must be carried out according to the protocol, which must be reviewed and approved by a properly constituted ethics committee[2].
- Only properly qualified physicians may provide medical care to trial subjects, and all other staff involved in clinical trials must be appropriately educated, qualified and experienced for the tasks they carry out.
- Human administration must be supported by the results of adequate preclinical testing in compliance with ICH guidelines for the administration of drugs to man.
- Data from clinical trials must be recorded, handled and stored in a way that allows accurate reporting, interpretation and verification.
- Trial subjects' privacy and confidentiality must be respected and assured.
- The material to be administered must be of acceptable quality and purity, as defined by the relevant ICH guidelines. This means both the drug substance and the formulated drug product must be manufactured in compliance with ICH Guidelines (2000) for good manufacturing practice (GMP) and used in accordance with the trial protocol.

Phase I

The first step in the clinical development of a new compound is to obtain preliminary information on its safety, tolerability, bioavailability and pharmacokinetics in man. The clinical investigators are normally clinical pharmacologists and the studies are carried out in specially equipped Phase I clinics.

Trial subjects are individuals who participate in clinical trials by receiving either the investigational drug or a control medication, such as placebo, and undergoing the assessments laid down in the trial protocol. Phase I trials are usually performed in healthy subjects rather than patients, as healthy subjects are more able to withstand any unexpected toxicity caused by the test drug and tend to show less intersubject variability than do patients. In Phase I trials there is no requirement or expectation that the medication will have a therapeutic effect or benefit in subjects in any way, and so the dosing regimen is designed to allow the collection of data relating to safety, tolerability and pharmacokinetics, rather than to efficacy. As they cannot gain any therapeutic benefit, healthy subjects can be paid for their participation in Phase I clinical trials. Nevertheless, guidelines prohibit excessive payments, which could induce subjects to participate in trials against their better judgement purely for financial gain.

Selection of subjects

What is a 'healthy subject'? Healthy does not necessarily mean normal, nor vice versa. Normality can be defined in a number of ways, but implies physiological characteristics at or close to the population mean. The term 'healthy', however, implies being in a state of disease-free good health, even if some physiological parameters deviate from the population mean. Otherwise healthy subjects are not excluded from Phase I clinical trials unless there is a specific reason to suspect that their abnormality puts them at risk. This allows populations of healthy people to be recruited that are representative of the variation in the population at large, without increasing the risk to their wellbeing. The definition of healthy subjects for a particular study is usually expressed in the inclusion and exclusion criteria set out in the trial protocol. On that basis, subjects volunteering to participate in clinical trials are carefully screened before they are allowed to participate.

The healthy subjects taking part in Phase I studies are volunteers. The definition of 'volunteer' in the context of clinical trials is a person who is capable of understanding the risks, purpose and requirements of the trial, and who is legally competent to freely consent to take part in it. Although the subjects participating in Phase I studies are usually healthy subjects, the requirement for informed consent is exactly the same for any subject in a clinical trial, whether healthy volunteer or patient.

Most volunteers in Phase I trials are young healthy males. This is because in order to administer experimental drugs to a woman, care must be taken that the drug will not impair her fertility nor cause harm to her unborn child if she becomes pregnant during the trial.

---

[2]The principal concern of the ethics committee is with the *safety* of trial participants, not with the purpose and design of the trial. Thus, the broader ethical issue of ensuring that effective treatments are made available for general use as quickly as possible is not normally considered. Some commentators argue that ethics committees should take into account the potential societal benefit, as well as the risk to trial participants. This arose recently in the case of a new orally active iron chelator, deferiprone, intended for the treatment of thalassaemia, a common life-threatening genetic disorder (see Savulescu, 2004). Trials of the drug were delayed for many years following concerns about toxicity, which surfaced in the initial trials but were subsequently refuted. The drug is now licensed for use in Europe and Asia, but not in the USA. Because of the delays, it is still uncertain whether thousands of European and Asian patients are being put at risk, or whether thousands of US patients are being denied treatment that could benefit them.

However, as most drugs will be used by women as well as men, and some drugs are exclusively for use by women, it is not possible to exclude women from all trials. Prior to entering women into any clinical trial the risks must have been evaluated by means of the reproductive toxicity studies described in Chapter 16. Full reproductive toxicity testing must usually be performed prior to submission of an application for approval to market a new drug (ICH, 1995), but Phase I studies take place much earlier in development, when the extent of the risk to female fertility or the unborn child is unkown. In that case, women of child-bearing potential may not usually be recruited. In Europe, women may only be recruited into Phase I studies if they have been surgically sterilized or are postmenopausal. Such women may be included if there are no signs of toxicity to the female reproductive organs in the repeated-dose general toxicity tests. Therefore, although the effects of new drugs on the fertility of both sexes need not be fully explored before Phase I studies, if any effects on the reproductive organs are observed in the repeat-dose toxicology studies these must be fully investigated before the drug is given to man.

Certain defined groups of volunteers are occasionally required for more specific Phase I trials. These include elderly volunteers, specific ethnic groups and, increasingly, volunteers belonging to a defined genetic subgroup for metabolism (fast or slow metabolizers). Elderly volunteers may be required in order to assess drugs for the elderly in a group of healthy subjects more representative of the target patient population. Specific ethnic groups, on the other hand, will be required when a drug being developed in Caucasian populations is also being submitted for approval in a different population, e.g. Japanese. In this case, it is to determine whether significant differences exist in the pharmacokinetics and pharmacodynamics of the two ethnic groups, and whether different dosage regimens will be necessary. Lastly, specific genetic metabolic subtypes might be selected in order to ensure that where slow metabolizer subtypes exist this does not cause accumulation of the drug and related toxicity in those individuals[3].

Sometimes, for example with anticancer drugs, the inherent toxicity of the test drug precludes giving it to healthy people, and Phase I trials of cytotoxic drugs are usually performed in cancer patients, so as to balance the risk with the possible benefits.

---

[3]Asian races, for example, are more sensitive to the antihypertensive and adverse effects of β_1-adrenoceptor antagonists, such as metoprolol, because the incidence of certain polymorphisms in the genes for cytochrome P450 and the α_1-adrenoceptor are much commoner than they are in Caucasians. In all these cases the definition of healthy volunteer is still applicable, though the evaluation of elderly subjects usually takes account of the normal ageing process and aims to select individuals who are healthy for their age.

Lastly, groups of subjects are sometimes required who are healthy except for one specific – usually mild – chronic medical condition, e.g. mild asthma. Because they only suffer mildly from the condition at which the drug is targeted, a potential therapeutic effect can be demonstrated in these subjects, e.g. a reduction in allergen or exercise-induced bronchoconstriction. This allows early investigation of the relationship between the dose of drug and the observed response in the target organ. Such dose–response testing is important for preliminary proof that the drug has a relevant pharmacological effect in man, and for the selection of appropriate dose levels for later efficacy trials. However, subjects selected on the basis of a medical condition relevant to the test drug can also be viewed as patients, and this raises some issues. For instance, whereas healthy subjects have no need or expectation of therapeutic benefit from any of the medications they may receive during a clinical trial, and can be paid for their time and inconvenience, the situation pertaining to patients is different. They have consulted their physicians in the expectation of treatment, and it is the responsibility of those physicians to act in the best interests of their patients' wellbeing at all times. They must therefore be satisfied that there is at least the possibility of therapeutic benefit for their patients before inviting them to participate in the trial. As physicians are themselves paid for the work they undertake in carrying out clinical trials, usually in the form of a fixed fee per completed patient, it is not acceptable for them to influence their patients' decision whether or not to participate by offering payment for taking part. Instead, they are expected to explain the possible benefits to the patient and to future sufferers of the same condition, along with the risks and procedures, and to allow the patient to decide on that basis alone. Attitudes do differ from country to country, however, regarding payment to patients participating in clinical trials, and although local guidelines may exist the ethics committee concerned should be informed and consulted on this issue. Before doing so, it is therefore important to consider carefully whether, in the context of the study design, the subjects are healthy volunteers or patients, and to provide the ethics committee with the rationale for that view. In certain borderline cases this judgement can be very difficult to make, but ultimately the regulatory authority and/or the ethics committee makes the binding ruling on this issue (WHO, 2000).

Regulatory procedures

The safety of subjects is always the paramount consideration in Phase I trials. There are two main bodies responsible for evaluating proposals for trials: the national drug regulatory authority in the country where the trial will take place, and the local ethics committee (EC) or, in the USA, the institutional review board (IRB) of the clinic in which the study will be performed. All clinical trials, irrespective of the degree of regulatory authority involvement, must be approved by a properly convened and correctly functioning EC or IRB before they can be initiated. Ethics committees are composed of independent experts and lay members, who review the proposed study (protocol, investigator's brochure, informed consent documentation, insurance arrangements etc.) and decide whether it is justified on ethical grounds. They evaluate the study in terms of the risk to the subjects, the appropriateness of any remuneration offered to both subjects and the clinical investigator, the design of the study and its ability to fulfil its primary objective(s), the qualifications, experience and clinical trial performance of the clinical investigator, the text of any advertising used to recruit subjects etc., and approve or reject the proposed trial on the basis of these ethical considerations. If it is approved, the EC/IRB remains involved with the trial until it is completed: for example, it must be informed of any serious adverse events (see below) that occur, and of any other major issues that cause concern during the study. Changes to an approved protocol may not normally be implemented without the EC/IRB approval.

In the case of regulatory authorities the degree of involvement varies from country to country (see Chapter 20), some reviewing all of the available data on the drug and some only requiring notification that EC/IRB approval has been given and that the trial will take place.

Recruiting volunteers

Once a trial protocol is approved by the EC/IRB and, if applicable, the regulatory authority, recruitment of healthy subjects can begin, and this can be done in a variety of ways. Advertising is permitted in most countries, within certain constraints and with prior approval of the advertising copy by the EC/IRB, but healthy subjects are also frequently recruited by word of mouth. Irrespective of how they are recruited, before any healthy subject can undergo any procedure whatsoever in a Phase I trial, he/she must first give informed consent. This is given in writing and follows an explanation of the risks, benefits, procedures, remuneration, insurance, volunteers' rights etc., both oral and written, in language appropriate for laypersons to understand. Volunteers must be allowed adequate time to consider their decision, and may not be pressured or otherwise influenced to participate. Consent signatures are normally witnessed and are held on file by the investigator, whose responsibility it is to ensure that the volunteers fully understand and consent to all of the procedures and constraints of the trial.

Eligibility criteria

Once informed consent is signed, subjects may be screened for eligibility to enter the trial. Screening aims

to ensure that all subjects are healthy within the context of the study, and will typically include:

- A full physical examination
- Documentation of the subject's full medical history
- 12-lead ECG
- Vital signs (blood pressure, heart rate, respiration rate and temperature)
- Height, weight and body mass index (BMI)
- Haematology, blood biochemistry and urine analyses
- Serology testing for hepatitis and HIV infection
- Urine screen for drugs of abuse
- Alcohol breath-testing
- Nicotine/cotinine testing (if non-smokers are required)

It may also include study-specific assessments. For instance, if the drug is known to be metabolized by a specific cytochrome P450 isoenzyme, its pharmacokinetic (PK) characteristics may be affected by genetic variations in the expression of that enzyme, i.e. individuals might be fast or slow metabolizers. Subjects may therefore be selected on the basis of their metabolic subtype to ensure that either or both groups are fully investigated.

Blood sampling for PK evaluation and for routine safety testing typically means that a total blood volume of between 250 and 450 mL will need to be taken from each volunteer in a Phase I trial. To avoid causing anaemia it is important to check that subjects entering the study have normal haemoglobin levels, and to exclude subjects who have recently given blood or taken part in another study requiring significant blood sampling.

In addition, if – exceptionally – female subjects of childbearing potential are to be included, a pregnancy test will be performed.

The investigator will then evaluate the subjects' screening results against the inclusion/exclusion criteria set out in the protocol. These are intended to identify the exact type of subject to be recruited and to exclude those who may be particularly at risk of adverse reactions, who are unable to give properly informed consent, who are likely to be atypical of the population in the way that they respond to drugs, who may find it difficult to comply with the study protocol, or whose response to the test medication might be difficult to interpret because of very recent participation in another trial. The exclusion criteria commonly include:

- Significantly high or low body weight in relation to height, age and sex;
- Clinically relevant cardiovascular abnormality (ECG, blood pressure or heart rate);
- Allergies relevant to the study situation (e.g. known drug hypersensitivity, skin allergies etc.);
- Medical history of conditions relevant to the study situation;

- Clinically relevant signs or symptoms at screening examination;
- Evidence or relevant history of drug or alcohol abuse;
- Evidence or history of any condition that could adversely affect absorption of the drug, if administered orally;
- Clinically relevant haematological, biochemical or urine abnormality at screening;
- Insufficient intellectual capacity to understand the information given about the study, and consequent inability to give legally valid informed consent;
- Participation in another study or blood donation in the previous 3 months;
- Any other specific condition, abnormality or characteristic that would increase the subject's risk.

Phase I trial design

- Phase I safety evaluation is usually divided into two parts, namely:
- Phase Ia (single-dose trials)
- Phase Ib (repeated-dose trials).

Phase Ia trials involve the drug's *first dose in man* (FDIM) – a red-letter day for the drug development team – when single doses of the drug are given to small cohorts of subjects. Usually four to eight cohorts of six to eight subjects are given the drug, each cohort receiving a higher dose than the last. If safety or tolerability issues arise during this dose escalation then the escalation will be stopped. In this case the *maximum tolerated dose* (MTD) in man has been determined, i.e. it is the highest dose that was given before safety/tolerability issues arose. This is important information for estimation of the therapeutic window, which is the dose range within which the drug is effective but safe and well tolerated. For some drugs with very low toxicity it may not be possible to escalate to the MTD, and the dose is increased to the highest practicable, or which is expected to be used in future clinical studies.

The choice of doses to be administered in Phase Ia trials should be based on the highest dose at which no adverse effects were seen in the most sensitive species tested in toxicology studies (the *no observed adverse effect level*, or NOAEL; see Chapter 16) and on the nature of the toxicity observed. Often, a single starting dose designed to deliver 1/50–1/100 of the NOAEL is considered an appropriate safety margin, but specific guidelines exist for the accurate determination of the starting dose on a case-by-case basis (FDA; http:www.fda.gov/cber/gdlns/dose.htm).

The dose escalation plan will depend on the characteristics of the drug and its metabolites, and especially on the nature of any toxicity seen in preclinical toxicology testing at doses above the NOAEL. It will also be influenced by the relationship between dose, systemic exposure as determined by its pharmacokinetic (PK) profile in animals, and the pharmacodynamic (PD) effects observed in efficacy pharmacology studies. Each dose escalation step will be dependent on satisfactory safety data from the previous dose level, according to the clinical judgement of the investigator.

Usually the drug is administered only once to each volunteer. Sometimes, however, it may be appropriate for each volunteer to receive two or three of the planned doses at successive visits, with the proviso that each dose is administered only after the response to the preceding dose in the series has been evaluated. In this way the required number of volunteers is reduced, but each has to attend more than once.

Although some Phase Ia studies only involve administration of the test drug, it is usual also to include a placebo, as this allows for more objective assessment of whether any adverse events are actually due to the test drug. Furthermore, to eliminate subject and observer bias, the trial is usually performed 'double-blind', meaning that although the investigator and the volunteers will be aware the doses are escalating in successive cohorts, within each cohort neither volunteer nor investigator will know which has been administered until after the results have been analysed and the study is 'unblinded'.

Typical dose escalation schedules from a starting dose of X are:

Dose escalation schedule 1:   X, 2X, 4X, 8X, 16X, 32X
Dose escalation schedule 2:   X, 2X, 4X, 6X, 8X, 10X

The dose escalation schedule and the dosing plan are elements of the study design that are mainly guided by safety considerations. Dose escalation schedule 1, where the dose is increased exponentially, would be appropriate for a drug that has shown low toxicity in animal testing. Schedule 2, where the dose increments are constant, is more conservative and might be more appropriate for a drug which has a toxicology profile that calls for a more cautious approach to dose escalation in man. There are many other possible dose escalation patterns, and each drug is considered on its own merits. If safety considerations permit, the dose should be increased beyond the level predicted from preclinical pharmacology studies to have the required therapeutic effect in man. Clearly, a drug that displays significant toxicity before it reaches therapeutic levels at the target site is unlikely to be successful.

Throughout the study, for an appropriate period after each dose, the volunteers are intensively monitored for signs and/or symptoms of toxicity (adverse events). This includes effects on heart rhythm and other ECG parameters, blood pressure, heart rate, respiration rate, body temperature, liver function and renal function, as well as observation for any other unwanted effects. All adverse events must be recorded, categorized by severity, duration, outcome and causality, analysed, tabulated, and included in the final report at the end of the study. If an adverse event meets certain specific criteria (for instance if it is life threatening or necessitates hospitalization) it is classified as a *serious adverse event* (SAE) and must be reported without delay to the ethics committee, and usually also to the regulatory authority.

Whereas assessment of safety and tolerability is the primary objective, pharmacokinetic evaluation is the secondary objective of a Phase Ia study. Blood samples will normally be taken before dosing and at specified intervals after dosing to measure the amount of drug in the blood or plasma at various time points after each dose. A typical sampling schedule is shown in Figure 18.1A.

In addition, urine and/or faeces may be collected to measure the excretion of the drug via the kidneys and/or liver (in bile). The results enable the rate of absorption, metabolism and excretion of the drug to be explored, and the PK parameters to be estimated.

It is common for the PK profiles of orally administered drugs to be affected by the presence or absence of food in the stomach at the time of dosing. Usually, this 'food effect' is also investigated in Phase Ia. At the end of the dose escalation schedule a safe and well tolerated dose level is selected and given to another cohort of subjects on two occasions, once 'fed' (immediately after a standard breakfast) and once 'fasted' (after an overnight fast), so that the PK parameters can be compared. The doses are usually given with an appropriate 'washout period' between them to ensure that the first dose has been completely eliminated from the body before the second dose is given. To eliminate any possible bias, these volunteers will be randomly allocated to have the 'fed' or 'fasted' dose first. The results of the fed/fasted comparison will form the basis of the dosing instructions for all future studies with the drug.

The plasma or serum PK parameters usually derived from Phase Ia studies are:

- C_{max}: peak drug and/or metabolite(s) concentration;
- T_{max}: time to peak drug and/or metabolite(s) concentration;
- $AUC_{0-\infty}$: area under the concentration–time curve of the drug and/or metabolite(s), extrapolated to infinity;

A Single-dose study

Time	0	10 min	20 min	30 min	1h	1½h	2h	4h	6h	8h	12h	24h	48h
Dose	↑												
Blood sample	●	●	●	●	●	●	●	●	●	●	●	●	●

B Repeat-dose study

Day 1	0	10 min	20 min	30 min	1h	1½h	2h	4h	6h	8h	12h
	↑										
	●	●	●	●	●	●	●	●	●	●	●

Days 2–7	0	10 min	20 min	30 min	1h	1½h	2h	4h	6h	8h	12h
	↑										↑
	●										●

Day 8	0	10 min	20 min	30 min	1h	1½h	2h	4h	6h	8h	12h	24h	48h
	↑												
	●	●	●	●	●	●	●	●	●	●	●	●	●

Fig. 18.1
Typical dosing and blood sampling schedules for Phase I studies.

- AUC_{0-T}: area under the concentration–time curve of the drug and/or metabolite(s), calculated to a specific time point T;
- $T_{1/2}$: time taken for levels of drug and/or metabolite(s) to decrease by half (a measure of the rate of elimination of the drug from plasma).

Other PK parameters may also be determined, including:

- V_D: volume of distribution of drug and/or metabolite(s);
- Cl: clearance of drug and/or metabolite, i.e. the volume of plasma/serum cleared of drug and/or metabolite(s) per unit time, e.g. mL/min, L/h;
- MRT: mean residence time, i.e. the average time a drug molecule remains in the body after rapid IV injection.

Specialist pharmacokineticists perform the calculation of these parameters.

A comparison of the PK parameters at each dose level, e.g. AUC_∞, C_{max}, will indicate whether they increase proportionally (linear kinetics) or disproportionately (non-linear kinetics) with increasing dose. This information will influence the selection of dose levels, regimen and duration of dosing for the Phase Ib repeated-dose study. The single-dose PK data can also be used to predict the drug/metabolite(s) concentrations expected on repeated dosing, based on the assumption that the kinetics do not change with time.

After review of the safety data and the single-dose PK profile, two or three safe and well-tolerated dose levels are chosen and the Phase Ib (repeated-dose) study is designed. Its purpose is to test safety, tolerability and PK when the drug is given repeatedly. The regimen is designed to give the PK profile necessary to allow the drug to exert its therapeutic effect. The single-dose PK characteristics are used to predict the likely PK profile with repeated dosing, including the time taken to reach the 'steady state' in which the drug's input rate is balanced by its rate of elimination. This will determine the frequency and duration of dosing required. The design of Phase Ib studies therefore generally involves a two- or three-step dose escalation, with successive groups of 12–24 subjects taking the drug repeatedly for several days at each dose level. Dose escalation is again dependent on satisfactory safety data from the previous dose level.

Safety assessment is necessary under these conditions, as steady-state blood levels are usually higher than peak blood levels following a single administration. It is also important to know whether the PK of the drug and/or metabolite(s) changes on repeated dosing. For instance, saturation of elimination pathways (e.g. metabolizing enzyme systems) could cause the drug to accumulate to toxic levels in the body, or alternatively stimulation (induction) of drug-metabolizing enzymes systems could cause the levels of drug and/or metabolite(s) to decrease to subtherapeutic levels. A comparison of the predicted and observed plasma–serum concentration time curves will provide evidence of any such non-linear or time-dependent kinetics for the drug and/or metabolite(s).

In addition to PK evaluation, pharmacodynamic (PD) assessments may be included in Phase Ib studies (and occasionally even in Phase Ia studies) to look for preliminary evidence of the required pharmacological activity in man. Such studies are termed PK/PD studies and, when possible, they offer an early means of exploring the relationship between dose and effects (dose–response curve) and concentration and effects (concentration–response curve). This can greatly assist the design of the early efficacy studies in patients, as the magnitude of effect can be plotted against the blood levels of the drug and an optimal dosing regimen chosen for early patient studies.

This approach must still be treated with some caution, as the physiology in patients may differ from that in healthy volunteers, and clinical efficacy may therefore not be reliably predicted from Phase I results. It is not uncommon for drugs that are highly effective in patients suffering from a certain condition to have little or no effect on the same body system in healthy volunteers. The meaningful addition of PD assessments in Phase I depends on the existence of biological or surrogate markers that are measurable in healthy volunteers and known to have relevance to the drug's mechanism of action and/or therapeutic effect. For example, the ability of a β-adrenoceptor antagonist to inhibit exercise-induced tachycardia, or the effect of a proton pump inhibitor on acid gastric secretion are relevant effects that can easily be measured in volunteers. However, such markers are not always available (e.g. in the case of many psychiatric diseases) or may be misleading, and the interpretation of such data is usually approached with care. Nonetheless, Phase I PK/PD studies can, in certain cases, be of great importance in confirming that a new drug is actually having the pharmacological effect in man that was predicted from animal studies.

The general requirements and procedures for Phase Ib studies are the same as those for Phase Ia, except that the subjects usually have to agree to reside in the clinic while they are taking the study medication, for safety reasons. A typical Phase Ib blood sampling schedule is shown in Figure 18.1B. Blood samples for PK profiling will generally be taken on the first and last days of dosing, with additional single samples taken immediately before the first morning dose each day, to measure the levels of drug remaining in the blood immediately before the next dose is administered.

The results of the Phase Ia and Ib studies together support the decision as to whether to administer the drug to patients and, if so, at what dose and regimen and for how long.

Phase II: Early efficacy and dose-finding trials in patients

New drugs can only reliably be tested for therapeutic efficacy in patients suffering from the diseases that they are designed to treat. Even if it has been possible to obtain some PK/PD and dose–response data from healthy volunteers, efficacy needs to be explored in an appropriate patient group in order to assess a new drug's potential for full development. The same requirements for ethical and regulatory approval apply to Phase II trials as to Phase I (see above). Phase II trials are typically performed in a hospital clinic setting, by experienced clinical investigators who specialize in the disease area involved and can closely monitor the patients and accurately assess any drug effects observed.

Phase II is divided into:

- *Phase IIa*   Exploratory trials in small groups of patients designed to give preliminary evidence of efficacy and safety;
- *Phase IIb*   Trials in sufficiently large groups of patients to confirm efficacy with statistical significance, and to determine the optimal dose and dosing regimen.

The transition from Phase IIa to IIb represents a particularly important decision point in any development programme. Phase I and IIa trials are designed to provide the pharmaceutical company's management with the information it needs in order to decide whether a compound satisfies the criteria for full development and stands a reasonable chance of being approved by regulatory authorities. This decision point is referred to as proof of concept (POC), or sometimes proof of principle (POP).

If POC is achieved in Phase IIa and a decision is taken to enter full development, Phase IIb studies mark the beginning of a confirmatory, registration-focused stage of clinical development. Together with the even larger Phase III trials required to prove efficacy and safety they provide pivotal data in support of marketing applications.

Phase IIb and III trials require major investment. The quality of the data obtained from early exploratory Phase IIa studies is therefore critically important in selecting good drug candidates and minimizing the risk of investing in new compounds that later prove to be ineffective or unsafe, or both.

Phase IIa: Proof of concept and go/no-go decision making

Phase IIa trials are kept as small as possible but are designed with great care in order to maximize the reliability of the decision-focused data they generate. Because the studies may lack the statistical power to draw inferences from the data with confidence, the interpretation of Phase IIa results requires experience and objectivity. In order to ensure a balanced evaluation of the drug's performance, criteria for progressing or halting its development are usually established in advance and are used to guide the study design, focusing clearly on generating the specific, decision-focused data required, taking account of the specific characteristics of the compound and the clinical situation in which it is intended to be used.

In addition to pharmacodynamic/efficacy outcome measures, Phase IIa studies frequently include PK sampling and analysis, as in many disease states the PK profile in patients differs from that in healthy individuals. The absorption of drugs, for instance, is often impaired in AIDS patients. Also, if no meaningful pharmacodynamic assessment was possible in Phase I, this may be the first opportunity to explore the PK/PD relationship and the dose–response curve.

The dosing regimen for Phase IIa studies will be chosen on the basis of the PK profiles generated in Phase I and the drug's mechanism of action. In addition, the duration of dosing will be influenced by the indication being treated. In some cases it is possible to show efficacy in days or weeks (e.g. asthma) or even less (e.g. post-operative pain), whereas in others it may be necessary to administer the drug for months before clinical effects can be reliably assessed (e.g. peripheral vascular disease, osteoporosis). The duration of treatment in Phase IIa is a critical issue in the design of early development programmes, as it dictates the duration of pre-clinical toxicology testing required (see Chapter 20). For this reason, a development programme requiring 6 months' dosing in Phase IIa will take about a year longer than one requiring only 28 days' dosing.

In setting the criteria for POC many other factors must be taken into account, as several approaches can be adopted depending on the setting. Two situations commonly occur, requiring different approaches.

'First in class' drug

A first-in-class drug is one that is entirely innovative and has a novel mode of action that has never been demonstrated to have a therapeutic effect in man. In this context, POC is for the new class of drugs rather than for a specific drug entity. The discovery team will want to know as quickly as possible if their hypothetical therapeutic effect is actually seen in man, and they may therefore choose an initial drug candidate with optimal pharmacodynamic characteristics, irrespective of its other properties, so as to maximize the chance of demonstrating its therapeutic effect. The compound tested may, in fact, have shortcomings that preclude it as a candidate for full development. Once the concept of its mechanism has been proved by observing its therapeutic effect in man, the discovery team will aim to modify the molecule in such a way as to preserve the desired pharmacological activity but improve other characteristics, such as pharmacokinetic properties or receptor selectivity. A new lead candidate will then be chosen from an array of optimized molecules, and again enter early development and POC testing. In this context, the POC studies serve essentially to confirm a hypothesis which, if substantiated, provides a sound basis for designing a truly innovative new drug – with luck, a blockbuster, the Holy Grail of the pharmaceutical industry. Alternatively, if the POC studies give negative or equivocal results, the discovery team may reluctantly decide to drop that particular line of research. Occasionally, teams lack such objectivity and remain determined to press on, insisting that the design of the studies was at fault rather than their hypothesis.

The preferred strategy for POC testing in this scenario may be to minimize cost by undertaking only those preclinical studies that are absolutely necessary to allow the drug to be administered to man as quickly as possible. This may mean, for instance, that rather than spend time and money on sophisticated oral formulation development, the drug may be given in the simplest possible way in Phase IIa. For instance, if it is reasonably water soluble it might be given orally or intravenously as a simple solution, even though the future marketed product would be a tablet formulation of a different, fully optimized compound.

Similarly, the indication chosen for POC testing of a first-in-class drug may differ from the indication envisaged for the marketed product. Consider, for example, a novel drug intended as an oral tablet for treatment of *intermittent claudication* (a condition in which peripheral vascular disease leads to insufficient blood flow to the leg muscles, causing pain on walking which gradually progresses to more serious ischaemia and ulceration). The clinical outcome measure in this indication (maximum walking distance) is notoriously variable, and large numbers of patients, typically many hundreds, have to be treated for up to 6 months in order to show a statistically significant effect compared to placebo[4].

One strategy to overcome this may be to test the drug first in a population relevant to, but different from, the actual target population. In this case, patients with ischaemic leg ulcers may offer an alternative, quicker and more reliable population in which to look for proof of pharmacological effect. The clinical outcome measure, reduction of ulcer size, is less variable than walking distance and could show a measurable response to treatment after only 4 weeks' dosing. The extrapolation from ischaemic ulcer patients to intermittent claudication patients would still need to be tested, but the answer to the primary question of pharmacological effect in peripheral ischaemia per se could be answered on the basis of 28-day repeated-dose toxicology testing, a standard Phase Ia/Ib programme and a Phase IIa study with 28 days' drug administration in this patient group. This compares favourably with the 6-month repeated-dose toxicology and 6-month duration of treatment required for a Phase IIa study in intermittent claudication, and shortens the time to POC for the mechanism by approximately a year.

In contrast to the use of a more severe manifestation of peripheral vascular disease for POC testing as described above, it would also be possible to test a new mechanism of action in mildly affected patients or healthy subjects who do not have the disease at all by using biological or (if they exist) clinical surrogate markers to prove the mechanism. In the peripheral vascular disease example, this might involve assessing the direct effect of the drug on the circulation in the affected leg by measuring blood flow before and after treatment. Alternatively, and even less directly, the effect on platelets or other blood parameters could be measured ex vivo in healthy volunteers in Phase I, if that was relevant to the mechanism. Such an approach is quick, relatively cheap, and allows POC to be achieved in Phase I. However, there are significant drawbacks to using it as the basis for decision making. Even assuming that relevant biological markers exist in healthy subject for the disease in question, the correlation between effects on those markers and clinical outcomes is often unknown. Unless validated surrogate markers exist for a particular condition, the extent to which Phase I data are predictive of clinical efficacy provable in large-scale clinical trials is questionable, and the interpretation of such data is extremely difficult. In most cases, therefore, it is necessary to conduct a Phase IIa study in patients using clinical outcome measures.

'Follower drug'

The second scenario for Phase IIa POC testing relates to a drug of an existing class. In this case the mechanism has already been proven and the therapeutic effect of the class established. Instead of 'first-in-class', this drug may be targeting 'best-in-class'. Such follower products are frequently even more successful than the 'first-in-class', and need to reach the market quickly to capitalize on the market created by the innovator and win market share. The criteria for POC in this case will focus on commercially important improvements over the first-in-

---

[4]This is because the variability of the disease between individuals and within individuals from day to day causes excessive 'noise' in the data. Such 'noise' might swamp the therapeutic effect of the drug, making it impossible to say with confidence that there is a beneficial effect. Statistical techniques exist for calculating the numbers of subjects required to provide specified levels of confidence in the reliability of results inferred from clinical trials. These 'power calculations' take into account the variability of the outcome measures and the magnitude of the therapeutic effect required, and predict how many subjects must be enrolled to test the drug's effect with a predefined level of confidence in the results, e.g. 80% confidence, 90% confidence etc.

class product, and will therefore be dictated by its short-comings. For instance, the first-in-class drug may be highly effective but have a poor safety/tolerability profile and/or unsatisfactory PK characteristics, requiring dosing three or four times daily. In order to compete successfully with it, the follower drug must be at least as effective and at the same time improve on its weaknesses

In this case the criteria for POC will focus not only on confirmation of the predicted efficacy of the compound, but equally on its safety/tolerability profile and its PK characteristics. This will drive the design of the Phase I programme, which may include the first-in-class drug as a comparator. Similarly, the Phase I programme may entail the investigation of a variety of oral formulations and dosing protocols to ensure that adequate exposure can be achieved with a regimen more acceptable than that of the innovator. Lastly, the probability of the compound going forward into full development is greater than that of a 'first-in-class' drug. It may therefore be considered less risky to invest early in formulation development to design oral forms that will allow the drug to move rapidly into full evaluation for once- or twice-daily dosing in Phase IIb. The Phase IIa POC testing in this situation may therefore take longer and cost significantly more than for a 'first-in-class' compound.

Whatever strategy is adopted, the objective of Phase IIa is to prove the basic concept of the drug and on that basis make an accurate go/no-go decision as to its further development.

Phase IIb: Dose-finding studies

Whereas early clinical development can be viewed as exploratory, late development should ideally be confirmatory. Phase IIb and III trials are designed to confirm, rather than explore, efficacy and safety, and surprises at this stage are seldom good news. Currently, it is not possible to eliminate risk in go/no-go decision making entirely, and attrition still occurs in late development, as discussed earlier. However, if the exploratory development plan and POC testing of a drug have been well designed, and assessment of the drug's performance has been objective and rigorous, the decision to move into confirmatory development (Phase IIb/III) can be made with the minimum of risk.

In order to grant market approval for a new drug, the licensing authorities in the region concerned will require extensive data to support its safety, its efficacy in the target indication, and the claims the company intends to make for it, once marketed. Exploratory trials therefore give way to large, fully statistically powered clinical trials designed to provide this. Usually the first step, Phase IIb, is to conduct a study specifically to confirm the preliminary safety and efficacy data generated in Phase I and IIa, and to explore the dose–response relationship in detail, to ensure that the correct dose is selected for large-scale Phase III efficacy studies.

These trials must include sufficient patients to allow inferences to be drawn from the results with confidence, i.e. the study must have sufficient statistical power to support extrapolation of the results obtained from the test patients to the patient population at large. As discussed earlier, the size of the population to be tested will therefore be carefully calculated (power calculation) by a biostatistician, who will take into account the variability of the primary outcome measure and the magnitude of the effect required to give a clinically significant improvement in the condition being treated. Typically, these trials involve several hundreds of patients.

The standard design of Phase IIb dose-finding studies is parallel-group randomized double-blind and, if possible, placebo controlled. The inclusion of a placebo group, when feasible in patients, allows more accurate evaluation of efficacy and safety than is possible when only the test drug, or test drug and active comparator, is used. (Studies involving the administration of test drug only are termed 'open label' and are performed in very specific indications, e.g. some types of cancer, when it is unethical to use placebo and there is no comparator.) Placebo-controlled trials allow absolute efficacy and safety to be assessed, whereas only relative values can be inferred from active comparator trials. In many disease states the mind plays an important part in the patient's (and often the physician's) perception of the severity of symptoms. The patient's belief that treatment is being given, coupled with faith in the physician administering it, can result in an apparent improvement irrespective of the effectiveness of the therapeutic agent used. This effect, known as the 'placebo effect', is well documented in the literature (Beecher, 1955)[5].

The physician's desire to see the patient improve can also influence his or her judgement when assessing the patient's condition. These effects justify the use of the randomization of trial subjects in a double-blinded manner, to remove patient or observer bias.

The design of clinical efficacy trials must therefore be sufficiently robust to ensure that any effects attributed to the test drug are not in fact placebo effects or spontaneous improvement, and the addition of a placebo arm allows a direct comparison to be made between patients receiving the test drug and those receiving dummy tablets. Some designs, however, eliminate patients who

---

[5]The magnitude of the placebo effect has recently been called into question. It is usually measured by comparing the difference between measures of severity before and after a course of active or placebo medication, and it is often found that significant improvement occurs in the placebo group. However, as pointed out by Hrobjartsson and Grotzche (2001) few trials had compared placebo with 'no treatment', and much of the apparent placebo effect may simply reflect spontaneous improvement, since trials that did include a no-treatment group showed, in most cases, a similar degree of improvement.

display a placebo response of sufficient magnitude to swamp any true drug effect. Such designs may incorporate a 'placebo run-in' period, i.e. a period at the beginning of the trial during which all patients receive placebo under single-blind conditions, where the physician knows they are receiving placebo but the patients do not. The protocol will specify a certain change from baseline response as the primary outcome measure, which, if it occurs on placebo treatment, disqualifies the patient from receiving active treatment on the basis that he/she is a placebo responder or a spontaneous recoverer. Exclusion of these patients, followed by double-blind randomization of the remaining patients to active or placebo treatment, strengthens the inferences that can be drawn from clinical trials with respect to efficacy.

In all cases, the objective in Phase IIb is to find the optimum dose for most patients, combining maximum efficacy with a satisfactory tolerability profile and an acceptable safety margin. At this stage, selection of the dose range to be tested in Phase IIb will be based on the results of the preliminary efficacy assessment in Phase IIa, and on the safety and tolerability profiles in preclinical testing and Phase I and IIa human trials.

Once the range of doses has been selected and the design of the study agreed, a decision needs to be taken as to where to carry out the trials. This should take into account the number and type of patients needed, the prevalence of the disease, the likely rate of recruitment and the regulatory requirements of the various country options. Phase IIb trials will form part of the dossier to be submitted for marketing approval, and if the submission is to be made in an ICH region or any other country that recognizes ICH guidelines, the study must be fully compliant with ICH as well as local rules. These rules place a large organizational and administrative burden on the trial centres, which need to be selected with care, based on inspection of their facilities and an assessment of the investigator's qualifications, experience and availability to carry out the study to the standard required.

Once the site is selected, it is the responsibility of the sponsoring pharmaceutical company, or its subcontractor, to train those involved in the trial in the requirements of the study protocol and ICH GCP standards, and then to monitor the project on site to ensure compliance. Clinical monitors are specially trained for this task and are instrumental in maintaining high standards of clinical research in the ICH regions, and in any sites in non-ICH countries where studies are being carried out in compliance with ICH guidelines. Further, to ensure compliance, an additional quality assurance (QA) step is carried out, involving the inspection of some or all of the sites by auditors independent of the project team. Auditors are responsible for thoroughly inspecting the data and documentation files to validate the site and the data it produces in terms of ICH compliance.

The wider objectives of monitoring and audit are the assurance of reliable, high-quality data and the prevention of fraud. Occasionally, the monitor may have concerns either that the data are not being obtained in accordance with the protocol or ICH GCP or even that they are being generated fraudulently. In this case, a 'for cause' audit will be carried out on the site and an audit report will detail any shortcomings in the conduct of the trial there, so that appropriate action can be taken by the study sponsor. Because of the critical role played by clinical monitors in the prevention of fraud, they usually have specific communication procedures that must be followed to ensure that any suspicions they may have about a particular site are adequately investigated and resolved.

All of these checks and controls on the quality and validity of data add substantially to the cost of clinical trials, but are essential because the complete dossier of information, including quality control checks, will be submitted to a regulatory authority in order to obtain approval to market the drug, and regulatory authorities must be confident that the data they are basing their decisions on are valid. The regulatory authority itself may choose to inspect one or more clinical sites and/or the files of the sponsoring company or its subcontractor, as a final check on data quality. Issues arising at this late stage cast suspicion on the whole dossier and can delay or prevent the granting of marketing approval. A detailed overview of the regulatory requirements for product development and licensing are given in Chapter 20.

Successful completion of Phase IIb and clarification of the optimal dose level allows the project to progress to the pivotal Phase III large scale efficacy trials required for marketing approval.

Phase III: Large-scale efficacy studies in patients

When new drugs are submitted to drug licensing authorities for marketing approval, the assessors review the supporting data package in great detail to ensure that the drug is safe, well tolerated and efficacious. Normally, it will be necessary to demonstrate absolute efficacy (compared with placebo) at some point during clinical development, but in cases where standard treatments already exist it is also necessary to demonstrate quantifiable advantages over them in order to obtain marketing approval. These advantages may be related to safety, tolerability, efficacy, patient acceptability and compliance or cost-effectiveness. Phase III trials are therefore planned with these factors in mind, and will usually be designed to compare the new drug's performance on each of them with the most commonly used or standard treatment in the chosen indication. The choice of the comparator drug is driven by a variety of considerations, depending on the particular claims the sponsor wishes to make for the product and the price it wants to command. The future marketing strategy for the product, when licensed, is therefore a strong element in the design of the programme of Phase III studies.

A Phase III programme will normally comprise several studies, usually carried out in the regions in which the drug will be sold. Occasionally all of the Phase III data will be generated in one region, e.g. in the USA, even though the drug is to be submitted for registration in another, e.g. Europe or Japan. As long as the data have been generated in compliance with ICH GCP this is possible, provided that ethnic differences in the populations in each region have been taken into account. These differences can be intrinsic (e.g. genetic) or extrinsic (e.g. diet, medical practice), and when using data from one population to support registration for use in another, the degree to which intrinsic and extrinsic ethnic factors might affect the drug's safety and efficacy must be taken into account. When data are being generated in the USA for submission to the European regulatory authority (European Medicines Evaluation Agency, EMEA) or vice versa, intrinsic ethnic factors are usually not an issue because both populations are predominantly Caucasian, but extrinsic ethnic factors also need to be taken into account. This means, for instance, that the diagnostic criteria used for patient enrolment and the method of evaluating the effects of the drug must be consistent in all regions in which the data will be submitted, and also that the selection of the comparator drugs must take into account the standard treatments used in different regions. Because of the pivotal nature of Phase III studies, and their importance not only for securing marketing approval but also for underpinning the claims upon which the marketing strategy will be based, the company's regulatory affairs and marketing groups, as well as the clinical research team, must be closely involved in their design.

Bridging studies

Data generated in the USA and used to support marketing approval of the drug in Japan present more problems, owing to the more significant intrinsic (e.g. genetic) differences between Caucasian and Japanese populations. An example is the greater frequency of polymorphisms in the cytochrome P450 enzyme CYP2A6 (Oscarson, 2001) seen in Chinese and Japanese populations, and the related differences in nicotine metabolism. It is therefore usually necessary for a study to be carried out to 'bridge' Caucasian data into Japan, i.e. to test the validity of Caucasian data in a Japanese population. This is done by studying the drug's phar-

macokinetics, and usually its pharmacodynamic properties, in both populations and comparing the results to determine whether they are comparable.

In considering the issue of extrapolating drug safety and efficacy data from one population to the other, the objective is to do this safely while not repeating clinical trials unnecessarily. Specific ICH guidelines exist for the extrapolation of data from one ethnic group to another (ICH, 1995). There are several strategies and approaches for exploring ethnic differences in drug response, but none is appropriate for all circumstances and each situation must be carefully evaluated, with a detailed understanding of the requirements of the target regulatory authority and its acceptance of foreign data.

Overall, the strategic planning and design of bridging studies can be one of the most challenging aspects of clinical development, as scientific knowledge in this field is rapidly increasing and regulatory requirements are still evolving and subject to change. However, it is an issue of great importance, as medical and commercial considerations increasingly call for new drugs to be developed globally and made available to patients wherever they need them.

Organizational issues

The ethical considerations described earlier apply with equal force to Phase III trials, as do the requirements for strict compliance with ICH GCP if the data are to be accepted as the basis for marketing approval in any of the ICH regions. The trials are large and typically performed across several countries; they therefore present an organizational challenge, and require expert project management if they are to be completed on time, within the allocated budget and to the required quality standards. It is not unusual for a Phase III pivotal study to involve more than 100 clinical investigator sites in more than a dozen countries.

By the time a drug reaches Phase III, a few hundred subjects have been exposed to it and the sponsor has gained experience with its safety profile. As each trial is completed, the summary information on the drug (investigator brochure) is updated, including the safety summary. If the results are satisfactory, this growing data package justifies testing of the drug in a wider population that is more representative of the patient population in which the drug will be used in the future. Indeed, one of the aims of Phase III is to expose sufficient numbers of patients to the drug to allow the detection of relatively rare adverse effects, and regulatory authorities sometimes specify how many patient-years of safety data must be submitted in order for approval to be considered. It is not feasible to perform clinical trials large enough to detect very rare idiosyncratic adverse events, but regulatory authorities need to be reassured that any serious toxicity likely to affect significant numbers of patients would have been identified in Phase III, before the drug reaches the market.

Drug interaction studies

When the drug is approved it may be given to patients who are taking other medications, and one of the aims of Phase III clinical research is to build experience with the drug in combination with others. In parallel with Phase IIb/III, in preparation for submission of the dossier the sponsor will have considered the theoretical risk of drug–drug interactions and will have carried out preclinical in vitro metabolic screening experiments to assess the potential for interaction. Where there is a theoretical risk or expectation of a drug interaction (e.g. where two drugs are metabolized by the same cytochrome P450 isoenzyme), specific drug interaction studies will be required to quantify the effect. These studies can be carried out in healthy volunteers, who take both drugs simultaneously so that the pharmacokinetics of the each new drug can be determined in the presence of the other, in order to detect any interference.

Trial design and outcome measures

The design of Phase III studies can vary, but is commonly a straightforward randomized double-blind comparison with standard treatment. Eligible patients will be allocated at random to one of the test treatments, and neither they nor the investigators will know which they have received until the trial has finished and the results have been analysed. In most cases the primary outcome measure is a clearly defined level of improvement in the patient's disease state. This may be straightforward; for example, relief of asthma can be demonstrated by measuring the effects on lung function parameters such as forced expiratory volume, peak expiratory flow etc. However, some drugs are designed to prevent the long-term effects of conditions that have few or no symptoms early on in the disease, such as hypertension. The rationale for treatment of hypertension is therefore to reduce the risk of cardiovascular morbidity and mortality. However, this is very difficult to demonstrate in clinical trials because in order directly to measure the effects of a new antihypertensive drug on cardiovascular morbidity/mortality huge populations have to be studied and followed up for many years, and the cost and time are prohibitive. Furthermore, modern antihypertensive therapy involves the use of several drugs in combination, and the trial would

need to test the new drug in combination with various others, further adding to its complexity. In this case the regulatory authorities acknowledge that lowering blood pressure reduces the risks, and therefore accepts blood pressure lowering as a surrogate for reduction in cardiovascular risk. Reimbursement agencies also accept this rationale, and it is common for pharmacoeconomic data demonstrating the cost-effectiveness of a drug that reduces cardiovascular risk to form part of the supporting information submitted to them.

Phase IV: Post-marketing studies to monitor safety in very large numbers of patients

As we have seen, the development of drugs is a lengthy and expensive process, but even the most extensive and costly clinical development process cannot guarantee that all adverse effects will be revealed before a drug reaches the market. However, it is not in the interests of patients to hold promising new medicines back for many years of safety testing, denying them the possibility of effective treatment. Caution must therefore be balanced against the possible benefits to patients. An increasingly common strategy is for regulatory authorities to grant marketing approval on the basis of a predefined number of patient-years' safety data, on condition that the manufacturer continues to collect safety data on their product after it is actually on the market. Typically, such data collection takes the form of a post-marketing surveillance study, involving thousands of patients actually being prescribed the drug in question. Basic data are collected with very simple documentation, often electronically, and specially trained and medically experienced pharmacovigilance groups monitor the safety of the drug. Periodically after launch, the safety data are analysed and scrutinized for patterns suggestive of previously unreported toxicity to ensure that the drug is withdrawn from the market at the earliest possible opportunity if such toxicity is observed. The importance of post-marketing surveillance is supported by the fact that around a fifth of new drugs may ultimately be recalled or cause serious side effects.

Trials in children

Drugs are of course used in children as well as adults, and there is increasing pressure from regulatory authorities to test them in this population instead of relying on extrapolation from adult data. There are many examples of drugs that show different pharmacokinetic or pharmacodynamic properties in children, or which differ in their clinical efficacy profile. Furthermore, possible effects of drug treatment on growth and development need to be taken into account (balanced, of course, against the effects of the untreated disease condition on growth and development). Until recently, very few drug trials were performed in children, and prescribing information did not cover paediatric use, despite the fact that many conditions such as epilepsy, asthma, allergies and infectious diseases that require drug treatment are common in children. Paediatric treatment therefore usually involved 'off-label' prescription, made more difficult by the fact that no formulations designed for children were available. Pharmaceutical companies were reluctant to carry out trials in children, partly for fear of arousing public opposition, and partly because the likely commercial returns seldom justified the cost. On the other hand, paediatricians argued that drug treatment in children was often clinically indicated, but – as in adult medicine – needed to be objectively assessed in relation to benefit and risk by properly controlled trials. The FDA recognized the need, and the 1997 FDA Modernization Act (FDAMA) incorporated specific incentives, in the form of a 6-month extension of patent protection, for certain drugs that had been tested in children according to the FDA guidelines. In some cases the FDA insists on trials in children before granting marketing approval (even for use in adults) if a new drug is considered likely to be useful in children. A draft ICH guideline (E11) covering the conduct of trials in children has been produced (see http://www.ich.org). The ethical issues (Smyth and Weindling, 1999) surrounding the participation of children in clinical trials are complex, and this specialist area is outside the scope of this chapter. There is no doubt, however, that there will be mounting pressure to carry out properly controlled trials in children (see Chapter 20) as a condition of registration of new drugs, in an effort to reduce the need for off-label prescribing.

Issues of confidentiality and disclosure

In the USA and Europe clinical trials approved by the regulatory authorities are now logged in publicly accessible databases (see http//www.clinicaltrials.gov, http//pharmacos.eudra.org), which provide details of the purpose and plan of the trial, the clinical centres and investigators involved, and the stage the trial has reached. This important recent development, supported by the World health Organization, is intended to cover all randomized controlled trials (Antes, 2004; www.controlled-trials.com). For every trial a registra-

tion number (International Standardized Randomized Controlled Trial Number, ISRCTN) is assigned, and it will allow public access to information on all prospective studies involving experimental and registered compounds. Its main aim is to avoid unnecessary repetition of clinical trials. These databases do not, however, include the *results* of completed trials, which frequently remain unpublished.

Regulatory authorities (see Chapter 20) require detailed results of all clinical trials approved by them – including trials of marketed compounds – to be reported to them, but this information is not, in general, publicly accessible, except to the extent that the Summary Basis of Approval (US) or Centralized Evaluation Report (EU) that is published when a drug is approved, includes a summary of the clinical trials results on which the approval was based. Clinical trial sponsors are under an obligation to report to the regulatory authority any safety issues that come to light, and the regulatory authority may respond by altering the terms of the marketing approval (for example by including a warning in the package insert, or, in an extreme case, by withdrawing the approval altogether). Publication of trial results in the open literature is not obligatory, and Dickersin and Rennie (2003) cite evidence suggesting that at least one-third of clinical trials performed since 1996 have remained unpublished; they argue that this lack of disclosure has left prescribers unaware of important information relating to drug safety and efficacy, and has been harmful to the interests of patients. Trial sponsors will, of course, often choose to publish their data in refereed journals, although they are not obliged to do so, and both they and journal editors will tend to give preference to positive rather than negative findings. Publication bias inevitably means that good news receives more publicity than does bad news.

There is growing pressure for obligatory publication of the results of all clinical trials, and it is likely that ethical committees will increasingly include a commitment to publish as a condition for approving new studies. One major drug company, GlaxoSmithKline, has recently announced that it is setting up a public database which will give the protocols and results of all the trials the company sponsors.

Concluding remarks

It will be seen from this chapter that conducting clinical trials on new drugs is a complex and costly business, which becomes more complex and more costly as development proceeds and as the emphasis shifts from providing the company's management with the information needed for it to make decisions, to providing the regulatory authorities with data needed for marketing approval. The end of Phase IIa, when management has to make the decision to move the project into full development, is a critical transition point.

The conduct of clinical trials must take into account the thorny ethical issues that have to be faced, in particular the need to balance the risk to the individual against the potential benefit to humanity at large of a successful scientific study.

The results of clinical trials have huge financial consequences for pharmaceutical companies, so there is a need for stringent safeguards to ensure their quality and reliability. In Phase III, when many trial centres in different countries are likely to be involved, considerable manpower and resources are needed to establish the training programmes, monitoring and audit that are needed to meet the data quality standards regulatory authorities demand.

References

Antes G (2004) Registering clinical trials is necessary for ethical, scientific and economic reasons. Bulletin of the World Health Organization 82: 321.

Beecher HK (1955) The powerful placebo. Journal of the American Medical Association 159: 1602–1606.

Cadman PE, O'Connor DT (2003) Pharmacogenomics of hypertension. Current Opinion in Nephrology and Hypertension 12: 61–70.

Dickersin K, Rennie D (2003) Registering clinical trials. JAMA 290: 516–523.

FDA Guidance for industry and reviewers: estimating the safe starting dose in clinical trials for therapeutics in adult healthy volunteers.

Hrobjartsson A, Grotzche P (2001) Is the placebo powerless? An analysis of clinical trials comparing placebo with no treatment. New England Journal of Medicine 344: 1594–1602.

ICH Topic E5 Ethnic factors in the acceptability of foreign clinical data. CPMP/ICH/289/95.

ICH Topic Q7A Step 5 Note for guidance good manufacturing practice for active pharmaceutical ingredients. (www.CPMP/ICH/4106/00 - released for consultation July 2000).

ICH Topic S5A Reproductive toxicology: detection of toxicity to reproduction for medicinal products. (www.CPMP/ICH/386/95).

Kuhlman J (1997) Drug research: from the idea to the product. International Journal of Clinical Pharmacology and Therapeutics 35: 541–552.

Lasser KE, Allen PD, Woolhandler SJ, Himmelstein DU, Wolfe SM, Bor DH (2002) Timing of new black box warnings and withdrawals for prescription medications. Journal of the American Medical Association 287: 2215–2220.

Oscarson M (2001) Nicotine metabolism by the polymorphic cytochrome P450 2a6 (cyp2a6) enzyme: implications for interindividual differences in smoking behaviour. Psycholoquy 12: (3).

Peck R W (1997) Strategies for selecting an agent for clinical trials. Annals of the New York Academy of Sciences 823: 319–327.

Pharma 2005. (1998) An industrial revolution in R&D. PriceWaterhouseCoopers.

PriceWaterhouseCoopers (1995) Strategic management of R&D in the pharmaceutical industry. London. PJB Publications.

Savulescu J (2004) Thalassaemia major: the murky story of deferiprone. British Medical Journal 328: 358–359.

Smyth RL, Weindling AM (1999) Research in children: ethical and scientific aspects. Lancet 354(Suppl II): 2124.

World Health Organization (2000) Operational Guidelines for ethics committees that review biomedical research. Geneva: WHO.

World Medical Association (2000) Declaration of Helsinki. Ethical principles for medical research involving human subjects. 52nd WMA General Assembly, Edinburgh, Scotland, October 2000; Note of Clarification on Paragraph 29 added by the WMA General Assembly, Washington 2002. http://www.wma.net/e/policy/pdf/17c.pdf.

19

Protecting the assets: patenting and intellectual property

P Grubb

When a pharmaceutical company makes an invention, it will usually wish to protect it by means of a patent. In this chapter we will look at what patents are, what kinds of inventions can be patented, and how a patent may be obtained and enforced.

Patents are not the only form of intellectual property (IP), but they are by far the most important for the pharmaceuticals industry. Many patents that are filed and granted prove to be worth nothing, but a patent protecting a blockbuster drug against generic competition may be worth one or two million dollars for each day that it is in force. An unexpected loss of patent protection may have a much larger effect upon the market value of the company holding the patent. In August 2000, when a US patent covering Prozac was held invalid by the Court of Appeal for the Federal Circuit, thereby reducing by about 3 years the term of exclusivity for this drug, 29% of the value of Eli Lilly stock was lost in 1 day – over $35bn. This is serious money by any standards.

What is a patent?

A patent is the grant by a nation state of the exclusive right to commercialize an invention in that state for a limited time. During that time (the 'term' of the patent, usually 20 years from the filing date) the patent owner can go to the courts and enforce his rights by suing an infringer. If he wins he can get damages or other compensation, but what is most important is that he can obtain a court order (an injunction) to stop any further infringement. Note that although the state grants the patent right, the state does not check whether the right is being infringed – the patent owner must do that.

It is important to realize that the rights given by a patent do not include the right to practise the invention, but only to exclude others from doing so. Many inventors and business managers think that having a patent gives them freedom to operate, but this is not so. The patentee's freedom to use the invention may be limited by laws or regulations having nothing to do with patents, or by the existence of other patents. For example, owning a US patent for a new drug does not give the right to market that drug in the USA without permission from the FDA (see Chapter 20).

What is less obvious is that having a patent does not give the right to infringe an earlier existing patent. To take a simple example, if A has a patent for a process using an acid catalyst, and B later finds that nitric acid (not disclosed in A's patent) gives surprisingly good results, B may be able to get a patent for the process using nitric acid as catalyst. However, because this falls under the broad description of acid catalysis covered in A's patent, B is not free to use his invention without the permission of A. On the other hand, A cannot use nitric acid without a licence from B, and in this situation, cross-licensing may allow both parties to use the improved invention.

Patents are important to industry because they give the innovator a period during which imitations can be excluded and the investment in R&D can be recovered. They are of particular importance to the pharmaceutical industry because once the chemical structure of a drug is published it is usually rather easy to copy the product, and because the manufacturing cost of a pharmaceutical is only a small part of the selling price, an imitator who has no R&D costs to recover can sell the product cheaply and still make a profit.

The patent specification

A patent (which strictly speaking is just a one-page certificate of grant) is in most countries published with a printed *patent specification*, which typically will be 10–100 pages long, or even more. The patent specification consists of three parts, the bibliographic details and abstract, the description, and the claims. Each part has a different purpose.

Bibliographic details

The title page usually sets out the bibliographic details, giving information such as the names of the inventors, the owner or assignee of the patent, the title, the dates of priority, filing, publication and grant, and the name of the attorney, if any, who acted for the patentee. It may also give the international search classification, and a list of prior published documents considered by the Patent Office when examining the application. Generally it will also have an abstract summarizing the invention; this is meant as a tool for searching purposes and is not used in determining the scope of protection given by the patent.

Description

The longest part of the specification is the description, the purpose of which is to give enough information about the invention to enable a reader who is technically qualified in the relevant field to reproduce it. This ensures that when the patent is no longer in force the invention will be fully in the public domain and able to be used by anyone having the necessary skills. The description will usually start with a brief account of the background to the invention, followed by a summary of the invention, then present full details, with actual examples where appropriate. There may also be figures (drawings, structural formulae, graphs, photographs etc.), and if DNA or amino acid sequences are disclosed there will be sequence identifiers in standard form.

Claims

At the end of the specification come one or more claims, which have the legal purpose of setting out exactly what is covered by the scope of the exclusionary right. If the reader sees that what he wishes to do clearly falls within the claims of someone else's patent, then he is put upon notice that if he goes ahead he may be sued for infringement, and will have to stop his activities unless he can prove that the patent is invalid. Unfortunately the reverse situation is not so clear. In many countries, particularly the USA, even an activity that does not fall within the literal wording of a patent claim may nevertheless be held to infringe by 'equivalence'. The consequence is that before doing anything in the USA that is even close to the claims of a granted US patent, you must make sure that you get a written opinion from a US patent attorney that you are not infringing any valid claims. If you do not, and infringement is found, you may find yourself having to pay triple damages for 'willful infringement'.

What can be patented?

There are basically only two categories of subject matter that can be patented – *products* and *processes*. Products are broadly anything having physical reality, including machines, manufactured articles, chemical compounds, compositions comprising a mixture of substances, and even living organisms. A process may be a process for manufacturing an article or synthesizing a compound, or may be a method of using or testing a product. However, a patent for a process for making something, for example a chemical compound, also covers the direct product of that process. A patent claiming simply 'the compound of formula X' covers X however it is made, but a process claim to 'a method of production of X by reacting Y and Z' covers X only when made by that process, and not in any other way.

There are also some types of subject matter for which the grant of patents is specifically excluded, and these exclusions vary from country to country. For example, some countries do not grant patents on any plants or animals, whereas in Europe only specific plant and animal varieties are excluded, and in the USA there is no such restriction. Similarly, the USA allows patents for methods of surgical or medical treatment or diagnosis, whereas most other countries do not. Nevertheless, the invention that a known drug may be used for a new indication may usually be protected in these countries by patents having a different form of claim. Generally, patents will not be granted in any country for aesthetic creations, mathematical and scientific theories, and discoveries without any practical application.

Pharmaceutical inventions

Within the pharmaceutical field, patentable inventions may include not only new chemical compounds of known structure, but also, for example, biopolymers and mixtures the structure of which has not been fully elucidated. Isolated DNA sequences and genes are also patentable as chemical compounds, albeit complex ones. Even if a chemical compound is already known, it may be possible to patent variants, such as new optical isomers and crystal forms of the compound, as well as new galenic formulations, mixtures with other active ingredients, manufacturing and purification processes, assay processes etc.

If a known compound, not previously known to have any pharmaceutical use, is found to be useful as a drug, this invention may be protected by claiming a pharmaceutical composition containing the compound, or, in Europe, the use of the compound as a pharmaceutical. Such claims will cover all pharmaceutical uses of the compound, not only the one found by the inventor. If the invention is that a known drug has a new and unexpected indication, such an invention may be protected in the USA by a 'method of medical treatment' claim ('method of treating a human suffering from disease Y by administering an effective amount of a compound X'), or in Europe by a so-called 'Swiss-type claim' ('use of compound X in the manufacture of a medicament for treating disease Y'), or (once the revision of the European Patent Convention comes into force) a use claim ('use of compound X for the treatment of disease Y').

Requirements for patentability

For an invention in any of the above categories to be patentable, it must meet three basic criteria:

- It must be *novel*.
- It must involve an *inventive step* (must not be obvious).
- It must be *industrially applicable* (must have utility).

Novelty

The first and clearest requirement is that nothing can be patentable which is not new. If a patent were to be granted for something already known, then the grant of a patent in respect of this information would violate the fundamental principle that a patent cannot deprive the public of rights that it already has. There are, however, different definitions of 'novelty'. The most straightforward is that of 'absolute novelty' applied in Europe and the majority of other countries, which provides that an invention is new if it is not part of the 'state of the art', the state of the art being defined as everything that was available to the public by written or oral publication, use or any other way, in any country in the world, before the priority date of the invention. In other words, if it could be proved that the invention had been described before that date in a public lecture given in the Mongolian language in Ulan Bator, a European patent application for the invention would lack novelty even if no European had heard or understood the lecture.

A few countries still have the system of 'local novelty', under which a disclosure of the invention before the priority date destroys novelty only if it is available within that country. Rather more countries, including the USA, have an intermediate 'mixed novelty' system, according to which a later patent application is invalidated by written publication anywhere in the world, but by oral publication or use of the invention only in the home country. Thus a US patent would not be invalidated by the lecture in Ulan Bator, but would be by an account of it published in a newspaper there. Similarly, prior use in a country outside the USA would not invalidate a US patent if there was no written description, whereas a European patent would be invalidated by prior use anywhere in the world, so long as the use made the invention available to the public – for example the sale of a chemical compound that could be analysed.

Novelty in the USA

A more basic difference between the USA and all other countries is that all countries other than the USA have a 'first-to-file' system, whereby if two persons make the same invention the first one to file a patent application gets the patent. The US system is 'first-to-invent', so that irrespective of who files the first application, the person who can prove the earlier invention date gets the patent. A consequence of this is that in most countries, prior art is what is published before the first filing date (the priority date). In the USA, however, prior art is what is published before the invention date. Since by definition an inventor cannot publish his or her invention before it is invented, self-publication cannot normally be prior art. However, if an invention has been published, by the inventor or by another person, after the invention date, a US patent application for the invention is regarded as lacking novelty unless it is filed within 12 months of the date of publication. This means that an inventor may publish the invention and still obtain a valid US patent so long as a US application is filed within this 12-month period. In the past, many US inventors, particularly those working in universities, sought to take advantage of this so-called grace period, only to find that by so doing they had destroyed their chances of getting any protection in other countries. Now most US inventors are aware of the dangers, and unless they are interested only in obtaining a US patent, they will adhere to the first-to-file principle and file an application before publishing their results.

Inventive step (non-obviousness)

Whereas the concept of novelty is (or should be) an objective matter, the question of whether or not something involves an inventive step is intrinsically much more difficult, as subjective judgement is involved. The basic principle to remember is that the reason for requiring the presence of an inventive step is that the ordinary worker in that field should remain free to apply his normal skills to making minor variations of old products.

Thus the person to whom the invention must be non-obvious in order to be patentable is the 'person skilled in the art', i.e. a worker who is competent but lacks imagination or inventive capability. In the days when the most patents were for simple mechanical devices the person skilled in the art was usually described as an 'ordinary workman'. However, for complex inventions in pharmaceutical chemistry and biotechnology, the 'person skilled in the art' may be considered to be a team of highly qualified scientists.

It is a legal fiction to suppose that such a team could be competent but non-inventive, considering that its members would, if employed in industry, be expected by their company to make inventions, and if academic scientists, would be expected by their university to produce original scientific work, which amounts to much the same thing. The point is that obviousness should be judged by a person with qualifications and imagination that are average for those in the field. It is tempting for a party attacking a patent on the ground of obviousness to use an expert witness with the highest possible qualifications, but it is not very helpful to have a Nobel laureate testify that something is obvious. It may be obvious to a genius, but the real question is whether it is obvious to the normal worker in the field.

It is often very easy to reconstruct an invention with the benefit of hindsight, as a series of logical steps from the prior art, but it does not necessarily follow that the invention was obvious, especially if there is evidence that the invention was commercially successful, or satisfied a need. The question 'If the invention was so obvious, why did no one do it before?' is usually a relevant one to ask.

Industrial applicability (utility)

In Europe it is a requirement that the invention should be capable of industrial application, which is broadly defined and includes making or using the invention in any kind of industry, including agriculture. In the USA, patentable inventions are defined as any new and useful process, machine, manufacture or composition of matter, or any new and useful improvement thereof. The US requirement that the invention be useful has generally been applied no more strictly than the corresponding European requirement, but recently US examination guidelines have been tightened up so as to make more difficult the patenting of DNA sequences for which no real function is known. At one time any trivial use (e.g. use as cat food, on the basis that you can always feed it to a cat) was enough to establish utility; now a specific, credible and practical utility must be alleged. Nevertheless, you can allege any number of specific utilities, and it is enough if only one of them is correct.

Filing a patent application

When to file

Given that in most countries the first to file an application gets the patent, it would seem to make sense to file as early as possible as soon as an invention is made. It is not quite as simple as this, however. For one thing, the earlier a patent is filed the earlier it will expire, and particularly in the pharmaceutical field, the last year or two of patent life for a major product can be worth hundreds of millions of dollars. For another, a patent application filed at a very early stage may lack sufficient enabling disclosure to support claims of the desired scope. Too much delay, however, and another party may have filed an earlier application or published a paper that destroys the novelty of the invention.

For pharmaceutical inventions, the decision when to make a first filing will depend on a number of factors, including the intensity of competition in the relevant field. As a general rule, however, it is generally best to wait at least until one or more lead compounds within the scope have shown clear activity in a validated in vitro assay, or in an animal model, i.e. close to the point at which a drug candidate (see Chapter 4) is identified.

Where to file

Normally a single filing in one country will be made, which under the Paris Convention for the Protection of Industrial Property can form the basis for a claim to priority in other countries. Some national laws, such as those of the USA, the UK and France, require that, for reasons of national security, an application for any invention made in that country must first be filed in that country (unless special permission is obtained). Other countries, for example Switzerland, are less paranoid, and allow a first filing to be made in any country.

The Paris Convention, now adhered to by the great majority of countries, provides that a later application filed for the same invention in another Convention country within 12 months of the first filing in a Convention country may claim the priority of the original application. This means that the first filing date (the *priority date*) is treated for prior art purposes as if it were the filing date of the later application, so that a publication of the invention before the later application but after the priority date does not invalidate the later application. If it were not for the Paris Convention, it would be necessary to make simultaneous filings in all the countries of interest at a very early stage, which would be extremely wasteful of time and money. Instead, a single priority filing may be made and a decision taken before the end of the priority year on what to do with the application.

During the priority year, work on the invention will normally continue, and for example further compounds will be made and tested, new formulations compounded, or new process conditions tried. All this material can be used in preparing the patent applications to be filed abroad, and, where possible, a subsequent application in respect of the country of first filing. It is also possible to file new patent applications for further developments made during the priority year, and then at the foreign filing stage to combine these into a single application. The advantage of this is that the new developments will then have an earlier priority date (the date of filing of the new application) than they otherwise would have (the date of filing of the foreign text).

The foreign filing decision

There are four options to be considered:

- Abandon
- Abandon and refile
- Obtain a patent in the country of first filing only

- File corresponding applications in one or more foreign countries.

Abandonment

If there is no commercial interest in the invention at all, or if a search has shown that it lacks novelty, one can simply do nothing. Sooner or later a fee must be paid or some action taken to keep the application in being, and when this is not done the application will lapse. It is best not to withdraw the application explicitly, as such a positive abandonment is usually irrevocable and applicants have been known to change their minds.

If the applicant wants to ensure that he retains freedom to operate and that no one else can patent the invention, he should have it published, either by continuing an application in his home country long enough for it to issue as a published application (see below) or by sending it to a journal such as *Research Disclosure*, in which any disclosure may be rapidly published for a reasonable fee.

Refiling

It frequently happens that by the time the foreign filing decision must be taken it is not yet possible to decide whether or not to invest time and money in foreign patenting. Commercial interest may be low but could increase later, more testing may have to be done, or the inventors may not have done any more work on the invention since the first application was filed. In such cases the best solution is to start from the beginning again. The existing application is abandoned, a new application is filed, and the 12-month countdown starts all over again. In this case it is essential to meet the requirements of the Paris Convention that the first application be explicitly abandoned before the second application is filed.

Of course, refiling always entails a loss of priority, usually of 8–10 months, and if someone else has published the invention or filed a patent application for it during this time, the refiled application cannot lead to a valid patent. Consequently, in a field where competitors are known to be active refiling may involve an unacceptable risk, and naturally if there has been any known publication of the invention since the priority date, abandonment and refiling is ruled out. Such publication most frequently arises from the inventor himself. Most inventors know that they should not publish inventions before a patent application is filed; it is not so generally realized that publication within the priority year can also be very damaging.

Home-country patenting

If the applicant is an individual or a small company having no commercial interests or prospects of licensing outside the home country (which will usually be the country in which the first filing is made), the expense of foreign filing would be wasted, and the applicant will wish only to obtain a patent in the home country. Even where the applicant is a larger company that would normally file any commercially interesting case in several countries, individual applications may be of such low interest that protection in the home country is all that is needed. This option is of course more attractive if the home country is a large market such as the USA, rather than a small country such as Switzerland.

Foreign filing

Finally, if an invention appears likely to be commercially important, the decision may be to file corresponding applications in a number of other countries. For the pharmaceutical industry one can assume that the costs of patent protection would be small compared with the value of protection for any compound that actually reaches the market, but at the time when a foreign filing decision must be taken, it is usually impossible to estimate the chance that the product in question will progress that far. Accordingly, one must rely upon some rule of thumb such that if the product is being developed further, foreign filing should be carried out as a matter of course. High patenting costs are a necessary part of the high research overheads of the pharmaceutical industry.

Procedures on foreign filing

National filings

It is possible to file patent applications (in the local language) in the national patent offices of each selected country individually. This involves a large outlay of money at a relatively early stage, and also means that all necessary translations must be prepared in good time before the end of the priority year. It is also very labour-intensive, as the application must be prosecuted separately before each national patent office. Fortunately, there are ways to simplify the procedure.

Regional patent offices

One is that there are certain regional patent offices by which patents in a number of countries can be granted based on a single application filed and prosecuted in one patent office. By far the most important of these is the European Patent Office, which as of May 2004 grants patents for a total of 28 countries. These are all the 25 current EU states except for Latvia, Lithuania and Malta, plus Bulgaria, Romania, Switzerland, Liechtenstein, Monaco and Turkey. The European application can be filed in English, French or German, and translations into other languages are required only at the time of grant. Once the European patent is granted, opposition to the patent may be filed by any other party within 9 months of the date of grant. If the opposition is wholly or partly successful, the patent is invalidated or limited in scope for all of the designated countries.

Although the European Patent Convention provides for a central filing, grant and opposition procedure, once

the European patent is granted it is treated as if it were a bundle of national patents in the designated contracting states, so that for example the European patent may be invalidated by the courts in one country without directly affecting its validity in other countries. Proposals have recently been made by the European Commission for a single unitary patent to cover all EU countries, just as a single US patent covers all 50 States.

Other regional patent offices are the Eurasian Patent Office (Russia and certain ex-Soviet countries), and ones for English-speaking and French-speaking African countries.

Patent Cooperation Treaty (PCT)

The PCT allows rights to be established in a large number of countries (126 as of April 2005) by a single international application. Search and optional preliminary examination are carried out before the application goes to the national or regional patent offices. This system gives the maximum flexibility and allows the costs associated with translations etc. to be significantly postponed. There are now only a few economically significant countries that are not members of the PCT, of which the most important are Argentina, Chile and Taiwan. An initial international phase, in which a search and possibly also a preliminary examination is carried out, is followed after 18 months by a national phase, in which selected national or regional patent offices conclude the examination process and grant (or refuse) the patent. The PCT procedure is described in more detail in Box 19.1.

Selection of countries

In deciding the list of countries in which patent protection should be obtained, the main criteria are the strength of patent protection in the country and the size of the market. Now that most countries have joined the World Trade Organization and are obliged by the TRIPs (Trade-Related Aspects of Intellectual Property Rights) agreement to introduce strong patent protection, the most important criterion has become market size. There is no point in filing patents in a country if the size of the market does not justify the costs, no matter how strong its patent laws may be. Nevertheless, for a new chemical entity that may become a market product, filing in 40–60 countries is normal practice. To avoid long discussions each time a decision must be taken, the use of standard filing lists to cover most situations makes a lot of sense.

Maintenance of patents

In nearly all countries, periodic (usually annual) renewal fees must be paid to keep a patent in force. These generally increase steeply towards the end of the patent term, thus encouraging patent owners who are not making commercial use of their patents to make the invention available to the public earlier than would otherwise be

International phase

Filing
An international application can be filed by any national or resident of a PCT country, at a national or regional patent office competent to act for that applicant, or at the International Bureau (World Intellectual Property Office, or WIPO) in Geneva. There are no longer separate designation fees for individual countries, and a single filing fee can give rights in all Contracting States.

International publication and search report
The PCT application is published 18 months from the first priority date, and the search report drawn up by the International Searching Office (selected from one of a number of patent offices including the USPTO and the EPO) is published at the same time or as soon as possible afterwards. At the same time, a Written Opinion on Patentability is drawn up, indicating on the basis of the search report whether or not the invention appears to be new and non-obvious. If no further steps are taken, this will be issued as the International Preliminary Report on Patentability (IPRP).

International preliminary examination
If the applicant wishes to contest the findings of the Written Opinion, he may within 22 months from the priority date file a *Demand for International Preliminary Examination*, pay a fee and respond to the Written Opinion, possibly also making amendments. This will then be taken into account in the final form of the IPRP.

National phase

After 30 months from the priority date the application may be sent to any of the national or regional patent offices, translated into the local language as necessary. The individual patent offices may rely on the international search and examination reports to any extent they choose in deciding whether or not to grant a patent. This varies from offices which usually ignore the IPRP altogether (e.g. the USPTO), to those which will grant a patent without further examination only if the IPRP is positive (e.g. Turkey), to Singapore, which will automatically grant a patent on any PCT application with an IPRP, whether it is positive or negative. Singapore very sensibly puts the burden on the applicant, who, if he wishes to enforce the patent, would have to prove to the court that the negative IPRP was incorrect.

the case. To save costs, pharmaceutical patents should be abandoned as soon as they no longer provide protection for a compound that is on the market or is being developed.

Extension of patent term

The standard patent term provided in the TRIPs agreement is at least 20 years from the filing date. However, because it takes a long time to bring a drug to market, the effective term (the term during which a drug is sold with patent protection) is much less than this. To compensate for these regulatory delays, a number of countries, including EU states, the USA, Switzerland and Japan, allow for patent term extensions of up to 5 years for pharmaceutical (and sometimes agricultural) products. In the USA, patent term extension is one part of the Hatch–Waxman Act, in which the interests of the innovative companies are balanced against those of the generic companies. The former get a longer patent term, the latter are allowed to do testing for FDA approval during the patent term, so that they can come on the market as soon as patent protection expires. In Europe, extension is provided by means of a separate form of intellectual property right known as a Supplemental Protection Certificate (SPC).

Enforcement of patent rights

Governments grant patents, but do not enforce them. The patent owner must take action against infringement by suing an infringer in the civil courts. If successful, the patentee can obtain an injunction to restrain further infringement, as well as other remedies such as damages and costs. Usually the alleged infringer will counterclaim that the patent is invalid, and if the patentee loses the case the patent may be revoked. This risk, as well as the high cost of litigation, must be weighed against the benefit gained if the infringer is forced out of the market. As an alternative to litigation, the patentee may choose to exploit the patent by granting exclusive or non-exclusive licences for royalties or other forms of compensation, or in exchange for a cross-licence.

Although the procedure for obtaining a patent has been harmonized to a large extent by the PCT and other means, the procedure for enforcement, as well as the cost and the chance of success, varies enormously from one country to another. In the USA, patent cases are heard at first instance in the Federal District Courts, in which the judges are not specialized in intellectual property law and in which many cases are decided by jury verdicts. At the appeal stage, however, the Court of Appeal for the Federal Circuit is a specialized and technically competent court. In England (a separate jurisdiction from Scotland!), on the other hand, patent cases are heard either in the Patents County Court or, more usually, in the Patents Court, which is part of the High Court. Both of these are specialized courts with technically literate judges, but appeals from them go to the general Court of Appeal, where the majority of the judges are not patent experts. Which of these two systems gives the best results is a matter of debate.

In both the US and the English systems issues of patent validity are dealt with by the same court that deals with the issue of infringement, and this is also the case in the majority of European and Asian countries. In Germany, Japan and Korea, however, these issues are kept separate, and a patent may be invalidated only by a special court or by a branch of the patent office.

It is a problem in many parts of the world that even if the country has a good patent law on paper, enforcement of patent rights may be very difficult for a number of reasons, ranging from lack of experienced judges to inefficiency and even corruption.

Other forms of intellectual property

A *trademark* is a word, design, shape or colour used to distinguish the goods of the trademark owner from those of another manufacturer. Unlike patents, registered trademarks may be renewed at the end of their term and may be kept alive indefinitely, although they may be liable to cancellation if they are not used. Thus once a patent for a drug has expired a competitor will be able to sell a generic version, but must sell it under the International Non-proprietary Name (INN) or his own trademark, not that of the originator.

Additional forms of IP include *copyright* (e.g. for the text of advertisements and package inserts), and *Internet domain names*, which may for example incorporate the name of a product and may be a useful marketing tool.

Further reading

Dutfield G (2003) Intellectual property rights and the life science industries. Aldershot: Ashgate Press.

Grubb P (2004) Patents for chemicals, pharmaceuticals and biotechnology: fundamentals of global law, practice and strategy, 4th edn. Oxford: Oxford University Press.

Kleemann A, Engel J (2001) Pharmaceutical substances: syntheses, patents, applications. New York: Thieme Medical.

Old F (1993) Inventions, patents, brands and designs. Sydney: Patent Press.

Reid B (1999) A practical guide to patent law. London: Sweet & Maxwell.

Rosenstock J (1998) The law of chemical and pharmaceutical invention: patent and nonpatent protection. New York: Aspen Publishers.

Useful websites
Patent Offices

EPO	http://www.european-patent-office.org
UK	http://www.patent.gov.uk or www.ukpats.org.uk
USA	http://www.uspto.gov
WIPO	http://www.wipo.int

Professional organizations

Chartered Institute of Patent Attorneys:http://www.cipa.org.uk
European Patents Institute:http://www.patentepi.com
American Intellectual Property Law Association: http://www.aipla.org

Lists of links

http://www.epo.co.at/online/index.htm
http://portico.bl.uk/collections/patents/html

I Hägglöf
Å Holmgren

20 Regulatory affairs

Introduction

This chapter introduces the reader to the role of the regulatory affairs department of a large pharmaceutical company, outlining the process of getting a drug approved, and emphasizing the importance of interactions of regulatory affairs with other functions within the company, and with the external regulatory authorities.

To keep this chapter to a reasonable size the typical examples refer to the first registration of a new chemical compound. The same way of reasoning always applies, however, to any subsequent change to the approval of products. Depending on the magnitude of the change, the new documentation that needs to be compiled, submitted and approved by health authorities is variable, ranging from a few pages of pharmaceutical data (e.g. for an update to product stability information) to a complete new application for a new clinical use in a new patient group in a new pharmaceutical form.

It needs also to be said that, as every drug substance and every project is unique, the views expressed represent the opinion of the authors and are not necessarily shared by others active in the field.

Brief history of pharmaceutical regulation

Control of pharmaceutical products has been the task of authorized institutions for thousands of years, even in ancient Greece and Egypt.

From the Middle Ages, control of drug quality, composition purity and quantification was achieved by reference to authoritative lists of drugs, their preparation and their uses. These developed into official Pharmacopoeias, of which the earliest was probably the New Compound Dispensatory of 1498 issued by the Florentine Guild of physicians and pharmacists.

The pharmacopoeias were local rules, applicable in a city or a district. During the 19th century national pharmacopoeias replaced the local ones, and since the early 1960s regional pharmacopoeias have successively replaced the national ones. Now work is ongoing to harmonize – or at least mutually recognize – interchangeable use of the US Pharmacopeia, the European Pharmacopoeia and the Japanese Pharmacopoeia.

As described in Chapter 1, the development of experimental pharmacology and chemistry began during the second half of the 19th century, revealing that the effect of the main botanical drugs was due to chemical substances in the plants. The next step, synthetic chemistry, made it possible to produce active chemical compounds. Other important scientific developments, e.g. biochemistry, bacteriology and serology, during the early 20th century accelerated the development of the pharmaceutical industry into what it is today (see Drews, 1999).

Lack of adequate drug control systems or methods to investigate the safety of new chemical compounds became a great risk as prefabricated drug products were broadly and freely distributed. In the USA the fight against patent medicines led to the passing of the US Pure Food and Drugs Act against misbranding as long ago as 1906. The act required improved declaration of contents, prohibited false or misleading statements, and required content and purity to comply with labelled information. A couple of decades later, the US Food and Drug Administration (FDA) was established to control US pharmaceutical products.

Safety regulations in the USA were, however, not enough to prevent the sale of a paediatric *sulfanilamide* elixir containing the toxic solvent diethylene glycol. In 1937, 107 people, both adults and children, died as a result of ingesting the elixir, and in 1938 the Food Drug and Cosmetics Act was passed, requiring for the first time approval by FDA before marketing of a new drug product.

The *thalidomide* disaster further demonstrated the lack of adequate drug control. Thalidomide (Neurosedyn®, Contergan®) was launched during the last years of the 1950s as a non-toxic treatment for a variety of conditions, such as colds, anxiety, depression, infections etc., both alone and in combination with a number of other compounds, such as analgesics and sedatives.

The reason why the compound was regarded as harmless was the lack of acute toxicity after high single doses. After repeated long-term administration, however, signs of neuropathy developed, with symptoms of numbness, paraesthesia and ataxia. But the overwhelming effects were the gross malformation in infants born to mothers who had taken thalidomide in pregnancy: their limbs were partially or totally missing, a previously extremely rare malformation called *phocomelia* (seal limb). Altogether around 12 000 infants were born with the defect in those few years. Thalidomide was withdrawn from the market in 1961/62.

This catastrophe became a strong driver to develop animal test methods to assess drug safety before testing compounds in humans. Also it forced national authorities to strengthen the requirements for control procedures before marketing of pharmaceutical products (Cartwright & Matthews, 1991).

Another blow hit Japan between 1959 and 1971. The SMON (*subacute myelo-optical neuropathy*) disaster was blamed on the frequent Japanese use of the intestinal antiseptic *clioquinol* (Entero-Vioform®, Enteroform® or Vioform®). The product had been sold without restrictions since early 1900, and it was assumed that it would not be absorbed, but after repeated use neurological symptoms appeared, characterized by paraesthesia, numbness and weakness of the extremities, and even blindness. SMON affected about 10 000 Japanese victims, compared to some 100 cases in the rest of the world (Meade, 1975).

These tragedies had a strong impact on governmental regulatory control of pharmaceutical products. In 1962 the FDA required evidence of efficacy as well as safety as a condition for registration, and formal approval was required for patients to be included in clinical trials of new drugs.

In Europe, the UK Medicines Act 1968 made safety assessment of new drug products compulsory. The Swedish Drug Ordinance of 1962 defined the medicinal product and required a clear benefit/risk ratio to be documented before approval for marketing. All European countries established similar controls during the 1960s.

In Japan, the Pharmaceutical Affairs Law enacted in 1943 was revised in 1961 and 1979 to establish the current drug regulatory system, with the Ministry of Health and Welfare assessing drugs for quality, safety and efficacy.

The 1960s and 1970s saw a rapid increase in laws, regulations and guidelines for reporting and evaluating the risks versus the benefits of new medicinal products. At the time the industry was becoming more international and seeking new global markets, but the registration of medicines remained a national responsibility.

Although different regulatory systems were based on the same key principles, the detailed technical requirements diverged over time, often for traditional rather than scientific reasons, to such an extent that industry found it necessary to duplicate tests in different countries to obtain global regulatory approval for new products. This was a waste of time, money and animals' lives, and it became clear that harmonization of regulatory requirements was needed.

European (EEC) efforts to harmonize requirements for drug approval began 1965, and a common European approach grew with the expansion of the European Union to 15 countries, and then 25. The EU harmonization principles have also been adopted by Norway and Iceland. This successful European harmonization process gave impetus to discussions about harmonization on a broader international scale (Cartwright & Matthews, 1994).

International harmonization

The harmonization process started in 1990, when representatives of the regulatory authorities and industry associations of Europe, Japan and the USA (representing the majority of the global pharmaceutical industry) met, ostensibly to plan an International Conference on Harmonization (ICH). The meeting actually went much further, suggesting *terms of reference* for ICH, and setting up an ICH Steering Committee representing the three regions.

The task of the ICH was '...increased international harmonization, aimed at ensuring that good quality, safe and effective medicines are developed and registered in the most efficient and cost-effective manner. These activities are pursued in the interest of the consumer and public health, to prevent unnecessary duplication of clinical trials in humans and to minimize the use of animal testing without compromising the regulatory obligations of safety and effectiveness.' (Tokyo, October 1990).

ICH has remained a very active organization, with substantial representation at both authority and industry level from the European Union, the United States and Japan. The input of other nations is provided through World Health Organization representatives, as well as representatives from Switzerland and Canada.

ICH conferences held every 2 years have become a forum for open discussion and follow-up of the topics decided. The important achievements so far are the scientific guidelines agreed and implemented in the national/regional drug legislation, not only in the ICH territories but also in other countries around the world. So far more than 40 guidelines have reached ICH approval and regional implementation, i.e. steps 4 and 5 (Figure 20.1). For a complete list of ICH guidelines and their status, see the ICH website (website reference 1)

The process described in Figure 20.1 is very open, and the fact that health authorities and pharmaceutical industry collaborate from the start increases the efficiency of work and ensures mutual understanding across regions and functions; this is a major factor in the success of ICH.

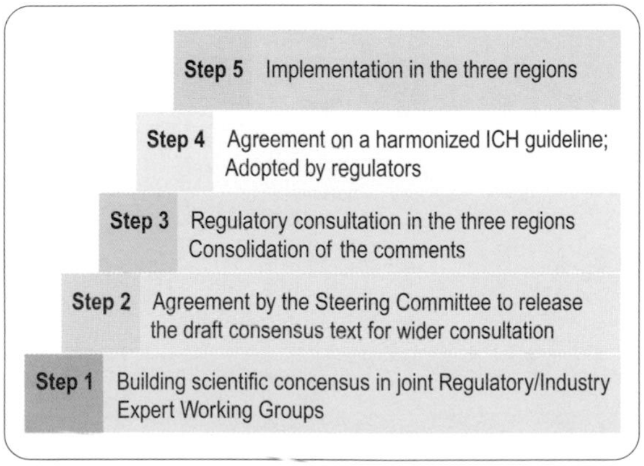

Roles and responsibilities of regulatory authority and company

The basic division of responsibilities for drug products is that the health authority is protecting public health and safety, and the pharmaceutical company is responsible for all aspects of the drug product. The approval of a pharmaceutical product is a contract between the regulatory authority and the pharmaceutical company. The conditions of the approval are set out in the dossier and condensed in the prescribing information. Any change that is planned must be forwarded to the regulatory authority for information and, in most cases, new approval before being implemented.

To protect the public health, regulatory authorities also develop regulations and guidelines for companies to follow in order to achieve a balance between the possible risks and therapeutic advantages to the patients.

The regulatory authority:

- Approves clinical trial applications;
- Approves for marketing drugs that have been scientifically evaluated to provide evidence of a satisfactory risk/benefit ratio;
- Monitors the safety of the marketed product, based on (a) reports of adverse reactions from healthcare providers, and (b) from compiled and evaluated safety information from the company that owns the product;
- Can withdraw the licence for marketing in serious cases of non-compliance (e.g. failure on inspections, failure of adequate additional warnings in prescribing information after clinical adverse reactions are reported, or failure of the company to consider serious findings in animal studies).

The company:

- Owns the documentation that forms the basis for assessment, is responsible for its accuracy and correctness, for keeping it up to date, and for ensuring that it complies with standards set by current scientific development and the regulatory authorities;
- Collects, compiles and evaluates safety data, and submits reports to the regulatory authorities at regular intervals – and takes rapid action in serious cases. This might involve the withdrawal of the entire product or of a product batch (e.g. tablets containing the wrong drug or the wrong dose), or a

Fig. 20.1
Five steps in the ICH process for harmonization of technical issues.

Within the figure:

Step 5   Implementation in the three regions

Step 4   Agreement on a harmonized ICH guideline; Adopted by regulators

Step 3   Regulatory consultation in the three regions Consolidation of the comments

Step 2   Agreement by the Steering Committee to release the draft consensus text for wider consultation

Step 1   Building scientific concensus in joint Regulatory/Industry Expert Working Groups request to the regulatory authority for a change in prescribing information;

● Has a right to appeal and to correct cases of non-compliance.

The role of the regulatory affairs department

The regulatory affairs (RA) department of a pharmaceutical company is responsible for obtaining approval for new pharmaceutical products and ensuring that approval is maintained for as long as the company wants to keep the product on the market. It serves as the interface between the regulatory authority and the project team, and is the channel of communication with the regulatory authority as the project proceeds, aiming to ensure that the project plan correctly anticipates what the regulatory authority will require before approving the product. It is the responsibility of RA to keep abreast of current legislation, guidelines and other regulatory intelligence. Such rules and guidelines often allow some flexibility, and the regulatory authorities expect companies to take responsibility for deciding how they

should be interpreted. The RA department plays an important role in giving advice to the project team on how best to interpret the rules. Networks between companies in different countries are a valuable source of informal information.

The RA department is responsible for all communications with regulatory authorities, including face-to-face meetings. During the development process sound working relations with some important authorities are essential, e.g. to discuss such issues as divergence from guidelines, the clinical study programme, and formulation development.

The RA department reviews all documentation from a regulatory perspective, ensuring that it is clear, consistent and complete, and that its conclusions are explicit. The department also drafts the core prescribing information that is the basis for global approval, and will later provide the platform for marketing. The documentation includes clinical trials applications, as well as regulatory submissions for new products and for changes to approved products. The latter is a major task and accounts for about half of the work of the RA department.

An important proactive task of the RA is to provide input in the planning stage when legislative changes are being discussed and proposed. In the ICH environment

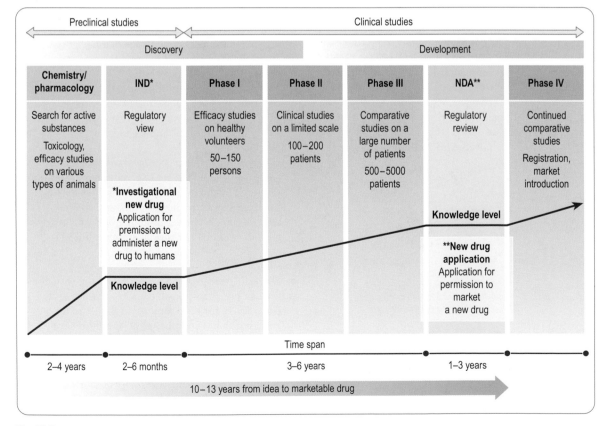

Fig. 20.2
The drug development process.

there is a greater possibility to exert influence at an early stage.

Overall, there has been a significant and beneficial change in recent years from a somewhat adversarial relationship between regulators and companies, towards a much more open and cooperative one.

The drug development process

An overview of the process of drug development is given in Chapters 15–18 and summarized in Figure 20.2. As already emphasized, this sequential approach, designed to minimize risk by allowing each study to start only when earlier studies have been successfully completed, is giving way to a parallel approach in order to save development time.

All studies in the non-clinical area – chemistry, pharmacology, pharmacokinetics, pharmaceutical development and toxicology – aim to establish indicators of safety and efficacy sufficient to allow studies and use in man. According to ICH conventions, documentation of chemical and pharmaceutical development relates to *quality* assessment, animal studies relate to *safety* assessment, and studies in humans relate to *efficacy*.

Quality assessment (chemistry and pharmaceutical development)

The *quality module* of a submission documents purity and assay for the drug substance, and purity data for all the inactive ingredients. The formulation must fulfil requirements for consistent quality and allow storage, and the container must be shown to be fit for its purpose. These aspects of a pharmaceutical product have to be kept under control throughout the development process, as toxicology and pharmacology results are reliable only for substances of comparable purity. Large-scale production, improved synthetic route, different raw material supply etc. may produce a substance somewhat different from the first laboratory-scale batches. Any substantial change must be known and documented.

The formulation of a product is a challenge. For initial human studies, simple i.v. and oral solutions are needed for straightforward results, whereas for the clinical programme in patients, bioequivalent formulations are essential for comparison of results across studies, and so it is preferable to have access to the final formulation already during Phase II.

If the formulation intended for marketing cannot be completed until late in the clinical phase, bioequivalence studies showing comparable results with the pre-liminary and final market formulations will be necessary to support the use of results with the preliminary formulation. There may even be situations when clinical studies must be repeated.

The analytical methods used and their validation must be described. Manufacturing processes and their validation are also required to demonstrate interbatch uniformity. However, full-scale validation may be submitted when sales production has eventually started.

Studies on the stability of both substance and products under real-life conditions are required, covering the full time of intended storage. Preliminary stability data are sufficient for the start of clinical studies. The allowable storage time can be increased as data are gathered and submitted. Even marketing authorizations can be approved on less than real-time storage information, but there is a requirement to submit final data when available.

Inactive ingredients as well as active substances need to be documented, unless they are well known and already documented. Even then it may become necessary to perform new animal studies to support novel uses of commonly used additives.

Although the quality module of the documentation is the smallest, the details of requirements and the many changes needed during development and maintenance of a product make it the most resource intensive module from a regulatory perspective. Also, legislation differs most in this area, so it will almost always be necessary to adapt the documentation for the intended regional submission.

Safety assessment (pharmacology and toxicology)

Next we consider how to design and integrate pharmacological and toxicological studies in order to produce adequate documentation for the first tests in humans. ICH guidelines define the information needed from animal studies in terms of doses and time of exposure, to allow clinical studies, first in healthy subjects and later in patients. The principles and methodology of animal studies are described in Chapters 11 and 16. The questions discussed here are *when* and *why* these animal studies are required for regulatory purposes.

Primary pharmacology

The primary pharmacodynamic studies provide the first evidence that the compound has the pharmacological effects required to give therapeutic benefit. It is a clear regulatory advantage to use established models and to be able at least to establish a theory for the mechanism of action. This will not always be possible and is not a firm requirement, but proof of efficacy and safety is helped by a plausible mechanistic explanation of the drug's effects, and this knowledge will also become a very powerful tool for marketing. For example, understanding the mechanism of action of proton pump inhibitors, such as *omepreazole* (see Chapter 4), was important in explaining their long duration of action, allowing once-daily dosage of compounds despite their short plasma half-life.

General pharmacology

General pharmacology[1] studies investigate effects other than the primary therapeutic effects. Safety pharmacology studies (see Chapter 16), which must conform to good laboratory practice (GLP) standards, are focused on identifying the effects on physiological functions that in a clinical setting are unwanted or harmful.

Although the study design will depend on the properties and intended use of the compound, general pharmacology studies are normally of short duration (i.e. acute, rather than chronic, effects are investigated), and the dosage is increased until clear adverse effects occur. The studies also include comparisons with known compounds whose pharmacological properties or clinical uses are similar.

When required, e.g. when pharmacodynamic effects occur only after prolonged treatment, or when effects seen with repeated administration give rise to safety concerns, the duration of a safety pharmacology study needs to be prolonged. The route of administration should whenever possible be the route intended for clinical use.

There are cases when a secondary pharmacological effect has, eventually, been developed into a new indication. *Lidocaine*, for example, was developed as a local anaesthetic agent and its cardiac effects after overdose were considered a hazard. Later that cardiac effect was exploited as a treatment for ventricular arrhythmia.

All relevant safety pharmacology studies must be completed before studies can be undertaken in patients. Complementary studies may still be needed to clarify unexpected findings in later development stages.

Pharmacokinetics: absorption, distribution, metabolism and excretion (ADME)

Preliminary pharmacokinetic tests to assess the absorption, plasma levels and half-life (i.e. exposure information) are performed in rodents in parallel with the preliminary pharmacology and toxicology studies.

---

[1]There are a number of widely used terms with similar meanings, e.g. secondary pharmacology, safety pharmacology, high-dose pharmacology, regulatory pharmacology and pharmacodynamic safety.

Studies in humans normally start with limited short-term data, and only if the results are acceptable are detailed animal and human ADME studies performed.

Plasma concentrations observed in animals are used to predict the concentrations that may be efficacious/ tolerated in humans, it being assumed that similar biological effects should be produced at similar plasma levels across species. This is a reasonable assumption provided the in vitro target affinity is similar.

Investigations during the toxicology programme give the bulk of the pharmacokinetic information due to the long-duration of drug exposure and the wide range of doses tested in several relevant species. They also give data about tissue distribution and possible accumulation in the body, including placental transfer and exposure of the fetus, as well as excretion in milk.

Metabolic pathways differ considerably between species, often quantitatively but sometimes also qualitatively. Active metabolites can influence study results, in particular after repeated use. A toxic metabolite with a long half-life may accumulate in the body and disturb results. The characterization and evaluation of metabolites are long processes, and are generally the last studies to be completed in a development programme.

Toxicology

The principles and methodology of toxicological assessment of new compounds are described in Chapter 16. Here we consider the regulatory aspects.

In contrast to the pharmacological studies, toxicological studies generally follow standard protocols that do not depend on the compound characteristics. Active comparators are not used, but the drug substance is compared at various dose levels to a vehicle control, given, if possible, via the intended route of administration.

Single and repeated-dose studies

The single-dose (acute) toxicity of a new compound must be evaluated prior to the first human exposure. Table 20.1 shows the duration of repeated-dose studies recommended by ICH, to support clinical trials and therapeutic use for different periods.

Genotoxicity

Preliminary genotoxicity evaluation of mutations and chromosomal damage (see Chapter 16) is needed before the drug is given to humans. If results from those studies are ambiguous or positive, further testing is required. The entire standard battery needs to be completed before Phase II.

Carcinogenicity

The objective of carcinogenicity studies is to identify any tumorigenic potential in animals, and they are required only when the expected duration of therapy, whether continuous or intermittent, is at least 6 months.

Table 20.1
Duration of repeated-dose toxicity studies

| Duration of Clinical trials | Minimum duration of repeated dose toxicity studies | | | |
| | To support Phase I and II trials in EU, also Phase III in USA and Japan | | To support phase III studies in EU and marketing in all 3 regions*** | |
	Rodents	Non-rodents	Rodents	Non-rodents
Single dose	2 weeks*	2 weeks		
Up to 2 weeks	2 weeks*	2 weeks	1 months	1 month
Up to 1 month	1 month	1 month	3 months	3 months
Up to 3 months	3 months	3 months	6 months	3 months
Up to 6 months	6 months	6 months**	6 months	Chronic**
>6 months	6 months	Chronic**		

*In the USA, as an alternative to 2-week studies, single-dose toxicity studies with extended examination can support single-dose human trials.
**Data from 6-month studies in non-rodents should be available before the start of clinical trials longer than 3 months. Alternatively, if applicable, data from a 9-month non-rodent study should be available before the treatment duration exceeds what is supported by the available toxicity studies.
***The marketing recommendations in the three regions are that a chronic toxicity study be performed for clinical use longer than 1 month.

Examples include treatments for conditions such as allergic rhinitis, anxiety or depression.

Carcinogenicity studies are also required when there is particular reason for concern, such as chemical similarities to known carcinogens, pathophysiological findings in animal toxicity studies, or positive genotoxicity results. Compounds found to be genotoxic by in vitro as well as in vivo tests are presumed to be trans-species carcinogens with hazards to humans.

Carcinogenicity studies normally run for the lifespan of the test animals. They are performed quite late in the development programme and are not necessarily completed when the application for marketing authorization is submitted. Indeed, for products for which there is a great medical need in the treatment of certain serious diseases, the regulatory authority may agree that submission of carcinogenicity data can be delayed until after marketing approval is granted.

Reproductive and developmental toxicity

These studies (see Chapter 16) are intended to reveal effects on male or female fertility, embryonic and fetal development, and peri- and postnatal development.

An evaluation of effects on the male reproductive system is performed in the repeated-dose toxicity studies, and this histopathological assessment is considered more sensitive in detecting toxic effects than are fertility studies. Men can therefore be included in Phase I–II trials before the male fertility studies are performed in animals.

Women may enter early studies before reproductive toxicity testing is completed, provided they are permanently sterilized or menopausal, and provided re-peated-dose toxicity tests of adequate duration have been performed, including the evaluation of female reproductive organs.

For women of childbearing potential there is concern regarding unintentional fetal exposure, and there are regional differences (Box 20.1) in the regulations about including fertile women in clinical trials.

Local tolerance and other toxicity studies

The purpose of local tolerance studies is to ascertain whether medicinal products (both active substances and excipients) are tolerated at sites in the body that may come into contact with the product in clinical use. This could mean ocular, dermal or parenteral administration.

> **Box 20.1 Requirement for reproduction toxicity related to clinical studies in fertile women**

EU: Embryo/fetal development studies are required before Phase I, and female fertility should be completed before Phase III

USA: Careful monitoring and pregnancy testing may allow fertile women to take part before reproduction toxicity is available. Female fertility and embryo/fetal assessment to be completed before Phase III

Japan: Assessment of female fertility and embryo/fetal development before inclusion of fertile women in any kind of clinical study and regardless of contraceptive measures

These studies need to be performed, using the proposed route of administration, prior to human exposure.

Other studies may also be needed. These might be studies on immunotoxicity, antigenicity studies on metabolites or impurities, and so on. The drug substance and the intended use will determine the relevance of other studies.

Efficacy assessment (studies in man)

When the preclinical testing is sufficient to start studies in man, the RA department compiles a clinical trials submission, which is sent to the regulatory authority and the ethics committee (see Regulatory procedures, below).

The clinical studies, described in detail in Chapter 18, are classified according to Table 20.2.

Human pharmacology

Human pharmacology studies refer to the earliest human exposure in volunteers, as well as any pharmacological studies in patients and volunteers throughout the development of the drug.

The first study of a new drug substance in humans has essentially three objectives:

- To investigate *tolerability* over a range of doses and, if possible, see the symptoms of adverse effects;
- To obtain information on *pharmacokinetics*, and to measure bioavailability and plasma concentration/effect relations;
- To examine the *pharmacodynamic activity* over a range of doses and obtain a dose–response relationship, provided a relevant effect can be measured in healthy volunteers.

Further human pharmacology studies are performed to document pharmacodynamic and pharmacokinetic effects. Examples of the data needed to support an application for trials in patients are the complete pharmacokinetic evaluation, and the performance of bioavailability/bioequivalence studies during the development of new formulations or drug delivery systems. Information is also obtained on the possible influence of food on absorption, and that of other concomitant medications, i.e. drug interaction. Exploration of metabolic pattern is also performed early in the clinical development process.

Special patient populations need particular attention because they may be unduly sensitive or resistant to treatment regimens acceptable to the normal adult population studied. One obvious category is patients with renal or hepatic impairment, who may be unable to metabolize or excrete the drug effectively enough to avoid accumulation. The metabolic pattern and elimination route are important predictors for such patients, who are not included in clinical trials until late in development

Gender differences may also occur, and may be detected by the inclusion of women at the dose-finding stage of clinical trials.

An interaction is an alteration in the pharmacodynamic or the pharmacokinetic properties of a drug caused by factors such as concomitant drug treatment, diet, social habits (e.g. tobacco or alcohol), age, gender, ethnic origin and time of administration.

Interaction studies can be performed in healthy volunteers looking at possible metabolism changes when co-administering compounds that share the same enzymatic metabolic pathway. Also, changed pharmacokinetic behaviour can be investigated in combinations of drugs that are expected to be used together. Generally, such human volunteer studies are performed when clinical findings require clarification.

Table 20.2
ICH classification of clinical studies

Type of study	Study objectives	Traditional terminology
Human pharmacology	Assess tolerance; describe or define pharmacokinetics/pharmacodynamics; explore drug metabolism and drug interactions; estimate activity	Phase I
Therapeutic exploratory	Explore use for the targeted indication; estimate dosage for subsequent studies; provide basis for confirmatory study design, endpoints, methodologies	Phase II
Therapeutic confirmatory	Demonstrate or confirm efficacy; establish safety profile; provide an adequate basis for assessing benefit/risk relationship to support licensing (drug approval); establish dose–response relationship	Phase III (a and b)
Therapeutic use	Refine understanding of benefit/risk relationship in general or special populations and/or environments; identify less common adverse reactions; refine dosing recommendations	Phase IV

Therapeutic exploratory studies

After relevant information in healthy volunteers has been obtained, safety conclusions from combined animal and human exposure will be assessed internally. If these are favourable, initial patient studies can begin. To obtain the most reliable results, the patient population should be as homogeneous as possible – similar age, no other diseases than the one to be studied – and the design should, when ethically justified, be placebo controlled. For ethical reasons only a limited number of closely monitored patients take part in these studies. Their importance lies in the assumption that any placebo effect in the group treated with active drug should be eliminated by comparison with blinded inactive treatment. They are used primarily to establish efficacy measured against no treatment.

Studies in special populations: elderly, children, ethnic differences

Clinically significant differences in pharmacokinetics between the elderly and the young are due to several factors related to ageing, such as impaired renal function, which can increase the variability in drug response, as well as increasing the likelihood of unwanted effects and drug interactions. Bearing in mind that the elderly are the largest group of consumers, this category should be studied as early as possible in clinical trials.

Clinical trials in children
Studies in children require experience from adult human studies and information on the pharmacokinetic profile of the substance. Because of the difficulties, and the often small commercial return, companies have seldom considered it worthwhile to test drugs in children and to seek regulatory approval for marketing drugs for use in children. Nevertheless, drugs are often prescribed 'off-label' for children, on the basis of clinical experience suggesting that they are safe and effective. Such off-label prescribing is undesirable, as clinical experience is less satisfactory than formal trials data as a guide to efficacy and safety, and because it leaves the clinician, rather than the pharmaceutical company, liable for any harm that results. During recent years, requirements to include a paediatric population early have forced the development of new guidance how to include children in clinical development. Market exclusivity prolongation has been successfully tried for some years in the USA, and in July 2003 the Federal Food Drug and Cosmetics Act was amended to request paediatric studies in a new submission unless omission is justified (see website reference 2). In Europe the Commission adopted a proposal for a similar regulation in September 2004 (see website reference 3). This stipulates that no marketing approval will be granted unless there is an agreed paediatric investigation plan in place or, alternatively, there is a waiver from the requirement because of the low risk that the product will be considered

for use in children. The paediatric studies may, with the agreement of the regulatory authority, be performed after approval for other populations. Marketing of the drug for paediatric use will be compulsory within 1 year of approval. For new compounds or for products with a Supplementary Protection Certificate (see p. 296), paediatric applications will be given a longer market exclusivity period, and off-patent products will be given a special paediatric use marketing authorization (PUMA); funds will be available for paediatric research in these products.

Ethnic differences

In order for clinical data to be accepted globally, the risk of ethnic differences must be assessed. ICH Efficacy guideline E5 defines a bridging data package that would allow extrapolation of foreign clinical data to the population in the new region. A limited programme may suffice to confirm comparable effects in different ethnic groups.

Ethnic differences may be genetic in origin, as in the example described in Chapter 18, or related to differences in environment, culture or medical practice.

Therapeutic confirmatory studies

The therapeutic confirmatory phase is intended to confirm efficacy results from controlled exploratory efficacy studies, but now in a more realistic clinical environment and with a broader population. An equally important function of this largest and longest section of the clinical documentation is to capture all adverse event information to enable evaluation of the relative benefit/risk ratio of the new compound, and also to detect rare adverse reactions that occur in less than 5% of the exposed population. For a reasonable evaluation, at least 2000 patients need to be included in the studies.

For a product intended for long-term administration, its performance must be investigated during long-term exposure. To document clinical safety, the ICH E1 guideline stipulates that 100 patients be treated for at least 1 year, and 300–600 treated for at least 6 months.

The clinical programmes for the relatively new COX-2 inhibitors, designed to show a lower incidence of the serious gastrointestinal adverse reactions caused by conventional NSAIDs, required more than 10 000 patients monitored during the therapeutic confirmatory phase. In general, proving the absence of an important side effect is much more demanding of resources than proving superior efficacy. This is also true for drugs in other therapeutic areas, in particular cardiovascular disorders.

Clinical safety profile

From each study performed, all adverse events (unintended events, not necessarily drug related) are collected and a preliminary evaluation is made; but not until several similar studies can be analysed together can a real estimate be made of the clinical safety of the product. To have statistical power in the evaluation, and to obtain a reasonable estimate of the nature and incidence of common and rare adverse reactions, it is usually necessary to collect data on at least 1500 patients.

The collected clinical database should be analysed across a sensible selection of variables, such as sex, age, race, exposure (dose and duration), as well as concomitant diseases and concomitant pharmacotherapy. This type of integrated data analysis is a rational and scientific way to obtain necessary information about the benefits and risks of new compounds, and has been required for FDA submissions for many years, though it is not yet a firm requirement in the EU or Japan.

Regulatory aspects of novel types of therapy

As emphasized in earlier chapters, the therapeutic scene is moving increasingly towards biological treatments, and this trend is likely to increase. The regulatory framework established to ensure the quality, safety and efficacy of conventional synthetic drugs is not entirely appropriate for many biopharmaceutical products, and even less so for the many gene- and cell-based products currently in development. Recombinant proteins have been in use since 1982, and the regulatory process for such biopharmaceuticals is by now well established. The regulatory framework for newer therapeutic modalities is, however, not yet clearly defined, and the regulatory authorities face a difficult task in keeping up with the rapid pace of technological change.

Biopharmaceuticals

Biopharmaceuticals account for an increasing share of all new molecular entities launched, representing around 30% of all new entities approved in the USA in 2001. Compared with synthetic compounds, biopharmaceuticals are by their nature more heterogeneous, and their production methods are very diverse, including complex fermentation and recombinant techniques, as well as production via the use of transgenic animals and plants, thereby posing new problems for quality control. This has necessarily led to a fairly pragmatic regulatory framework. Quality, safety and efficacy requirements have to be no less stringent, but procedures and standards are flexible and generally established on a case-by-case basis. Consequently, achieving regulatory approval can often be a greater challenge for the pharmaceutical company, but there are also opportunities to succeed with novel and relatively quick development programmes.

Published guidelines on the development of conventional drugs need to be considered to determine what parts are relevant for a particular biopharmaceutical product. In addition, there are to date seven ICH guidelines dealing exclusively with biopharmaceuticals, as well as numerous FDA and CPMP guidance documents (see websites 1 and 4, p. 297). These mostly deal with quality aspects, and in some cases preclinical safety aspects. The definition of what is included in the term 'biopharmaceutical' varies somewhat between documents, and therefore needs to be checked. The active substances include proteins and peptides, their derivatives, and products of which they are components. Examples include (but are not limited to) cytokines, recombinant plasma factors, growth factors, fusion proteins, enzymes, hormones and monoclonal antibodies.

Quality considerations

At the time when biopharmaceuticals first appeared, the ability to analyse and exactly characterize the end-product was very far from what could be done with small molecules. Therefore, their efficacy and safety depended critically on the manufacturing process itself, and emphasis was placed on 'process control' rather than 'product control'. It was also uncertain what level of potential risk contaminants such as residual DNA in a product might represent.

Since then, much experience and confidence has been gained. Bioanalytical technologies for characterizing large molecules have improved dramatically and so has the field of bioassays, which are normally required to be included in such characterizations, e.g. to determine the 'potency' of a product. As a result, the quality aspects of biopharmaceuticals are no longer as fundamentally different from those of synthetic products as they used to be. Today there is even talk of generic biopharmaceuticals, and the concept of 'comparability' has been established. Approaches for demonstrating product comparability after process changes have been outlined by regulatory authorities. There is, for example, the emerging ICH guidance Q5E on the comparability of biotechnological/biological products, which has currently reached step 5 of the ICH process, as well as draft FDA and final CPMP guidance. However, to make use of these provisions, very comprehensive knowledge of the process and product characteristics is crucial. Thereby the company may convincingly demonstrate which process parameters are likely to affect product quality, safety and efficacy, and may have the opportunity to optimize the manufacturing process without necessarily repeating clinical or non-clinical studies.

A unique and critically important feature for biopharmaceuticals is the need to ensure and document viral safety aspects. Furthermore, there must be a preparedness for potentially new hazards, such as infective prions. Therefore strict control of the origin of starting materials and expression systems is essential. The current battery of ICH quality guidance documents in this area reflects these points of particular attention (ICH Q5A-E, and Q6B).

Environmental risk assessment, focusing particularly on genetically modified organisms (GMOs), is another point that is attracting growing attention, similar to environmental risk in general (see Environmental considerations, below)

To conclude, it is still fair to say that regulatory requirements and review are focused on the quality of the manufacturing process, and rigorous process control for these products. The quality documentation will typically be more extensive than it is for a small-molecule product.

Safety considerations

The expectations in terms of performing and documenting a non-clinical safety evaluation for biotechnology-derived pharmaceuticals are very well outlined in the ICH guidance S6. It indicates a flexible, case-by-case and science-based approach, but also points out that a product needs to be sufficiently characterized to allow the appropriate design of a preclinical safety evaluation.

Generally, all toxicity studies must be performed according to GLP. However, for biopharmaceuticals it is recognized that some specialized tests may not be able to comply fully with GLP. The guidance further comments that the standard toxicity testing designs in the commonly used species (e.g. rats and dogs) are often not relevant.

To make it relevant, a safety evaluation should include a species in which the test material is pharmacologically active. Further, in certain justified cases one relevant species may suffice, at least for the long-term studies. If no relevant species at all can be identified, the use of transgenic animals expressing the human receptor, or the use of homologous proteins, should be considered.

Other factors of particular relevance with biopharmaceuticals are potential immunogenicity and immunotoxicity. Long-term studies may be difficult to perform, depending on the possible formation of neutralizing antibodies in the selected species. For products intended for chronic use, the duration of long-term toxicity studies must, however, always be scientifically justified. Regulatory guidance also states that standard carcinogenicity studies are generally inappropriate, but that product-specific assessments of potential risks may still be needed, and that a variety of approaches may be necessary to accomplish this.

Efficacy considerations

The need to establish efficacy is in principle the same for biopharmaceuticals as for conventional drugs, but there are significant differences in practice. The establishment of a dose–response relationship can be irrelevant, as there may be an 'all-or-none-effect' at extremely low

levels. Also, to determine a maximum tolerated dose (MTD) in humans may be impractical, as many biopharmaceuticals will not evoke any dose-limiting side effects. Measuring pharmacokinetic properties may be difficult, particularly if the substance is an endogenous mediator. Biopharmaceuticals may also have very long half-lives compared to small molecules, often in the range of weeks rather than hours.

For any biopharmaceutical intended for chronic or repeated use, there will be extra emphasis on demonstrating long-term efficacy. This is because the medical use of proteins is associated with potential immunogenicity and the possible development of neutralizing antibodies, such that the intended effect may decrease or even disappear with time. Repeated assessment of immunogenicity may be needed, particularly after any process changes.

To date, biopharmaceuticals have typically been developed for serious diseases, and certain types of treatments, such as cytotoxic agents or immunomodulators, cannot be given to healthy volunteers. In such cases, the initial dose-escalation studies will have to be carried out in a patient population rather than in normal volunteers.

Regulatory procedural considerations

In the EU, only the centralized procedure can be used for biopharmaceuticals (see Regulatory procedures, below).

In the USA, biopharmaceuticals are in most cases approved by review of Biologics License Applications (BLA), rather than as New Drug Applications (NDA). The FDA was partly reorganized in 2003, with the result that many biotechnologically derived products previously reviewed by the Center for Biologics Evaluation and Research (CBER) will now instead be handled by the Center for Drugs Evaluation and Research (CDER) which is responsible for small-molecule drugs. Depending on a product's target indication, different therapeutic review divisions within CDER will handle applications (including the first IND application). Other biopharmaceutical products (e.g. blood products and vaccines) remain the responsibility of CBER.

Individualized therapies

It is recognized that an individual's genetic makeup influences the effect of drugs. Incorporating this principle into therapeutic practice is still at a very early stage, and it presents a difficult problem for regulatory authorities, who are seeking ways to incorporate pharmacogenomics into the regulatory process, where appropriate and discussions with industry representatives are in progress with the aim of developing a concrete regulatory framework. Two issues of particular concern are *ethical* and *technical* aspects.

Ethical issues arise when deciding what patient group should be included in therapeutic clinical trials. Should it be the unselected population that is normally studied today, or the genetically defined group thought likely to benefit most?

Studying the general population provides safety information relevant to a broader population, as that may be how the drug will frequently be used in practice. On the other hand, can it be ethically justified to expose patients who are thought less likely to benefit to both the drug and its potential risks?

As regards *technical issues*, it is not yet clear to what extent the use of a drug can or should be linked to the performance of a particular pharmacogenomic test, or whether they need to be approved simultaneously. How should tests be validated, or data bridged when improved test methods become available? To date, there are very few approved products from which to learn. The FDA has, however, indicated that it would be unable to approve a drug for which the safety profile was predicated on a pharmacogenomic test that was not freely available.

Gene therapy

Gene therapy products are subject to the same regulatory controls as other medicinal products, and it is illegal in most countries to embark on human trials, or to sell a product, without first obtaining approval. Despite the great potential of gene therapy, and the large amount of research effort involved (see Chapter 12), no gene therapy product has yet (February 2004) received FDA approval (see websites 5 and 6, p. 297).

There is US (FDA) as well as European (CPMP) guidance addressing the regulatory aspects of human somatic cell therapy and gene therapy products, which follow the same principles of ensuring quality, safety and efficacy as are applied to any new medicinal product. More precise guidelines concerning issues specific to gene therapy products are under active discussion, and the development of gene therapy medicinal products, or gene transfer products, has been identified by the ICH as an area of particular importance that needs to be closely monitored.

Currently, approval of investigational gene therapy protocols is based on case-by-case evaluation, with close attention to safety issues, and such approvals are often subject to continuous regulatory monitoring. The main concerns at present are with the safety of the viral vectors commonly used for gene therapy, and the risk of disrupting the genome of somatic cells in ways that could lead to malignant transformation.

Orphan drugs

Orphan medicines are those intended to diagnose, prevent or treat rare diseases, in the EU further specified as life-threatening or chronically debilitating conditions. The concept also includes therapies that are unlikely to be developed under normal market conditions, where the company can show that a return on research investment will not be possible. To qualify for orphan drug status, there should be no satisfactory treatment available or, alternatively, the intended new treatment should be assumed to be of significant benefit (see website references 5 and 6)

In the USA the legislation also includes medical devices and medical food as possible orphan candidates, and medical devices are covered in Japan. To qualify as an orphan indication, the prevalence of the condition must be fewer than 5 in 10 000 individuals in the EU, fewer than 50 000 affected in Japan, or fewer than 200 000 affected in the USA. Orphan designation in Europe is granted by the European Commission; in Japan and the USA by the health authorities.

Financial and scientific assistance is made available for products intended for use in a given indication that obtain orphan status. Examples of financial benefits are a reduction in or exemption from fees, as well as funding provided by regulatory authorities to meet part of the development costs in some instances. Specialist groups within the regulatory authorities provide scientific help and advice on the execution of studies. Compromises may be needed owing to the scarcity of patients, although the normal requirements to demonstrate safety and efficacy still apply.

The most important benefit stimulating orphan drug development is, however, market exclusivity for 7–10 years for the product, for the designated medical use. In the EU the centralized procedure (see Regulatory procedures, below) will become the compulsory procedure for orphan drugs.

The orphan drug incentives are fairly recent. In the USA the legislation dates from 1983, in Japan from 1995, and in the EU from 2000. The US experience has shown very good results, with nearly 250 orphan drugs approved, the majority of which are intended to treat rare cancers or metabolic/endocrinological disorders.

Environmental considerations

Environmental evaluation of the finished pharmaceutical products is now required in the USA and EU, the main concern being contamination of the environment by the compound or its metabolites. Pesticide residues in the environment are believed to have estrogen-like actions which can affect both humans and wildlife, and urinary excretion of drugs and metabolites may have similar consequences. The environmental impact of the manufacturing process is a separate issue that is regulated elsewhere.

The US requirement for environmental assessment (EA) applies in all cases where action is needed to minimize environmental effects. An Environmental Assessment Report is then required, and the FDA will develop an Environmental Impact Statement to direct necessary action. Drug products for human or animal use can, however, be excluded from this requirement under certain conditions (see website 7, p. 297), for example if the estimated concentration in the aquatic environment of the active substance is below 1 part per billion, or if the substance occurs naturally. In Europe, a similar draft guidance paper (website 8, p.297) is under discussion.

The current diffuse requirements and the relative lack of knowledge about what impact drugs and/or active metabolites have on drinking water and soil has caused criticism from environmental experts. Resistant bacteria have been found in waterworks owing to pollution with antibiotics, and hermaphrodite fish have been discovered close to hospital sites, probably reflecting pollution of the water by steroid hormones. These examples are serious, and stricter requirements for environmental investigations are to be expected.

Regulatory procedures

Clinical trials

It is evident that clinical trials can pose unknown risks to humans: the earlier in the development process, the greater the risk. *Regulatory* and *ethical* approvals are based on independent evaluations, and both are required before investigations in humans can begin.

The ethical basis for all clinical research is the Declaration of Helsinki (website 9, p. 297), which states that the primary obligation for the treating physician is to care for the patient. It also says that clinical research may be performed provided the goal is to improve treatment. Furthermore, the subject must be informed about the potential benefits and risks, and must consent to participate. The guardians of patients who for any reason cannot give informed consent (e.g. small children) can agree on participation.

Ethical evaluation is made by an independent hospital ethics committee (known in the USA as the Institutional Review Board, IRB) composed of medical and legal professionals, as well as laypersons.

Regulatory authorities are concerned mainly with the scientific basis of the intended study protocol. Is the regulatory requirement to start the trial fulfilled? Is there a scientific need to perform this study, and will the information be needed when the drug is being considered for marketing approval? Regulatory authorities require all results of clinical trials approved by them to be reported to them.

All clinical research in humans should be performed according to the internationally agreed Code of Good Clinical Practice, as described in the ICH guideline E6 (see website 1, p. 297).

Europe

Until recently, the regulatory requirements to start and conduct clinical studies in Europe varied widely between countries, ranging from little or no regulation to a requirement for complete assessment by the health authority of the intended study protocol and all supporting documentation. All countries, however, required approval by an ethics committee.

The efforts to harmonize EU procedures has led to the development of a Clinical Trial Directive implemented in May 2004 (website 10, p. 297). The requirement for information to be submitted to regulatory authorities as well as to ethics committees is being defined and published in a set of guidelines. Much of the information submitted to the regulatory authority and ethics committee is the same, and the division of responsibility between them is currently unclear. The pharmaceutical industry is trying to avoid a situation where requirements from all national authorities will simply be combined, causing a large increase in the regulatory burden which would discourage the performance of clinical studies in Europe.

One great benefit will be that both regulatory authorities and ethics committees must respond within 60 days of receiving clinical trials applications. Another benefit will be that all data concerning European studies will be collected in a central database accessible to regulatory authorities. All adverse event reports from clinical trials will be similarly collected and made available.

USA

An Investigational New Drug (IND) application must be approved by the FDA before a new drug is given to humans. The application is simple (see website 11, p. 297), and to encourage early human studies it is no longer necessary to submit complete pharmacology study reports. The toxicology safety evaluation can be based on draft and unaudited reports, provided the data are sufficient for the FDA to make a reliable assessment. Complete study reports must be available in later clinical development phases.

If approved, the IND is considered opened and information (study protocol) is added to it for every new study planned. New scientific information must be submitted whenever changes are made, e.g. dose increases, new patient categories or new indications. The IND process requires an annual update report describing project progress during the year.

Approval from IRB is needed for every institution where a clinical study is to be performed.

Japan

Up to now, because of differences in medical culture, in treatment traditions and the possibility of significant racial differences, clinical trials in Japan have not been useful for drug applications in the western world. Also, for a product to be approved for the Japanese market, repetition of clinical studies in Japan has been necessary, often delaying the availability of products in Japan.

With the introduction of international standards under the auspices of ICH, data from Japanese patients will increasingly become acceptable in other countries. The guideline on bridging studies to compensate for ethnic differences (ICH E5; website 12, p. 297) may allow Japanese studies to become part of global development.

The requirements for beginning a clinical study in Japan are similar to those in the USA or Europe. Scientific summary information is generally acceptable, and ethics committee approval is necessary.

Application for marketing authorization

The application for marketing authorization (MAA in Europe, NDA in the USA) is compiled and submitted as soon as the drug development programme has been completed and judged satisfactory by the company. Different authorities have differing requirements as to the level of detail and the format of submissions, and it is the task of the RA department to collate all the data as efficiently as possible to satisfy these varying requirements with a minimum of redrafting.

The US FDA in general requires raw data to be submitted, allowing them to make their own analysis, and thus they request the most complete data of all authorities. European authorities require a condensed dossier containing critical evaluations of the data, allowing a rapid review based on conclusions drawn by named scientific experts. These may be internal or external, and are selected by the applicant.

Japanese authorities have traditionally focused on data generated in Japan, studies performed elsewhere being supportive only.

Below we describe the procedures adopted in these three regions in more detail.

Europe

Three procedures are available for marketing authorization in the EU (see website 13, p. 297).

- *National procedure*, where the application is evaluated by one regulatory authority. This procedure is allowed for products intended for that country only. Also, it is the first step in a mutual recognition procedure.

- *Mutual recognition* (Figure 20.3), whereby a marketing approval application is assessed by one national authority, the Reference Member State (RMS), which subsequently defends the approval and evaluation in order to gain mutual recognition of the assessment from other European authorities. The pharmaceutical company may select countries of interest. These, the Concerned Member States, have 90 days to recognize the initial assessment.
  - ○ After mutual recognition the final marketing authorizations are given as national decisions, but the scientific assessment is quicker and requires fewer resources from all national authorities.
  - ○ In the case of non-agreement, arbitration by the European Commission is possible as a last resort. It is, however, more common to withdraw the application before day 90 in the country that cannot agree. The worst case of an arbitration is that the marketing authorizations obtained are withdrawn in all EU countries, including the RMS.
- *Centralized procedure*. The centralized procedure is a 'federal' procedure carried out by EMEA, with scientists selected from CPMP to perform the review, the approval body being the European Commission. Since its introduction in 1995 the centralized procedure has been available for biotechnological products, new active substances or 'innovative medicinal products with novel characteristics'

The last two categories are admitted to the centralized procedure only after approval from EMEA. The revision of legislation in 2004 will result in the stepwise adoption of the centralized procedure as the sole approval procedure. Currently, biopharmaceuticals must use the centralized procedure, and applications for products intended to treat AIDS/HIV, cancer, neurodegenerative diseases and diabetes will follow.

The centralized procedure starts with the nomination of one CPMP member to act as *rapporteur*, who selects and leads the assessment team. A selected *co-rapporteur* and team make a parallel review. The European Commission approves the application based on a CPMP recommendation, which in turn is based on the assessment reports by the two rapporteur teams. Products approved in this way can be marketed in all EU countries with the same prescribing information, packs and labels.

CPMP is prepared to give scientific advice to companies in situations where published guidance on the European position is not available, or when the company need to discuss a possible deviation from guidelines. Such advice, as well as advice from national regulatory authorities, may be very valuable at any stage of the development programme, and may later be incorporated in new guidelines. Providing it requires

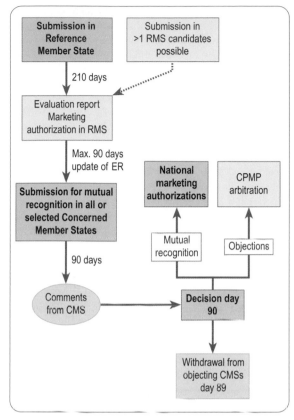

Fig. 20.3
Submission process for marketing approval by the ICH Mutual Recognition Procedure.

considerable effort from CPMP specialists, and fees have to be paid by the pharmaceutical company.

USA

The FDA is more willing than other large authorities to take an active part in planning the drug development process. Some meetings between the FDA and the sponsoring company are more or less compulsory (e.g. end-of-Phase II meeting) and it is important that the advice from FDA is followed. At the same time, these discussions may make it possible in special cases to deviate from guidelines by prior agreement with FDA. These discussion meetings ensure that the authority is already familiar with the project when the dossier is submitted.

The review time for the FDA has decreased substantially in the last few years (see Chapter 22) since an application fee was instituted in the USA. Standard reviews should be completed within 10 months, and priority reviews of those products with a strong medical need within 6 months.

The assessment result is usually communicated via an *FDA approvable letter*, meaning that the application can be approved provided some specified commitments are accepted by the applicant. Such commitments are

likely to include further studies that are not critical to the benefit/risk evaluation but are important for the total assessment of the product.

Japan

The Japanese health authority, the Ministry of Health Labor and Welfare (MHLW), was by tradition a very closed organization, whose scientific experts did not meet the pharmaceutical industry, all communication taking place through administrative officials. Prior to 1997, when a major reorganization of MHLW and a review of the approval process took place, Japan did not allow the kind of planning and discussion meetings with experts that are favoured by US and European authorities.

Since 1997, a non-governmental advisory organization, KIKO, has been available for consultation, allowing scientific discussion during the development phase. These meetings tend to follow a similar pattern to those in the rest of the world, and have made it much easier to address potential problems well before submission for marketing approval is made.

These changes have meant shorter review times and a more transparent process. The review in Japan is performed by an Evaluation Centre, and the ultimate decision is made by the MHLW based on the Evaluation Centre's report. Discussions between the company and the Evaluation Centre are possible and recommended.

It is worth mentioning that health authorities, in particular in the ICH regions, have well-established communications and often assist and consult each other.

The Common Technical Document

Following the good progress made by ICH in creating scientific guidelines applicable in the three large regions, discussions on standardizing document formats began in 1997. The aim was to define a standard format, called the Common Technical Document (CTD), for the application for a new drug product. It was realized from the outset that harmonization of *content* could not be achieved, owing to the fundamental differences in data requirements and work processes between different regulatory authorities. Adopting a common *format* would, none the less, be a worthwhile step forward.

The guideline was adopted by the three ICH regions in November 2000 and subsequently implemented, and it will most probably be accepted in most other countries. This will save much time and effort in reformatting documents for submission to different regulatory authorities. The structure of the CTD (see website 14, p. 297) is summarized in Figure 20.4.

Module 1 (not part of the CTD) contains regional information such as the application form, the suggested

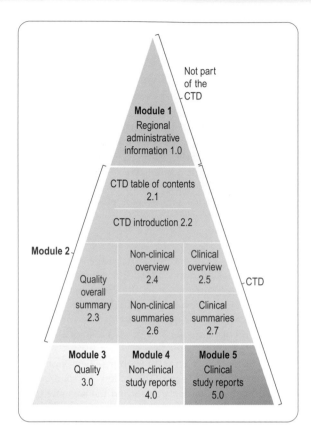

Fig. 20.4
Diagrammatic representation of the organization of the Common Technical Document (CTD).

The clinical summary is similar to what was required by the FDA, incorporating many features taken from the Integrated Summaries of Efficacy (ISE) and Safety (ISS). ISE will generally fit in the clinical summary document. The ISS document has proved very useful in drawing conclusions from the clinical studies by sensible pooling and integration, but is too large (often more than 400 pages in itself) to be accepted in the EU and Japan. This problem may be resolved by including the ISS as a separate report in Module 5.

Modules 3–5 comprise the individual study reports. Most reports are eligible for use in all three regions, possibly with the exception at present of Module 3, Quality, which may need regional content.

An initiative is also under way to switch to electronic submissions – known as e-CTD – in place of the large quantities of paper that now comprise an application for marketing approval. When this is implemented experimental data will be lodged mainly in databases, allowing the information to be exchanged between pharmaceutical companies and regulatory authorities much more easily than at present. Guidelines on the structure and interface between databases in the industry setting and those at the authorities are available.

Administrative rules

Patent protection and data exclusivity

Supplementary Protection Certificate

During the 1980s, the time taken to develop and obtain marketing approval for a new drug increased so much that the period of market exclusivity established by the original patent could be too short to allow the company to recoup its R&D costs. To overcome this problem (see Chapter 19), the EU Council in 1992 introduced rules allowing companies to apply for a Supplementary Protection Certificate (SPC), matching similar legislation in the USA and Japan. This can prolong market protection by a maximum of 5 years to give an overall period of exclusivity of up to 15 years.

The application for an SPC has to be submitted within 6 months of first approval anywhere in Europe, within or outside the EU, and from then on the clock starts. It is thus strategically important to obtain first approval in a financially important market for best revenue.

Data exclusivity

After the regulatory approval of a pharmaceutical product in an EU country the confidentiality of the data

prescribing information, the application fee, and also other information that is not considered relevant in all territories, such as environmental assessment (required in the USA and Europe, but not in Japan). Certificates of different regional needs are also to be found in Module 1, as well as patent information not yet requested in the EU.

Module 2 comprises a very brief general introduction, followed by summary information relating to quality, safety (i.e. non-clinical studies) and efficacy (i.e. clinical studies). Quality issues (purity, manufacturing process, stability etc.) are summarized in a single document of a maximum 40 pages. The non-clinical and clinical summaries each consist of a separate *overview* (maximum 30 pages) and *summaries of individual studies*. The overviews in each area are similar to the previous EU Expert Reports in that they present critical evaluations of the programme performed. Detailed guidelines (see website 14), based on existing US, European and Japanese requirements, are available to indicate what tabulated information needs to be included in these summaries, and how the written summaries should be drafted. The non-clinical section has been fairly non-controversial. The guidance is very similar to the previous US summary, with clear instructions on how to sort the studies regarding animals, doses, durations of treatment and routes of administration.

submitted will be protected for 6–10 years before it may be referenced as documentation by another company seeking marketing authorization for a copy of the same product. Within this period, even if the original patent has expired, a company wishing to sell a generic copy would have to repeat all of the trials at great expense in order to gain approval, so this rule effectively rules out generic copies until the exclusivity period ends.

Currently, the exclusivity rule does not apply uniformly across EU countries, but it is intended that they should be harmonized by 2006 to provide 8 years for regulatory data protection, another 2 years of market exclusivity, and 1 extra year possible for 'a significant new indication'.

Pricing of pharmaceutical products – 'the fourth hurdle'

The 'fourth hurdle' is an expression for the currently growing demand for cost-effectiveness in pharmaceutical prescribing. Payers, whether health insurance companies or publicly funded institutions, now require more stringent justification for the normally high price of a new pharmaceutical product. This means that, if not in the original application, studies have to demonstrate that the clinical benefit of a new compound is commensurate with the suggested price, compared to the previous therapy of choice in the country of application.

To address this concern, studies in a clinical trials programme from Phase II onwards now normally include health economic measures (see Chapter 18). In the USA, certainly, it is advantageous to include a statement of health economic benefit approved in the package insert, to justify reimbursement. Reference pricing systems are also being developed in Europe. A favourable risk/benefit evaluation is no longer sufficient: value for money must also be demonstrated.

References

Cartwright AC, Matthews BR (1991) Pharmaceutical product licensing requirements for Europe. London: Ellis Horwood.

Cartwright AC, Matthews BR (eds) (1994) International pharmaceutical product registration. London: Taylor and Francis.

CPMP Draft Guideline CPMP/SWP/4447/00: Environmental risk assessment of medicinal products for human use. 24 July 2003.

Drews J (1999) In quest of tomorrow's medicines. New York: Springer-Verlag.

Guidance for Industry: Environmental assessment of human drug and biologics applications (Final). July 1998 Code of Federal Regulations 21:25 A–E.

Meade TW (1975) Subacute myelo-optic neuropathy and clioquinol. An epidemiological case-history for diagnosis. British Journal of Preventive and Social Medicine 29: 157–169.

Website references

1. http://www.ich.org/
2. http://www.fda.gov/cder/guidance/pedrule.pdf
3. http://pharmacos.eudra.org/F2/paediatrics/index.htm
4. http://www.fda.gov
5. http://www.emea.eu.int/index/indexh1.htm
6. http://www.fda.gov/opacom/laws/orphandg.htm
7. http://www.fda.gov/cder/guidance/1730fnl.pdf
8. http://www.emea.eu.int.pdfs/human/swp/444700en.pdf
9. http://www.wma.net/e/ethicsunit/helskinki.htm
10. http://www.mca.gov.uk/ourwork/licensingmeds/types/clintrialdir.htm
11. http://www.fda.gov/cder/regulatory/applications/ind_page_1.htm
12. http://www.ich.org/MediaServer.jser?@_ID=481&@_MODE=GLB
13. http://pharmacos.eudra.org/F2/eudralex/vol-2/home.htm
14. http://www.aboutctd.com

List of abbreviations

CHMP	Committee for Medicinal Products for Human use, the new name to replace CPMP early 2004
CPMP	Committee for Proprietary Medicinal Products
CTD	Common Technical Document
EC	Ethics Committee (EU), known as Institutional Review Board (IRB) in USA
eCTD	Electronic Common Technical Document
EMEA	European Agency for the Evaluation of Medicinal Products
ERA	Environmental Risk Assessment (EU)
EU	European Union
FDA	Food and Drug Administration; the US Regulatory Authority
GCP	Good clinical practice
GLP	Good laboratory practice
GMP	Good manufacturing practice
ICH	International Conference on Harmonization
IND	Investigational New Drug application (US)
IRB	Institutional Review Board (US), equivalent to Ethics Committee in Europe
ISS	Integrated Summary of Safety (US)
MAA	Marketing Authorization Application (EU), equivalent to NDA in USA
MHLW	Ministry of Health, Labor and Welfare (Jpn)
MTD	Maximum tolerated dose
NDA	New Drug Application (USA), equivalent to MAA in Europe
NTA	Notice to Applicants; EU set of pharmaceutical regulations, directives and guidelines
SPC	Supplementary Protection Certificate
WHO	World Health Organization

Marketing the drug

R Howell

What is marketing?

What is marketing? Clearly, the role of marketing a drug involves optimizing the sales of that drug, but how? It involves more than just selling the drug, but what? When and how does marketing get involved in drug development? This chapter addresses these questions, first by defining what marketing is, then describing how marketing is applied at a local country level and at a global level.

Successful marketing, in any industry, encompasses the following three principles:

- Marketing is knowing your customer's needs.
- In a successful company everyone is involved in marketing.
- Marketing works by changing perceptions in the outside world.

Whatever your speciality in the pharmaceutical industry, having a good understanding of these three elements will ensure that the company maximizes every new opportunity. It will also help you in your dealings with marketing professionals – you may want to become one yourself!

'Just another name for selling'

Many people think that marketing and selling are the same, mainly because the activity of selling is what affects us visibly as consumers. Although retail stores have moved away from experienced sales staff towards self-service, the salesperson is still important in many businesses, from car sales, through life insurance to double glazing, all of which sell expensive products at sufficient profit to cover the commission due to the salesperson. Businesses of this sort have given a generally negative image to marketing and selling. However, not everything that we buy is expensive enough to warrant a salesperson's time to convince us to choose their product, and even businesses such as insurance, which can generate enough profit to support a sales force, are beginning to change as Internet and telephone advertising take over from door-to-door selling.

So, how can a company convince you to buy their product without a sales force? Why should you choose one brand of cereal, soap powder or car over another? What makes you buy a new gadget that you have happily managed without for years? The answer is marketing.

Definitions of marketing

Popular and *incorrect* definitions of marketing are:

● 'The art of selling people things that they don't need'
● 'Advertising'
● 'Product, Promotion, Place and Price'.

The first definition describes the insurance or double-glazing salesperson. Often the only long-term customer relationship here will be the resolution never to buy anything from that person or company again. For a company wishing to build their business this type of 'slash and burn' approach will not be a recipe for success. The second, advertising, covers only one limited aspect of marketing, a particular (though powerful) communication link between the company and its customers which is designed on the basis of the company's marketing strategy. The last description, known as the 'four Ps', is often quoted as a definition of marketing in some older marketing books. Obviously these elements are part of marketing, but they leave out a critical component: the customer's perception of the product and its competitors.

What we need is a definition that captures the relationship between the customer and the company: what marketing *is* rather than what marketing *does*.

Because the older definitions focus on what marketing does and ignore the customer aspects, there was a move towards completely redefining marketing, recognizing that the customer has to feel that they need the product or service, and that the company needs to make money. Consequently, more recent texts define marketing as: 'Meeting customer needs at a profit'.

This is all well and good as long as your company is the only one who can satisfy those needs and you don't care how much profit you make. In the 1990s the airline companies did some market research to find out what were the features of air travel that customers wanted most. They argued that if they asked their customers to identify their needs, and if the airline could satisfy those needs better than their competition, then it would be a simple job to become the market leader. In the event it turned out that what the average customer wanted was a business-class seat for an economy price. So even if the airline found a way to offer this, it would inevitably be at the expense of profit. Interestingly, the airlines have found ways to offer some of the benefits of higher-class travel to their customers travelling in lower classes. On the very competitive North Atlantic route some airlines

introduced the reclining bed/seat for first-class and business-class passengers. The business class is the most profitable section of the aeroplane, with a high number of 'chooser-users', who have the ability to exercise their choice of airline. Market research showed that the business user values very highly the ability to sleep on nocturnal long-haul flights, and the traveller's employer benefits from having an employee who is fresh on arrival. Introducing sleeper seats has a cost both in fitting the seats and in the reduction in the number of seats that will fit in the space, but this is more than offset by attracting more customers, enabling the airline to fill its capacity and charge a premium, thereby increasing its profits. The important factor was to place a value on the need by understanding the value to the customer, and to realize that this increased customer value could be balanced by a pricing structure that would increase the profit to the company. This comes closer to describing the role of marketing.

The best definition of marketing, in the author's view, comes from Davidson (1997): 'Offensive marketing involves every employee in building superior customer value, very efficiently for above average profits'. 'Offensive' (despite its double meaning) in this context means leading the market, rather than reacting to competition. Davidson indicates that this type of marketing, despite representing the best practice, is nevertheless rare. A good example of a company that uses offensive marketing effectively is Microsoft, a company that leads the market because it has a strong corporate vision of where it wants to be, and consistently strives to offer superior value. Microsoft's progress has been characterized by its creation of the industry standard for software, ensuring that competitors 'dance to the Microsoft tune'. However, even Microsoft has off days, and clearly underestimated the impact of the Internet because of its focus on personal computers; but was quick to realize its mistake and utilize its market leadership in other areas so as to dominate the Internet arena as well.

In his book, Davidson uses the acronym POISE to describe effective marketing:

P   Profitable
O   Offensive
I   Integrated
S   Strategic
E   Effectively implemented.

Davidson focuses mainly on 'consumer-oriented' industries, so how does POISE translate in the world of the pharmaceutical industry?

Profitable

How profitable should the pharmaceutical industry be? Critics of the industry would point to the huge profit margins for marketed drugs and imply that the sick are being exploited. However, industry professionals point out that – as emphasized throughout this book – developing drugs is an exceptionally risky and expensive business, and that the few successes have to pay for the many drugs that fail to reach the market. Pharmaceutical marketing is charged with ensuring that products quickly reach high peak sales, because products that are slow-growing with low sales will always be substantially less profitable, while consuming resources that could be used more profitably elsewhere. Marketing in the pharmaceutical industry needs to ensure that the products are fully optimized, using all the resources available during drug development to ensure that the resulting product is fully valued by the customers and thereby maximally profitable.

An example of this is in the importance of publications on the final value of the product. These can be generated thoughout the development of the product, from interesting findings in Phase I, through the results of dose-finding studies, small pilot studies, and finally the results of the larger product characterization and registration studies. In the cancer treatment area there is a clear correlation between the number of published studies and the value of the product, whether they are hormonal treatments or cytotoxic drugs.

Offensive

Offensive marketing is about leading the market, through innovation and vision. It is not the province of the marketing department alone, but requires everyone in the company to be innovative and visionary, and share their ideas. This requires taking risks: tackling new indications, speeding up development with short-cuts, and exploiting novel mechanisms of action of drugs. In the marketing department itself, this 'offensive' attitude involves taking risks with novel approaches to marketing.

Pharmaceutical marketing is dogged with a history of literal, factual marketing; with an over-reliance on market research and ignorance of the emotional drivers of prescribing practice. This leads to a monotonous similarity between the advertising of the products, heavily focused on 'safe and effective', resulting in campaigns that are safe but ineffective. Look through many of the medical journals and you will see that companies direct their advertising internally to keep the management happy, rather than engage the enthusiasm of their customers.

Changes in pharmaceutical marketing strategies, especially direct-to-consumer marketing (DTC) in the USA, are now having a profound impact on the marketing of pharmaceuticals. This has resulted in greater emphasis on the branding of products, ensuring that the brand captures both the literal scientific benefits of the drug and the implied emotional qualities that drive usage.

Integrated

Everyone is involved in marketing.

Many activities go towards creating a profitable brand, particularly if they raise the value of the brand to the customer. These include ensuring that the maximum number of publications are produced, that the product is developed in a timely fashion so that it is available as early as possible, and even that the formulation is optimized to make it simpler to take or less likely to interact with other medications. In large companies this function of integration is performed by project teams. Often these teams are based in the research and development departments and driven by project management, who ensure that the development targets are met. However, it is not uncommon for the focus to be on a single outcome – the registration of the product – and it becomes important that marketing encourages vision in the teams, so that they deliver not only a registrable compound, but a marketable product with maximum value for the customer. Unless the team embraces the marketing approach, its focus can shift to narrow internal targets, such as satisfying departmental performance criteria, which can, and does, result in products that obtain registration but fail in the market. There are many examples of products that were licensed specifically for patients resistant to other treatments, and then only later became used in less needy patients. If these products had been deliberately targeted on the less severe patients early on, they would have made substantially more money for the company and benefited many more patients. Fortunately, the increasing cost of product development and competition is encouraging companies to form 'heavyweight teams', teams who assume the budgets and risks of developing the brand, and are therefore encouraged to think like 'mini companies'. This process helps the members to better understand the activities of their colleagues, and has been shown to result in faster development of new products, particularly in the automobile industry.

Strategic

Marketing may be likened to warfare without the casualties. (Nowadays, the term 'campaign' is often used by pharmaceutical companies to describe what would hitherto have been called a project.) Like warfare, good marketing is about knowing the terrain and knowing the competition. It is based on considerable analysis of the environment, the customers and the competition. This analysis must also be forward-looking. How will the competition react to our campaign? What are our contingency plans if a planned clinical trial delivers better or worse results than expected? Marketing has to encompass good business and management skills, and marketers have to be able to present convincing arguments to support investment in their products. Often this is in the face of short-term thinking in the company, particularly where the annual profit targets for the company could be achieved by reducing investment. This is where marketing has to drive the management into taking a longer-term view for the health of the company.

Effectively executed

Sometimes marketing is executed less than effectively in pharmaceutical companies, particularly at the level of local affiliates. This is because marketing becomes preoccupied with delivering new materials to the sales force, forecasts, market planning, market research, reacting to customers and generalized firefighting, without stopping long enough to prepare a high-quality strategy. Marketers are not so much managers of their products as managed by them. The outcome can be that marketing starts to become an unenviable job – a 'rite of passage' to something less demanding and more rewarding. Fortunately, it does not need to be like that.

Some pharmaceutical companies are starting to introduce a more strategic role for their marketing departments, insisting that strategic plans should reflect all the options available in the market, and also the cost, feasibility and time required to deliver a result. This approach results in a much more efficient use of resources, clear deliverables, and raises the standard of marketing expertise. Marketers who use this approach claim that it empowers them in discussions with management, as well as helping them with their personal time management. This type of strategic planning also involves sales, clinical and other management functions, so that the resulting plan gives a clear direction to all the players in the product team.

Summary of marketing

We have described in simple terms what goes into excellent marketing. No one pharmaceutical company practises offensive marketing all the time with all their products, but some stand out as leaders in the field. A recent example includes Pfizer with *sildenafil* (Viagra), who launched a product into an area where there was no similar product and spent a large amount of money on prelaunch activities. The exceptional success of Viagra prompted a number of other companies, which had shown no interest previously, to explore the same condition of erectile dysfunction. These other companies are likely to have some success as followers, but will they be as successful as Pfizer?

Marketing at the local country level

What is the role of marketing in the countries?

Marketing at the local company level is an extremely important link between the 'grand strategy' of corporate marketing and the customers themselves. The job of the local organization is to ensure that the overall strategy for the product is effectively and profitably implemented in their country. This may require some slight modification of the corporate messages to maximize the local effect. In some companies this modification is strictly limited in order that international brands remain consistent (e.g. Coca-Cola); in others the branding may be 'localized (e.g. 'Jif' cleaner in the UK is known elsewhere as 'Cif' – although this has recently been changed to 'Cif' in the UK as well!). The tendency is towards increased central control of the branding and messaging of products, especially in pharmaceuticals, where there is considerable interaction between country affiliates and physicians. The same drug is very often marketed under different brand names in different countries. For example, the antipsychotic drug *clozapine* is marketed as Clozaril in the USA and UK, and as Leponex in most European and Middle Eastern countries, and under seven more brand names elsewhere. The antihypertensive drug *enalapril* (Vasotec in the USA, Innovace in the UK) is sold under no fewer than 63 different registered trade names in different parts of the world.

The marketers in the countries have another valuable role, that of helping to guide corporate strategy, as they are closest to the final customer. Consequently, most pharmaceutical companies have regular meetings of local and corporate marketing to ensure that this valuable dialogue continues.

The make-up of the country-based marketing department

A typical local company will have a marketing department split into groups of people for each product, who take the following roles:

- *Product manager* – the product 'champion', who produces the strategic and tactical plan, also 'project manages' the deliverables, ensuring that they happen on time;
- *Market researcher* – works with the product manager to find information about the current market, including customer opinions and feedback on the success of the promotion;
- *Publications planner* – creates the plan for turning the body of clinical and preclinical data into publications, ensuring that the messages are consistent;
- *Promotions planner* – organizes congresses, symposia and other promotional events, and may also have responsibility for liaison with advertising companies and suppliers;
- *Medical information* – ensures that the claims in the selling materials are consistent with the licence of the product, and also that they can be referenced.

In addition to these office-based staff, the *sales management team*, responsible for managing the travelling sales force, forms an essential part of the local marketing team:

- *Sales manager* – ensures that the sales force is effective and active;
- *Sales training* – ensures that the sales team is correctly educated on product and selling skills.

Typical activities

Sales forecasting and planning (including market research)

Sales forecasting is an essential and unloved part of marketing. Mark Twain once said: 'forecasting is difficult, especially concerning the future'; forecasts are generally unlikely to be correct – the art of forecasting is rather to manage expectations of the product. Sales forecasts from the countries are used as the basis for calculating the value of a product to the entire company, and so any errors need to be spotted and corrected at source. Forecasting is made easier when it is based on the strategic marketing plan: if there is a clear reason for the sales, such as a direct-to-consumer campaign, then this activity can be monitored to see if it is really performing as expected. Forecasts should also have a range if they are to be truly useful - a 'best case' and a 'worst case' scenario.

Developing the forecast usually requires a substantial amount of market research, which is divided into *primary* and *secondary* research. Secondary research is also known as 'table' research, because in the past it involved extracting the required information from existing documentation. This exists in the form of large compilations prepared by specialist pharmaceutical market research companies, the best known of which are IMS (international) and, in the USA, Scott Levin. These compilations are now available in computerized form, but still require a good deal of interpretation by experienced researchers. There are a number of data sets available. The *sales data* consist of sales figures for each of the 'bricks' or reporting areas in the country under study, which is collected from pharmaceutical wholesalers. Interpreting the data is complicated by the fact that it is historical, arriving about 3 months after the actual sales, and that hospital-based products, such as immuno-suppressants and oncological products, are poorly represented, often being under-reported and inconsistently reported. Consequently, pharmaceutical companies have to resort to primary research, which is customized research that they commission themselves. Another useful data set is the *medical indices*, comprising data on the actual prescribing habits of general practitioners. This gives an insight into what actually happens in the doctor's surgery, although because it is based on a limited sample it does not accurately reflect national prescribing habits. It is often used to guide the design and question the structure of primary research, as asking doctors direct

questions usually provides the answers they think that they should give, rather than what they actually do. Because the medical indices data do not cover hospital prescribing, primary research is also important in gathering information on hospital doctors' prescribing habits.

Market research is also used to fine-tune the messages from marketing to the doctors. Once the sales story has been developed, market researchers perform a closely monitored test of the promotional materials on the target customers, to discover their reaction to the promotion. This can be useful to ensure that the promotional material is clear in its messages, but care must be taken to avoid physicians being used as amateur art directors ('I think the name of the product would be much better in pink…').

Finally, another important role for market research is in monitoring the progress of the promotional campaign. They will have performed a usage and awareness study of target physicians prior to the campaign, by means of a series of questions designed to see if the physicians are already aware of the product and how they perceive it in comparison to the competition. This will be done again during the campaign to see if the promotional messages are being effectively delivered, and if there has been a change in prescribing habits. If the campaign is not going well for some reason then it can be modified to overcome the problem.

Leader development

Any product that hopes to be successful needs to have its supporters among the end users. Usually the company will develop certain triallists and opinion leaders to act as supporters for the product. These physicians will have been approached by the head office or the local office and will act as the 'key opinion leaders' – they will often be the lead authors on the pivotal clinical papers and form part of the advisory group who have worked with the company during the development of the product. In the country operation they will be used to lead regional meetings and help develop the local leaders who will guide local prescribing practice. Opinion leaders are usually physicians who have considerable experience in the therapeutic area; often they will have become well known because of their experience with the previous generation of drug treatments, or because they have a background of research into the disease area. These opinion leaders will travel extensively on behalf of the company to help present on their behalf, and are important to establishing the network of local opinion leaders at the country level. An important part of opinion leader development is their involvement in clinical studies (see below).

Tactics

Local marketing is all about effective implementation, and there are a number of important tactics that are key to success.

Local experience trials (Phase IV, clinical characterization trials)

'Try it, you'll like it' is the concept of this type of clinical study. Once the drug has been approved – or sometimes slightly earlier – the company will initiate experience trials. Sometimes these follow standard trials protocols and are either multicentred or single centre; often they will be initiated by the investigator with the cooperation of the pharmaceutical company. These studies enable the physicians to gain hands-on experience with the new product, which in turn may lead them to prescribe the drug outside the study. They are also important as a means to get the product accepted on to hospital formularies, which normally requires support from the local physicians to influence the formulary board. There is a strong correlation between the size and scope of this type of study and the success of the new product: the fastest-growing products usually have large Phase IV studies involving thousands of patients.

Sales force

This is the most expensive form of promotion – and probably the most effective. Because of the technical nature of pharmaceuticals, and their high price, face-to-face contact is still the first line of promotion. In recent years the size of the field force has been increasing in most companies, particularly in those that have increased in size through mergers and acquisitions. These large companies need one or more new 'blockbuster' products to be launched each year, and these products also need to be supported in the following years. Whereas 10 years ago companies would have one or two field forces, each selling three products, now there is a trend towards having perhaps three general practice/office forces, and perhaps two specialist or hospital forces. In addition, companies now have specialists who deal only with large accounts, negotiating with the buyers to ensure that non-promoted products are still purchased, particularly those that may have reached the end of their patent protection. Even with these sales forces, most companies still find that the need to support recently launched products, or older products in aggressive markets, requires still more sales people. This has led to an increase in the use of contract sales teams supplied by specialized contract companies, and in co-marketing arrangements with other companies, including the 'fostering' of older products to other companies, who adopt them as if they were their own. One problem with this expansion is that many physicians are being called on by seven or eight sales people per day, to which they react by rationing visits through appointment systems, or even refusing to see sales people at all. Pharmaceutical companies try to target their sales representatives to the most productive doctors, which exacerbates the problem. In the USA this has led pharmaceutical companies to consider other tactics to complement their sales forces, such as Internet detailing and DTC (direct-to-consumer) advertising (see below).

Internet detailing

A relatively new phenomenon, Internet detailing is a system whereby the sales call takes place over the Internet. There are various ways of encouraging physicians to access these Internet sites, the most common being physical incentives and information incentives. Physical incentive systems ask the physician to call in to a call centre about once or twice a month at a time to suit themselves, where they will be 'detailed' by a sales representative. Usually the physician gets the use of an ISDN line or computer in return for subscribing to this service. Such rewards are limited by government regulations that prohibit excessive gift-giving to physicians. Information-based schemes capture the physician's attention as he or she searches for information on a topic or issue, and direct them towards unbiased information sites (usually accredited by a medical association) where pharmaceutical companies have access buttons to their product sites. However, this type of scheme depends heavily on the physician having the curiosity to visit the pharmaceutical company site.

All these schemes are relatively new, many having been started during the recent 'dot.com' boom, and they may not turn out to be quite as useful as first thought.

DTC (direct to consumer) advertising

Between 1999 and 2004 marketing promotional budgets in the USA rocketed upwards. The reason was DTC, where companies discovered the value of approaching the end-user directly. In most countries the advertising of prescription drugs directly to the public is forbidden. However, over the past 10 years the US pharmaceutical industry has been focusing on the patient, or the potential patient. Initially the programmes that were introduced were awareness-raising activities, such as publishing articles on the disease area in magazines, or presenting information on television. This then moved to actual television advertising directed at patients who have a certain symptom, or who are in a high-risk group for certain diseases; they were told that they should see their physician because there were new treatments available. This escalated to direct product advertising when the FDA, after continuous lobbying, allowed such advertising to go ahead. These advertisements are strictly controlled. They must have full information on side effects; they must not mislead or attempt to hide information (e.g. by playing music over it or showing a distracting visual); and they must insist that the patient sees a suitably qualified physician for advice. Despite all these restrictions the approach has been very successful. As an example, DTC enabled the proton pump inhibitor *omeprazole* (Prilosec, Losec, manufactured by AstraZeneca) to keep its rank in 2000 as the world's biggest-selling pharmaceutical product in value terms. Indeed, 'the purple pill' is now an extremely strong brand, well known throughout the USA. Unusually, the brand has proved to represent more than the product: since the launch of the isomer version of omeprazole, *esomeprazole* (NEXIUM), this brand has successfully been transferred to the new product, and AstraZeneca has been able to defend its market share.

No other country has gone as far as the USA in this area, but elsewhere companies are finding that the promotion of a disease area by DTC marketing accelerates the uptake of new products, particularly if they are for indications easily identified by patients themselves. In the UK Novartis has embarked on a 'fungal toenail infection' campaign, which has increased the total market for antifungal treatments such as *terbinafine* (Lamisil). This initially started as advertisements with a telephone hotline number in Sunday papers, and 3 years later is now a multimillion pound national campaign.

Congresses and symposia
Congresses and symposia often make up a significant part of the annual marketing budget, in some countries as much as 50%. Much of this cost is attributable to delegate travel and accommodation, and it is often criticized both within the company (how does this increase the business?) and externally. In the USA and France such expenditure is limited by law to physicians who are either speakers or participants in a recognized clinical study. Most congresses are organized by professional bodies representing physicians and biomedical scientists, and they are often supported by the pharmaceutical industry, which contributes to their running and organizational costs, although increasingly individual companies are sponsoring their own meetings and congresses. From a marketing perspective congresses give the company's representatives an opportunity to make contact both scientifically and socially with their customers, which has benefit in leader development. Congresses are also important places to showcase new science developed within the company, ranging from interesting preclinical findings to the results of clinical trials.

Next career steps for the local marketer
After working in a local marketing organization, many marketing personnel widen their experience by joining the global, or international, marketing team. Local experience in marketing and sales is extremely important as a preparation for a role in global marketing, which requires an excellent understanding of the needs of the local operations and customers.

International marketing
What is the role of international marketing?

International marketing, particularly new product marketing, provides the opportunity to change the world,

by taking a novel concept and developing it into a viable and top-selling product. Whatever the development stage of the product, international marketing is all about maximizing its potential in the most efficient manner.

For a newly discovered product this involves selecting the right strategy to develop the product (what claims do I need to be successful?), building a perception of the product (e.g. a superstatin, high affinity, anti-nephrotoxic), and gaining support for investing in the project. With a more mature brand it is a case of managing new indications and new formulations; coordinating the core advertising materials, congresses and training materials and messages; and anticipating and handling competitor messages. With a brand at the end of its patent life it may involve strategies to improve the product and sustain a new patent, or it could be designed to ensure that the product lives on as a consumer brand, despite the availability of cheaper generic products.

Many of the activities of international marketing are similar to those of the local marketer, but with less involvement in tactics and a much more important role in setting strategy. Probably the most important and unique role for international marketing is its direct involvement with the project team, helping it to define and achieve the vision of the ideal product.

Typical activities
Tactical activities
Certain promotional activities are more efficiently carried out from a central office, either because they are international in nature, such as congresses and symposia, or because they are an essential part of the implementation of the overall product strategy (branding, trademarks, promotional plans and launch plans). This last section looks briefly at branding.

Strategy
Marketing strategy is the backbone to the success of the product. At the international level the brand manager has to develop a vision of what the product will be and how he or she hopes to take it there. The manager has to use the expertise of the project team, the local marketing managers and external advisers, but must eventually define a clear route to success. (To get an idea of how difficult this is, refer back to the description of 'offensive marketing.') A well-executed and visionary strategy can certainly 'change the world': blockbuster drugs would not exist without it.

Changing the world: branding and trademarks

'A rose by any other name would smell as sweet.' This is no doubt the case, but it is necessary to appreciate the difference between a product and a brand: despite the scent, a rose variety called 'Titania' would almost certainly outsell one called 'Bottom'.

In the UK 70% of BMW cars are bought without a test drive. These drivers are buying something that is more than the car itself, that something being the added extra that turns a product into a brand. The brand values of BMW (quality, sporty, manly, sexy, success) are not intrinsic to the car, but are entirely the creation of marketing.

Conversely, the 2001 model of the Ford Mondeo was described by one magazine as having only one fault, namely the maker's badge on the front. General Motors decided to kill off its long-established Oldsmobile range of cars because of its indelible brand image – 'the kind of car my dad drove'.

One can see the value of brands by watching the financial news. Recently the brand 'Gatorade' came up for sale, and the considerable purchase price reflected the future value of the brand. The new owners assume that the public will continue for the foreseeable future to buy Gatorade in preference to other brands of similar soft drinks. If the brand had no value they would have paid a much lower price for the stock and production capability and then sold the same product under a different name.

The pharmaceutical industry has also realized that excellence is not enough, and that strong brand values add financial value to the product. Today's highly competitive market for pharmaceuticals, with many similar competitors offering similar benefits, means that the battle to be 'first to mind' (i.e. the first choice) requires that products be distinctive. As a consequence, branding the product well will ensure that it appeals to both the logical and the intuitive part of the customer's mind.

To do this the marketing team and the product team discuss both the possible clinical outcomes of studies and the intangible benefits the product might have. An example of this would be in cancer treatment, where it can often be shown that a new drugs slows down the progression of the cancer, but not often that it encreases patient survival, as this takes many years of follow-up in clinical trials. Consequently, the brand should reflect the qualities that the treating physician and the patient would hope for, namely an optimistic prognosis, improved quality of life etc.

How does a company go about developing a brand image for a new product? Most will involve a branding agency in the development of a new brand name (or trademark). To give some idea of the value of brand name development, the current fee for developing a brand name is about $100 000. To identify the new name the agency will coordinate meetings to extract the key benefits of the new product that will be the strongest emotional drivers. This involves producing a 'word bank' of nouns and verbs that describe the product, using allegories such as 'if the product was an animal,

what would it be?'. For a drug that treats cancer in men the word bank might contains the following:

Hope	Strength
Koala bear	Volvo
Masculine	Potency
Warm	Control.

This 'word bank' would then be used by the agency to develop a number of names – probably 60 or 70 – that capture the feeling of these words. The names will then be reviewed by a multinational team to exclude words that are too close to existing products, or which mean something unfortunate in another language. The surviving words will then be put through a checking process to eliminate any that are too similar to names already in use in pharmaceuticals, and finally there may only be two or three left. Once the final name is chosen it will be registered. The whole process can take up to 2 years or more, most of this time (about 9 months) being taken up with checking the name with the registration authorities.

Once the name of the product has been chosen, the advertising or branding company will produce a layout similar to the one shown in Figure 21.1, where 'logotype' is the new product name in its distinctive typeface, the symbol is a small diagram which captures the 'feeling' of the product, the 'crystallized product promise' is a simple phrase that captures the unique benefits of the product, and the eyebrow line is an 'introduction' to the product, such as 'In gastric reflux…'. Figure 21.1B shows a real example developed for the new antipsychotic drug *olanzapine* (Zyprexa). Even if you know nothing about this product, it is clear from this branding layout that the product should powerfully bring the patient back to 'normal'. Before this brand existed, there was nothing except a development code number and a collection of clinical data. The brand brings the whole project into one, clear, marketable message – the 'essence' of the product.

The excitement of marketing lies in creating an entirely new way for the world to think about a product.

A career in marketing

As emphasized many times in this chapter, in a successful company everyone is involved in marketing through their contribution to increasing customer value and company profitability. To become a marketing professional, probably the best way to start is as a sales representative. Sales representatives need to know their customers and to learn the important skill of anticipating their needs: bonuses depend on the salesperson's skill in generating sales.

Working in an international marketing organization entails participating in the drug development process itself, and a good knowledge of the scientific and technical basis of drug development is important. The marketing professional in this context serves as the link between

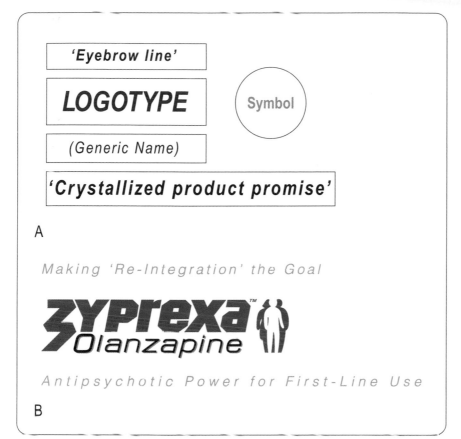

Fig. 21.1
(A) Typical branding layout for a pharmaceutical product (courtesy Clive Lewis). (B) A real example.

the scientific and technical operations of the development team and the commercial interests of the company. The interface can be a turbulent one, and negotiating it skilfully requires a good understanding of both worlds.

Reference

Davidson H (1997) Even more offensive marketing. London. Penguin Books.

SECTION 4
FACTS AND FIGURES

22 Drug discovery and development – facts and figures

H P Rang

In this chapter we present summary information about the costs, timelines and success rates of the drug discovery and development operations of major pharmaceutical companies. The information comes from published sources, particularly the Pharmaceutical R&D Compendium (2000), published by the Centre for Medicines Research, and the websites of the Association for the British Pharmaceutical Industry (www.abpi.org.uk) and the Pharmaceutical Research and Manufacturers of America (www.phrma.org). The information comes, of course, from the pharmaceutical companies themselves, who are under no obligation to release more than is legally required. In general, details of the development process are quite well documented, because the regulatory authorities must be notified of projects in clinical development. Discovery research is less well covered, partly because companies are unwilling to divulge detailed information, but also because the discovery phase is much harder to codify and quantify. Development projects focus on a specific compound, and it is fairly straightforward to define the different components, and to measure the cost of carrying out the various studies and support activities that are needed so that the compound can be registered and launched. In the discovery phase, it is often impossible to link particular activities and costs to specific compounds; instead, the focus is often on a therapeutic target, such as diabetes, Parkinson's disease or lung cancer, or on a molecular target, such as a particular receptor or enzyme, where even the therapeutic indication may not yet be determined. The point at which a formal drug discovery project is recognized and 'managed' in the sense of having a specific goal defined and resources assigned to it, varies greatly between companies. A further complication is that, as described in Section 2 of this book, the scientific strategies applied to drug discovery are changing rapidly, so that historic data may not properly represent the current situation. For these reasons, it is very difficult to obtain anything more than crude overall measures of the effectiveness of drug discovery research. There are, for example, no published figures to show what proportion of drug discovery projects succeed in identifying a compound fit to enter development, whether this probability differs between different therapeutic areas, and how it relates to the resources allocated.

As will be seen from the analysis that follows, the most striking aspects of drug discovery and development are (a) that failure is much more common than success, (b) that it costs a lot, and (c) that it takes a very long time. By comparison with other research-based industries, pharmaceutical companies are playing out a kind of slow-motion and very expensive arcade game, with the odds heavily stacked against them but offering particularly rich rewards.

Spending

Worldwide, the R&D spending of the international pharmaceutical companies has soared, from roughly $5bn in 1982 to $40bn in 1998. Figure 22.1 shows total R&D expenditure for US-based companies. The R&D expenditure of the 10 largest pharmaceutical companies in 2003 averaged nearly $2bn per company, accounting between them for a budget close to the research budget of the US National Institutes of Health (approximately $21bn in 2003). Marketing and administration costs for these companies are about three times as great as R&D costs. The annual increase in R&D spending in the industry is in line with sales growth, reflecting the policy of most companies to invest a fixed percentage of revenues into research and development. Today 15–20% of sales are reinvested in R&D, a higher percentage than in any other industry (Figure 22.2). The overall cost of R&D covers discovery research as well as various development functions, described in Section 3 of this book. The average distribution of R&D expenditure on these different functions is shown in Table 22.1. Roughly one-quarter of this budget is allocated to discovery research, 40% goes on clinical studies, and the rest on preclinical development, regulatory submission and other functions. These proportions represent the overall costs of these different functions, and do not necessarily reflect the costs of developing an individual compound. As will be discussed later, the substantial drop-out rate of compounds proceeding through development means that the overall costs cover many failures as well as the few successes.

R&D spending according to therapeutic classes is shown in Figure 22.3, based on a survey of the American research-based pharmaceutical industry, and is dominated by four therapeutic areas, namely:

Table 22.1
R&D expenditure by function (1998)

Function	Total R&D costs (%)	
	UK	US
Discovery	25	33
Preclinical development	21	42
Clinical development	40	
Regulatory affairs	4	8
Others	11	17

Data from CMR Compendium (2000), PhRMA Survey (2002)

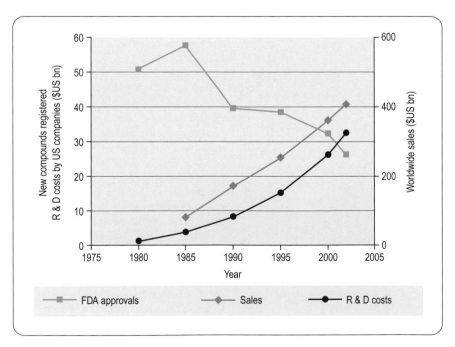

Fig. 22.1
R&D expenditure, sales and number of new compounds registered 1980–2002. (Source: CMR R&D Compendium, 2000.)

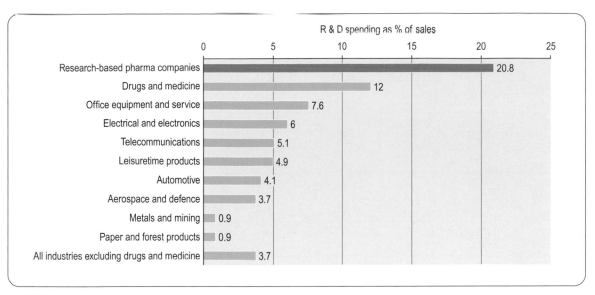

Fig. 22.2
R&D spending as percentage of sales of high-tech industries.

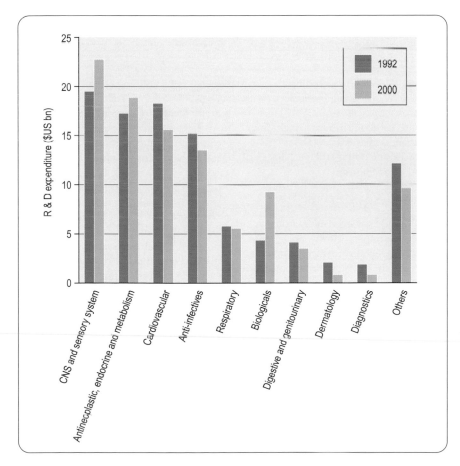

Fig. 22.3
Allocation of R&D expenditure in the USA by therapeutic class (1992 and 2000).

Table 22.2
Cost of developing a compound

	Discovery	Preclinical development	Phase I	Phase II	Phase III	Regulatory approval	Total
Number of compounds							
Number of compounds entering stage	Many projects	11.8	4.7	3.3	1.7	1.1	1
Number of compounds failing		7.1	1.4	1.6	0.6	0.1	11
Probability of passing (%)		40	70	50	67	90	
Costs (in 1995 $US, millions)							
Cost per compound completing stage		6	12	12	100	40	170
Cost of failures	230	65	44	28	70	4	441
Total cost	230	71	56	40	170	44	611

- Central nervous system disorders (including Alzheimer's disease, schizophrenia, depression, epilepsy and Parkinson's disease);
- Cancer, endocrine and metabolic diseases (including osteoporosis, diabetes and obesity);
- Cardiovascular diseases (including atherosclerosis, coronary disease and heart failure);
- Infectious diseases (including bacterial, viral and other infections such as malaria).

The trend in the last decade has been away from cardiovascular disease towards other priority areas, particularly cancer and metabolic disorders, and also a marked increase in research on biopharmaceuticals, whose products are used in all therapeutic areas.

How much does it cost to develop a drug?

From the global R&D spend of about $44bn in 2000 (CMR R&D Compendium, 2000) and the number of drugs registered in that year (32), one could conclude that each one cost about $1.3bn. This is misleading, however, as the R&D costs of these compounds will have accrued over the previous 15 years, during which costs were rising sharply.

Estimating the cost of developing a drug is not as straightforward as it might seem, as it depends very much on what is taken into account in the calculation. Factors such as 'opportunity costs' (the loss of income that theoretically results from spending money on drug development rather than investing it somewhere else) and tax credits (contributions from the public purse to encourage drug development in certain areas) make a large difference, and are the source of much controversy. A realistic estimate – $611m at 1995 prices – comes from the analysis shown in Table 22.2. In this analysis, the average cost of carrying out each stage of development on a single compound was estimated, and allowance made for the average drop-out rate of compounds at that stage. The analysis shows that the cost of all the studies performed on a single successful development compound averaged $170m, the remaining $441m representing money spent on compounds that never made it to registration.

Of this $441m, $230m represents the cost of discovery research leading up to the identification of a drug candidate that proceeds to preclinical development; the rest is made up by the development costs of unsuccessful drug candidates. The Tufts Centre for Drug Development Studies estimated the average cost of developing a drug in 2000 to be $802m, increasing to $897m in 2003[1]

[1]Quote from a commentary on this analysis (Frank RG (2003) Journal of Health Economics 22: 325): 'These are impressively large numbers, usually associated with a purchase of jet fighters – 40 F16s in fact'.

(DiMasi et al., 2003), compared with $318m (inflation adjusted) in 1987, and concluded that the R&D cost of a new drug is increasing at an annual rate of 7.4% above inflation.

Based on different assumptions, even larger figures – $1.1bn per successful drug launch over the period 1995–2000, and $1.7bn for 2000–2002 – were calculated by Gilbert et al. (2003).

The fact that more than 70% of R&D costs represents discovery and 'failure' costs, and less than 30% represents direct costs (which, being determined largely by requirements imposed by regulatory authorities, are difficult to reduce), has caused research-based pharmaceutical companies in recent years to focus on improving (a) the efficiency of the discovery process, and (b) the success rate of the compounds entering development.

Sales revenues

Despite the decline in compound registrations over the past 25 years (Figure 22.1), the overall sales of pharmaceuticals have risen steadily, at some 8% annually. The total global sales in 2002 reached $400.6bn. In western countries the cost of prescribed drugs accounts for some 10–15% of overall healthcare costs.

The revenue cycle

Figure 22.4 shows schematically the cash flow associated with the development and sales of a typical, aver-

agely profitable drug. The net income clearly exceeds the net costs, but two factors need to be taken into account when interpreting this. First, the R&D costs reflect only the work performed on the successful drug, not the costs of failures. Second, the costs are incurred many years before the revenues arrive, and no correction is made for the cost of capital. With such a correction, as is routinely incorporated in the *net present value* (NPV) calculation (see below), the balance will appear much less favourable.

Particular features to note on the cash flow diagram are:

- The steady and modest cost of discovery – hard to estimate with confidence – sometimes continuing for several years and thus requiring a significant cash outlay well in advance of revenues;
- The sharply increased costs associated with clinical development;
- The gradual build-up of sales, offset by marketing costs, which means that net revenues may not arise until about 2 years after launch;
- The abrupt decline in sales revenues associated with patent expiry and generic competition.

Profitability

For a drug to make a profit, sales revenue must exceed R&D, manufacture and marketing costs. Grabowski et al. (2002) found that only 34% of new drugs introduced between 1990 and 1994 brought in revenues that exceeded the average R&D cost (Figure 22.5). This quite surprising result, which at first sight might suggest that

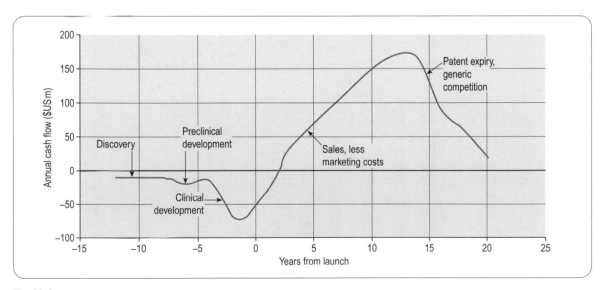

Fig. 22.4
Typical cash flow for a marketed drug. (Based on Grabowski et al., 2002.)

the industry is extremely bad at doing its sums, needs to be interpreted with caution for various reasons. First, development costs vary widely, depending on the nature of the compound, the route of administration and the target indication, and so a drug may recoup its development cost even though its revenues fall below the average cost. Second, the development money is spent several years before any revenues come in, and sales predictions made at the time development decisions have to be taken are far from reliable. At any stage, the decision whether or not to proceed is based on a calculation of the drug's 'net present value' (NPV) – an amortised estimate of the future sales revenue, minus the future development and marketing costs. If the NPV is positive, and sufficiently large to justify the allocation of development capacity, the project will generally go ahead, even if the money already spent cannot be fully recouped, as terminating it would mean that *none* of the costs would be recouped. At the beginning of a project NPV estimates are extremely unreliable – little more than guesses – so most companies will not pay much attention to them for decision-making purposes until the project is close to launch, when sales revenues become more predictable. Furthermore, unprofitable drugs may make a real contribution to healthcare, and companies may choose to develop them for that reason.

Even though only 34% of registered drugs in the Grabowski (2002) study made a profit, the profits on those that did so more than compensated for the losses on the others, leaving the industry as a whole with a large overall profit during the review period in the early 1990s. The situation is no longer quite so favourable for the industry, partly because of price control measures in healthcare, and partly because of rising R&D costs; nevertheless, pharmaceuticals remain one of the most consistently profitable industries.

Pattern of sales

Figure 22.6 shows the distribution of sales (1999 figures) by major pharmaceutical companies according to different therapeutic categories. The main changes since then

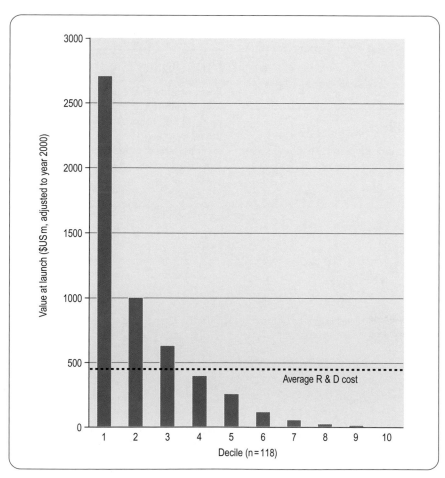

Fig. 22.5
Calculated values of 118 compounds launched 1990–1994. (Data from Brabowski et al., 2002.)

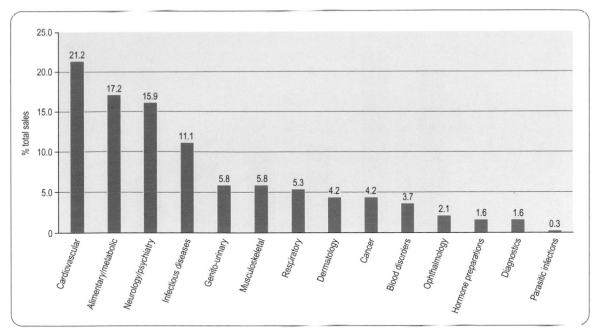

Fig. 22.6
Worldwide drug sales by therapeutic area (1999). (Source: CMR R&D Compendium, 2000.)

have been a substantial increase in sales of anticancer drugs and drugs used to treat psychiatric disorders. The relatively small markets for drugs used to treat bacterial and parasitic infections contrasts sharply with the worldwide prevalence and severity of these diseases, a problem that is currently being addressed at government level in several countries. The USA represents the largest and fastest-growing market for pharmaceuticals (48% of global sales in 2002). Together with Europe (24%) and Japan (16%), these regions account for 88% of global sales. Asia, Africa and Australia together account for only 6%, as does the whole of Latin America.

Blockbuster drugs

The analysis by Grabowski et al. (2002) showed that 70% of the industry's profits came from 20% of the drugs marketed, highlighting the commercial importance of finding 'blockbuster' drugs – defined as those achieving annual sales of $1bn or more – as these are the ones that actually generate significant profits. A recent analysis of pharmaceutical company pipelines suggested that 18 new blockbusters are likely to be registered in the period 2001–2006, roughly four per year globally among the 30 or so new compounds that are currently being registered each year. In 2000, a total of 44 marketed drugs (Figure 22.7, Tables 22.3, 22.4) achieved sales exceeding $1bn, compared with 17 in 1995 and 35 in 1999. The contribution of blockbuster drugs to the overall global sales has also increased from 18% in 1997 to 45%

in 2001, reflecting the fact that sales growth in the block-buster sector has exceeded that in the market overall. Interestingly, there are many quite old compounds on the list, including 15 that were first registered before 1990, whose original patents had expired before 2000. This highly beneficial extension of a drug's bestseller status is achieved mainly by developing new, advantageous and patentable dosage forms. One of the oldest drugs on the list, ciclosporin (Sandimmun), was registered in 1983, and given a new lease of life in a better-absorbed oral formulation (Neoral) in 1995. The 44 blockbusters came from 19 companies, only six of which had more than two block-busters to their name. Without one or more such drugs on the market or in prospect a large pharmaceutical company finds itself in trouble, and this has had a significant impact on company strategy. Drug discovery and development efforts have become increasingly focused on creating blockbusters, rather than on innovation (Drews, 2003a), despite the fact that the prediction of which development compounds will achieve such sales has been historically poor[2].

---

[2]Examples of drugs which turned out to be blockbusters against marketing expectations include tamoxifen, a drug widely used in the treatment of breast cancer; captopril, the first ACE inhibitor, used in treating cardiovascular disease; fluoxetine, the second SSRI antidepressant; and ciclosporin, the first of a novel class of immunosuppressants, used to prevent transplant rejection. There are doubtless many examples of predicted blockbusters that failed to make it, but these receive less publicity.

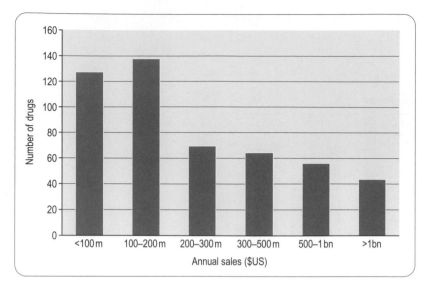

Fig. 22.7
Distribution of annual sales of 500 bestselling drugs (2000). No. 1 omeprazole ($6.3 bn); no. 500 ipriflixene ($40 m). (Data from Med Ad News (2000) 20(5).)

Table 22.3
Global sales of top ten drugs

Drug	Trade name	Type	Indication	Sales 1998 ($bn)	Sales 2002 ($bn)
Atorvastatin	Lipitor	HMG CoA reductase inhibitor	Cholesterol lowering	1.9	8.6
Simvastatin	Zocor	HMG CoA reductase inhibitor	Cholesterol lowering	4.9	6.2
Omeprazole	Losec	Proton pump inhibitor	Gastric ulcer	4.4	5.2
Olanzapine	Zyprexa	Atypical antipsychotic drug	Schizophrenia		
Amlodipine	Norvasc	Calcium channel inhibitor	Hypertension, heart failure	2.3	4.0
Erythropoietin	Erypo	Stimulant of red cell production	Anaemia		
Lansoprazole	Ogastro	Proton pump inhibitor	Gastric ulcer		
Paroxetine	Seroxat	Serotonin uptake inhibitor	Depressiom	1.7	4.0
Celecoxib	Celebrex	Cyclooxygenase-2 inhibitor	Inflammatory pain, arthritis		
Sertraline	Zoloft	Serotonin uptake inhibitor	Depression	1.7	3.8
Fluoxetine	Prozac	Serotonin uptake inhibitor	Depression	2.6	3.6
Enalapril	Renitec	ACE inhibitor	Hypertension, heart failure	1.8	3.3
Amoxycillin/ calvulanic acid	Augmentin	Antibacterial	Infectious diseases	1.5	3.1
Loratadine	Claritin	Antihistamine	Urticaria, itching	1.5	3.1

Source: IMS

The recent spate of pharmaceutical company mergers has also been driven partly by the need for companies to remain in blockbuster territory despite the low rate of new drug introductions and the difficulty of predicting sales. By merging, companies are able to increase the number of compounds registered and thus reduce the risk that the pipeline will contain no blockbusters.

Timelines

One important factor that determines profitability is the time taken to develop and launch a new drug, in particular the time between patent approval and launch, which will determine the length of time during which competitors are barred from introducing cheap generic copies of the drug. A drug that is moderately successful by today's standards might achieve sales of about

Table 22.4
Drugs exceeding $1bn sales worldwide (blockbusters) 2000

Drug	Trade name	Class	Launch year	Sales 2000 ($US bn)	Change since 1999 (%)
Omeprazole	Prilosec	Proton pump inhibitor	89	6.26	5.9
Simvastatin	Zocor	HMGCR inhibitor	91	5.21	17.5
Atorvastatin	Lipitor	HMGCR inhibitor	96	5.03	32.6
Amlodipine	Norvasc	Vasodilator	92	3.36	12.4
Loratadine	Claritin	Non-sedating antihistamine	93	3.01	12.6
Prevacid	Lansoprazole	Proton pump inhibitor	95	2.82	27.0
Epoetin-α	Procrit	Erythropoietic factor	90	2.71	29.4
Celecoxib	Celebrex	Cyclooxygenase 2 inhibitor	98	2.61	77.7
Fluoxetine	Prozac	SSRI	87	2.5	–0.6
Olanzapine	Zyprexa	Atypical antipsychotic	96	2.37	26.6
Paroxetine	Paxil	SSRI	92	2.35	19.0
Rofecoxib	Vioxx	Cyclooxygenase 2 inhibitor	99	2.16	358*
Sertraline	Zoloft	SSRI	91	2.14	7.2
Epoetin α	Epoetin	Erythropoietic factor	89	1.96	11.4
Conjugated estrogens	Premarin	Hormone replacement	95	1.87	5.3
Amoxycillin/clavulanic acid	Augmentin	Antibacterial	91	1.85	8.5
Pravastatin Na	Pravachol	HMGCR inhibitor	91	1.82	6.6
Enalapril	Vasotec	ACE inhibitor	85	1.79	–22.3
Metformin	Glucophage	Antidiabetic	88	1.73	31.5
Pravastatin	Mevalotin	Cholesterol reduction	88	1.72	44.5
Losartan	Cozaar	Angiotensin antagonist	95	1.72	23.8
Ciprofloxacin	Cipro	Antibacterial	87	1.65	17.5
Risperidone	Risperdal	Atypical antipsychotic	93	1.60	20.7
Paclitaxel	Taxol	Anticancer	92	1.59	7.6
Azithromycin	Zithromax	Antibacterial	91	1.38	5.6
Interferon-α/Ribavirin	Intron A	Antiviral	86	1.36	21.5
Sildenafil	Viagra	Phosphodiesterase inhibitor	98	1.34	32.3
Gabapentin	Neurontin	Antiepileptic	93	1.33	46.1
Fluticasone	Lovent	Antiasthmatic	96	1.33	32.1
Alendronate	Fosamax	Antiosteoporosis	91	1.28	22.2
Clarithromycin	Biaxin	Antibacterial	91	1.34	–3
Filgrastim	Neupogen	Haemopoietic growth factor	91	1.22	–3.2
Ciclosporin	Neoral/Sandimmun	Immunosuppressant	83	1.21	2.1

Table 22.4
Drugs exceeding $1bn sales worldwide (blockbusters) 2000—cont'd

Lisinopril	Zestril	ACE inhibitor	93	1.19	−2.7
Venlafaxine	Effexor	SSRI	97	1.16	48.5
Human insulin	Humulin	Recombinant insulin	82	1.14	6.8
Levofloxacin	Levagrin	Antibacterial	96	1.09	43.7
Fexofenadine	Allegra	Non-sedating antihistamine	96	1.08	59.9
Lisinopril/ hydrochlorothiazide	Prinivil	ACE inhibitor/diuretic	87	1.08	31.9
Sumatriptan	Imitrex	Antimigraine	92	1.07	8.0
Nifedipine	ADALAT	Vasodilator	85	1.07	13.1
Fluconazole	Diflucan	Antifungal	90	1.01	2.5
Ceftriaxone	Roceptin	Antibacterial	84	1.01	−2.8
Famotidine	Gaster	Histamine H_2 antagonist	85	1.01	1.7

ACE, angitensin-converting enzyme; HMGCR, HMG CoA-reductase; SSRI, selective serotonin reuptake inhibitor.
Source: MedAdNews, May 2001.
*Withdrawn 2004, because of increased cardiovascular risk.

$400m/year, so each week's delay in development, by reducing the competition-free sales window, will cost the company roughly $8m.

Despite increasing expenditure on R&D costs and decreased output, the mean development time from first synthesis or isolation (i.e. excluding discovery research preceding synthesis of the development compound) to first launch was over 14 years in 1999, having increased somewhat over the preceding decade (Figure 22.8). The time taken for different phases, based on a 1995 report on US-based pharmaceutical companies, is summarized in Figure 22.9. Development activities took on average about 13 years, half of which was taken up by discovery and preclinical development and half by clinical studies. A further 2 years was required for FDA review and approval. The long FDA review times during the 1980s have since come down substantially, averaging about 18 months in 2000/2001 (Reichert, 2003; Figure 22.10), mainly because user fees and fast-track procedures for certain types of drug were introduced.

There are, of course, wide variations in development times between individual projects, although historically there has been little consistent difference between different therapeutic areas (with the exception of anti-infective drugs, for which development times are somewhat shorter, and anticancer drugs, for which they are longer by about 2 years). During the 1990s, most biopharmaceuticals were recombinant versions of human hormones, and their clinical development was generally quicker than that of small molecules. More recently, biopharmaceuticals have become more diverse and many monoclonal antibodies have been developed, and these have generally encountered more problems in development because their therapeutic and unwanted effects are unpredictable, and so clinical development times for biopharmaceuticals have tended to increase.

Information about the time taken for discovery – from the start of a project to the identification of a development compound – is sparse in the public literature. Management consultants McKinsey and Arthur Andersen estimate that in 1995, the time taken from the start of the discovery project to the start of clinical studies was extremely variable, ranging from 21 to 103 months (Table 22.5). Both studies predicted a reduction in dis-

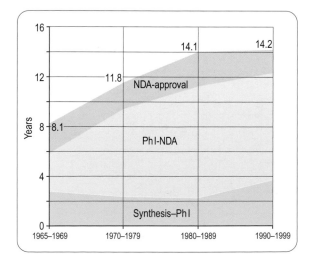

Fig. 22.8
Change in average drug development time in the USA 1965–2000. (Data from DiMasi (2001) Clinical Pharmacology and Therapeutics 69: 286–296.)

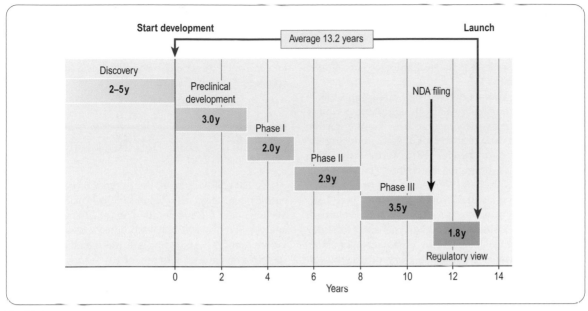

Fig. 22.9
Average times for development phases in the USA (mid-1990s). (Data from PhRMA website and DiMasi (2002) Clin Pharm Ther 69: 286–296.)

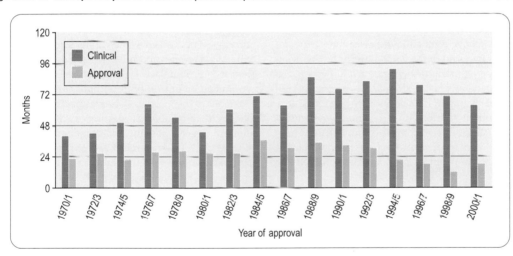

Fig. 22.10
Average clinical and FDA approval times for drugs approved in the USA.

Table 22.5 Discovery timelines	Target identification and validation	Screening	Lead optimization	Total discovery	Preclinical development	Total to clinic
McKinsey (1997)						
	10–36	1–3	7–14	18–53	8–16	26–69
2000 predicted	6–17	1	5–9	12–27	7–15	19–42
Andersen (1997)						
	10–24	6–24	24–36	40–84	6–30	46–114
2000 predicted	5–8	1–12	12–18	18–38	5–8	23–46

covery time by the year 2000 to 46 months or less, owing to improved discovery technologies. Although solid data are lacking, few believe that such a dramatic improvement has actually occurred, though, as discussed in Section 2, the technologies are indeed advancing rapidly.

Intensifying competition in the pharmaceutical marketplace also is demonstrated by the shrinking period of exclusivity during which the first drug in a therapeutic class is the sole drug in that class, thereby reducing the time a premium can be charged to recover the R&D expenditure. For example, cimetidine (Tagamet), an ulcer drug introduced in 1977, had an exclusivity period of 6 years before another drug in the same class, ranitidine (Zantac), was introduced. In contrast, celecoxib (Celebrex), the first selective cyclooxygenase-2 inhibitor (COX-2), which had a significant advantage over established non-steroidal anti-inflammatory drugs, was on the market only 3 months before a second, very similar, drug, rofecoxib (Vioxx), was approved (Figure 22.11). (Vioxx was withdrawn in 2004, because it was found to increase the risk of heart attacks: other COX-2 inhibitors are being investigated for this hazard).

Loss of patent protection opens up the competition to generic products (the same compound being manufactured and sold at a much lower price by companies that have not invested in the R&D underlying the original discovery), and the sales revenue from the branded compound generally falls sharply. Over the period 2001–2005 an average of 22 drugs each year will lose patent protection, resulting in a revenue loss averaging $4.4bn (CMR R&D Compendium, 2000). These global figures vary from year to year as individual high-revenue drugs drop out of patent protection, and the

revenue swings for an individual company are of course much more extreme than the global average, so maintaining a steady pipeline of new products and timing their introduction to compensate for losses as products become open to generic competition is a key part of a company's commercial strategy.

Pipelines and attrition rates

As we have already seen, the number of new chemical entities registered as pharmaceuticals each year has declined over the last decade (Figure 22.1), and various analyses (Drews, 2003b) have pointed to a serious 'innovation deficit'. According to these calculations, to sustain a revenue growth rate of 10% – considered to be a healthy level – the 10 largest pharmaceutical companies each needed to launch on average 3.1 new compounds each year, compared to 1.8 launches per company actually achieved in 2000 – a rate insufficient to maintain even zero growth.

The number of clinical trials being carried out (Figure 22.12) provides a measure of potential future launches. The figures shown may somewhat overestimate the numbers, because official notification of the start of clinical projects is obligatory, but projects may be terminated or put on hold without formal notification. Estimates of the number of active preclinical projects are even more unreliable, as companies are under no obligation to reveal this information, and the definition of what constitutes a project is variable. The number of clinical trials appears large in relation to the number of

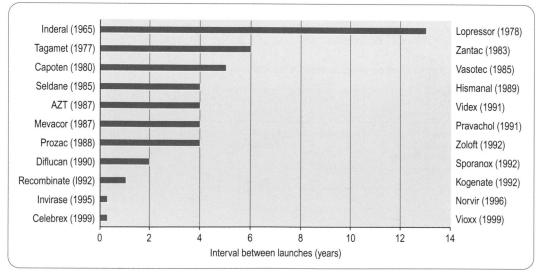

Fig. 22.11
Shrinking period of market exclusivity.

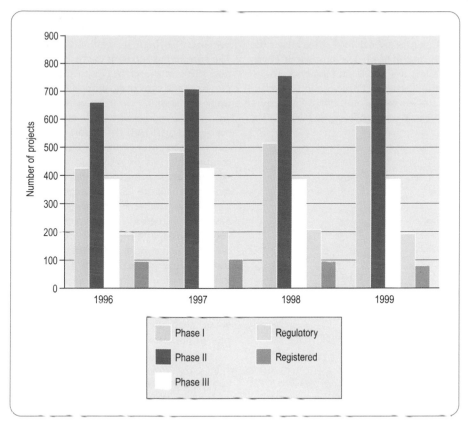

Fig. 22.12
Number of clinical projects (1996–1999). (Data from CMR R&D Compendium, 2000.)

new compounds registered in each year (Figure 22.1), partly because each trial usually lasts for more than 1 year, and partly because many trials (i.e. different indi-cations, different dosage forms) are generally performed with each compound, including previously registered compounds as well as new ones.

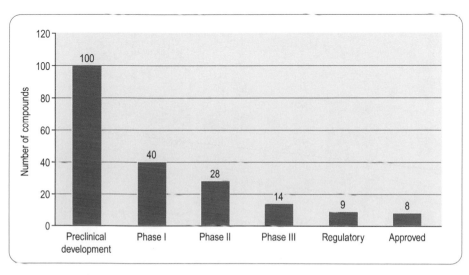

Fig. 22.13
Average attrition curve 1995–1997. Numbers represent the number of compounds entering the phase. One hundred drug candidates entering preclinical development resulted, on average, in eight approved drugs. (Data from CMR R&D Compendium, 2000.)

The fact that in any year there are more Phase II than Phase I clinical projects in progress reflects the longer duration of Phase II studies, which more than offsets the effect of attrition during Phase I. The number of Phase III projects is smaller, despite their longer duration, because of the attrition between Phase II and Phase III.

High attrition rates – which would horrify managers in most technology-based industries – are a fact of life in pharmaceuticals, and are the main reason why drug discovery and development is so expensive and why drug prices are so high in relation to manufacturing costs. The cumulative attrition curve, based on projects in the mid-1990s, is shown in Figure 22.13, the overall success rate from the start of preclinical development being 8%; from the start of clinical development (Phase I), the success rate increased to 20%. However, a recent analyses quoted by FDA (FDA Report, 2004) suggest a success rate of compounds entering Phase I trials of only 8%, compared to 14% in 1985.

The main reasons for failure of compounds are summarized in Figure 22.14, which shows that unsatisfactory pharmacokinetic properties and lack of therapeutic efficacy in patients were the commonest shortcomings. As discussed in Chapter 10, determined efforts have been made to control for pharmacokinetic properties in the discovery phase, and this appears to have reduced the failure rate during development. Accurate prediction of therapeutic efficacy in the discovery phase remains a problem, however, particularly in disease areas, such as psychiatric disorders, where animal models are unsatisfactory.

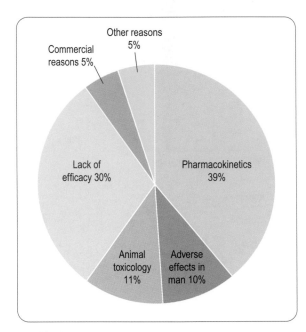

Fig. 22.14
Reasons for failure in development: causes of failure of 198 NCEs. (Data from Kennedy (1997) Drug Discovery Today 2: 436–444.)

Biotechnology-derived medicines

An increasing share of research and development projects is devoted to the investigation of therapies using biotechnology-derived molecules (see Chapter 12). The first such product was recombinant human insulin

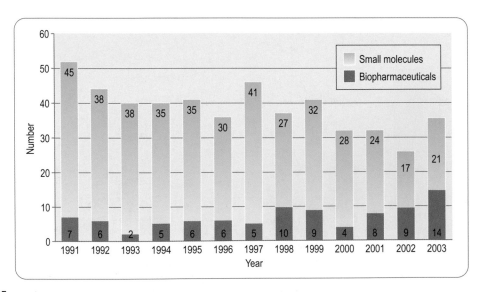

Fig. 22.15
Number of new molecules registered 1991–2001.

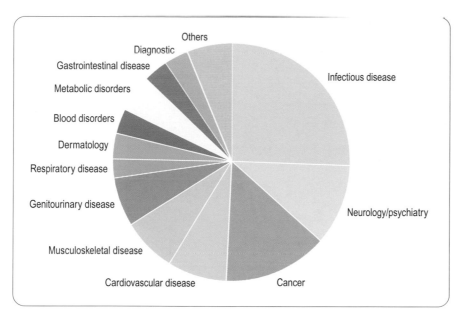

Fig. 22.16
Therapeutic areas covered by new drugs 2001–2002 (n = 58).

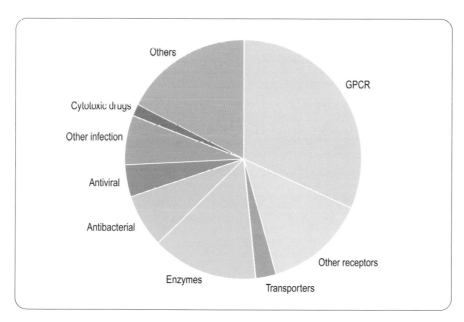

Fig. 22.17
Pharmacological targets of new compounds registered 2001–2002 (n = 41).

(Humulin), introduced by Lilly in 1982. Over the decade 1991–2003, 79 out of 469 (17%) new molecules registered were biopharmaceuticals (Figure 22.15). Recently (2002–2003) the proportion was around 30% – partly reflecting reduced numbers of small molecules registered in recent years – and this is predicted to increase to about 50% over the next few years. Nearly one-third of all projects currently in clinical trials in the USA involve biophar-

maceuticals; in 2002 an estimated 371 biopharmaceuticals were in clinical development (PhRMA Survey, 2002), with strong emphasis on new cancer therapies (178 preparations) and infectious diseases, including AIDS (68 preparations).

Many biotechnology-based projects originate not in mainstream pharmaceutical companies, but in specialized small biotechnology companies, which generally

325

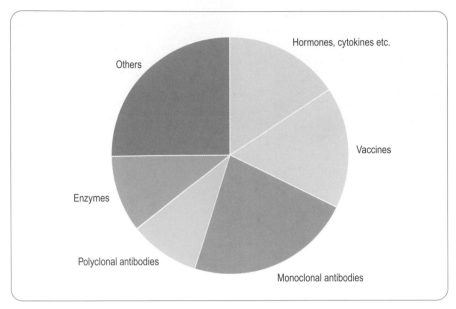

Fig. 22.18
Types of biopharmaceutical registered 2001–2002 (*n* = 17).

lack the money and experience to undertake development projects. This has resulted in increased in-licensing activities, whereby a large company licenses in and develops the substance, for which it pays fees, milestone payments, and eventually royalties to the biotechnology company.

Recent introductions

An analysis of the 58 new substances approved by the FDA in the period 2001–2002 is shown in Figures 22.16–22.18. It is striking that about half of the new synthetic compounds were directed at receptor targets (mostly GPCRs, and some steroid receptors), all of which had been identified pharmacologically many years earlier, as had the transporter and enzyme targets. Only a minority of the new compounds were 'first-in-class' drugs. The 20% of compounds directed at infectious agents were also mainly 'follow-up' compounds', directed at familiar targets, and so it is clear that during the 1990s, when these drugs were being discovered and developed, the industry was operating quite conservatively. Although, as described in Section 2, many new technologies were being applied in the hope of improving the speed and efficiency of drug discovery, drug targets and therapeutic approaches had not really changed. You are more likely to produce blockbusters, it was argued, by following the routes that produced blockbusters in the past than by trying new approaches with the aim of being 'first-in-class'.

Biopharmaceuticals registered during this period (Figure 22.18) include several protein mediators produced by recombinant methods – the approach that heralded the beginning of the biopharmaceutical era. There is a much larger proportion of 'first-in-class' therapeutics in the biopharmaceutical sector, perhaps reflecting a greater willingness to take risks than exists in small-molecule-based R&D. Monoclonal antibodies and vaccines are also strongly represented, representing the 'second wave' of biopharmaceutical products. Judging from the portfolio of new biotechnology products undergoing clinical evaluation in 2002, the trend towards biopharmaceuticals is set to continue, with cancer and viral infections as the main therapeutic targets.

What we have yet to see is the real impact of the genomic revolution on pharmaceutical R&D. The human genome sequence was published in 2001, so it is too early to expect a revolution in development and approval pipelines. Time alone will tell how radically the facts and figures of pharmaceutical R&D will be transformed.

References

Arthur Andersen Consultants (1997) Report on innovation and productivity.

Association of the British Pharmaceutical Industry (website: www.abpi.org.uk).

Centre for Medicines Research International (2000) Pharmaceutical research and development compendium. (website: www.cmr.com).

DiMasi JA, Hansen RW, Grabowski HG (2003) The price of innovation: new estimates of drug development costs. Journal of Health Economics 22: 151–185.

Drews J (2003a) Strategic trends in the drug industry. Drug Discovery Today 8: 411–420.

Drews J (2003b) In quest of tomorrow's medicines, 2nd edn. New York: Springer-Verlag.

FDA (2004) Report. Challenge and opportunity on the critical path to new medical products. (www.fda.gov/oc/initiatives/critical path/whitepaper.html).

Gilbert J, Hnaske P, Singh A (2003) Rebuilding big pharma's business model. InVivo, the Business & Medicine Report, 21(10). Norwalk, Conn: Windhover Information; Vol 21 No 10.

Grabowski H, Vernon J, DiMasi JA (2002) Returns on research and development for 1990s new drug introductions. Pharmacoeconomics 20(Suppl 3): 11–29.

McKinsey (1997) Report. Raising innovation to new heights in pharmaceutical R&D.

PhRMA Survey 2002 Biotechnology medicines in development. (www.phrma.org/newmedicines/surveys.cfm).

Pharmaceutical Research and Manufacturers of America. (www.phrma.com).

Reichert JM (2003) trends in development and approval times for new therapeutics in the United States. Nature Reviews Drug Discovery 2: 695–702.

Index

Index

333

Index

Index

Index

Index

trastuzumab (Herceptin)
  development and commercialization
    50
  discovery and commercialization,
    timeline 47f
  history 50
TrEMBL 93
tricyclic antidepressants, target 67t
trimethoprim 12
triptans 253
troglitazone 229
tubocurarine 8
tyrosine kinase inhibitors 201

U

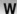

UK, reimbursement strategies 60
ultrasound imaging, in vivo profiling in
    animals 169
Unigene 93
unmet medical need 58
  assessment 58
urokinase 178, 181
US National Cancer Institute 46
US National Center for Biotechnology
    Information (NCBI) 90
US Public Health Service 30
USA
  direct-to-consumer advertising
    304–305
  drug development time requirement
    320, 321f
  environmental assessment 293
  life expectancy 23f
  Medicare 59
  orphan drug regulations 292
  patent court cases 279
  patents and novelty description
    275–276
  regulatory process development 14
  regulatory requirements for trials 293
  requirement for reproductive toxicity
    studies 287b

V

vaccination, disvalue 22
vaccines 35t, 36, 183
  genetic 183
  production 190
  progress and future prospects 36
vaginal administration 252
validated hits 117
  definition 123b
validation
  of drug targets see targets for
    therapeutic drugs, validation
  high-throughput screening 114f
'validation' of hits 52, 53f
validity
  animal models 173
  construct validity 173, 174t
  face validity 173, 174t
  predictive validity 173, 174t
valuation of project 211–212
  estimation parameters 211f
vanilloid receptor, TRPV1 74
variability in response to drugs 28, 241
  reduction by use of
    pharmacogenomics 88
vasopressin analogues 253
ventricular arrhythmias 233
verapamil 150
vertebrates, genome size 95t
Viagra 23, 30, 50, 226
vinblastine 8
vinca alkaloids 46t
  target 67t
viral infections, biopharmaceutical safety
    290–291
viral vectors
  concerns over use 238
  gene therapy 37, 38, 184t
Virchow, R. 5
virtual compound libraries 125, 129
'virtual ligands' 135
virtual screening 130

volunteers
  definition 258
  phase I trials 258–259
  recruitment for phase I trials 260

W

warfarin 46t
welfare economics 29, 30
Western blot 154
'white-powder' libraries 53, 54
withdrawal of drugs 229, 257, 322
Woods, D.D. 10
'word bank' 306
World Health Organization (WHO),
    definition of health 20
World Patent Index (WPI), patenting
    197

X

Xenopus laevis oocytes 150
xenotransplantation 39
X-ray crystal analysis, in proteomics 86
X-ray densitometry tomography, in vivo
    profiling in animals 169

Y

yeast
  artificial chromosome (YAC) 87
  complementation assay 111, 111f
  protein expression system 187t, 188
  two-hybrid systems 111, 111f

Z

z´-factor equation 103
zidovudine 12
Zollinger–Ellison syndrome 49

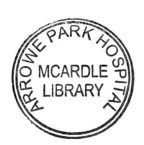